ONE Touch Surgery

For NEET/NEXT/FMGE/INI-CET

R Rajamahendran
MS, MRCS (UK), FMAS, MCh (Surgical Gastroenterology)
Senior Assistant Professor in Surgical Gastroenterology
Government Villupuram Medical College, Villupuram, Tamil Nadu
Consultant Surgical Gastroenterologist and Advanced Laparoscopic Surgeon
Director, RRM Gastro Superspeciality Clinic and Endoscopy Centre, Villupuram
Founder/Director – KONCPT PG Medical Coaching Centre, Tamil Nadu
Leading National Faculty Surgery for NEET PG and Surgical Gastroenterology for NEET SS
Author of more than 12 Medical Entrance and Clinical Examination Books

CBSPD
Dedicated to Education

CBS Publishers & Distributors Pvt Ltd
• New Delhi • Bengaluru • Chennai • Kochi • Kolkata • Lucknow
• Mumbai • Hyderabad • Nagpur • Patna • Pune • Vijayawada

ONE Touch
Surgery
For NEET/NEXT/FMGE/INI-CET

ISBN: 978-93-94525-19-1

First Edition: 2023

Published by **Satish Kumar Jain** and produced by **Varun Jain** for

CBS Publishers & Distributors Pvt Ltd
4819/XI Prahlad Street, 24 Ansari Road, Daryaganj, New Delhi 110 002, India.
Ph: +91-11-23289259, 23266861, 23266867 Website: www.cbspd.com
Fax: 011-23243014
e-mail: delhi@cbspd.com; cbspubs@airtelmail.in.

Corporate Office: 204 FIE, Industrial Area, Patparganj, Delhi 110 092
Ph: +91-11-4934 4934 Fax: 4934 4935
e-mail: feedback@cbspd.com; bhupesharora@cbspd.com

Branches

- **Bengaluru:** Seema House 2975, 17th Cross, K.R. Road, Banasankari 2nd Stage, Bengaluru-560 070, Karnataka
  Ph: +91-80-26771678/79 Fax: +91-80-26771680 e-mail: bangalore@cbspd.com
- **Chennai:** 7, Subbaraya Street, Shenoy Nagar, Chennai-600 030, Tamil Nadu
  Ph: +91-44-26680620, 26681266 Fax: +91-44-42032115 e-mail: chennai@cbspd.com
- **Kochi:** 68/1534, 35, 36-Power House Road, Opp. KSEB, Cochin-682018, Kochi, Kerala
  Ph: +91-484-4059061-65 Fax: +91-484-4059065 e-mail: kochi@cbspd.com
- **Kolkata:** Hind Ceramics Compound, 1st Floor, 147, Nilganj Road, Belghoria, Kolkata-700056, West Bengal
  Ph: +033-2563-3055/56 e-mail: kolkata@cbspd.com
- **Lucknow:** Basement, Khushnuma Complex, 7-Meerabai Marg (Behind Jawahar Bhawan), Lucknow-226001, Uttar Pradesh
  Ph: +0522-4000032 e-mail: tiwari.lucknow@cbspd.com
- **Mumbai:** PWD Shed, Gala No. 25/26, Ramchandra Bhatt Marg, Next to J.J. Hospital Gate No. 2, Opp. Union Bank of India, Noor Baug, Mumbai-400009, Maharashtra
  Ph: +91-22-66661880/89 Fax: +91-22-24902342 e-mail: mumbai@cbspd.com

Representatives

- **Hyderabad** +91-9885175004
- **Pune** +91-9623451994
- **Patna** +91-9334159340
- **Vijayawada** +91-9000660880

Printed at : Goyal Offset Works Pvt. Ltd. Haryana (INDIA)

Preface

I am ecstatic to write the preface of this book. It's not so tough to write books when you have complete freedom regarding the pages and contents, but when you are supposed to do a book in a concise form suitable for the students who are about to face their exams, you have to take lots of factors into consideration. Some of the difficulties I confronted with while compiling and making the book concise are to add all essential features without missing any important point. I tried my level best to include all the essential images needed for exam while updating the book to the latest editions of Bailey and Love, and Sabiston.

After completing the task of finalizing and making a concise and compact book like this, I can say with surety that the readers will love and appreciate it because of its beautiful color scheme and presentation, extremely useful content and stylist formatting.

I thank the entire team of CBS Publishers and Distributors for their tireless efforts and I am waiting eagerly to hear the response from the readers.

R Rajamahendran

Contents

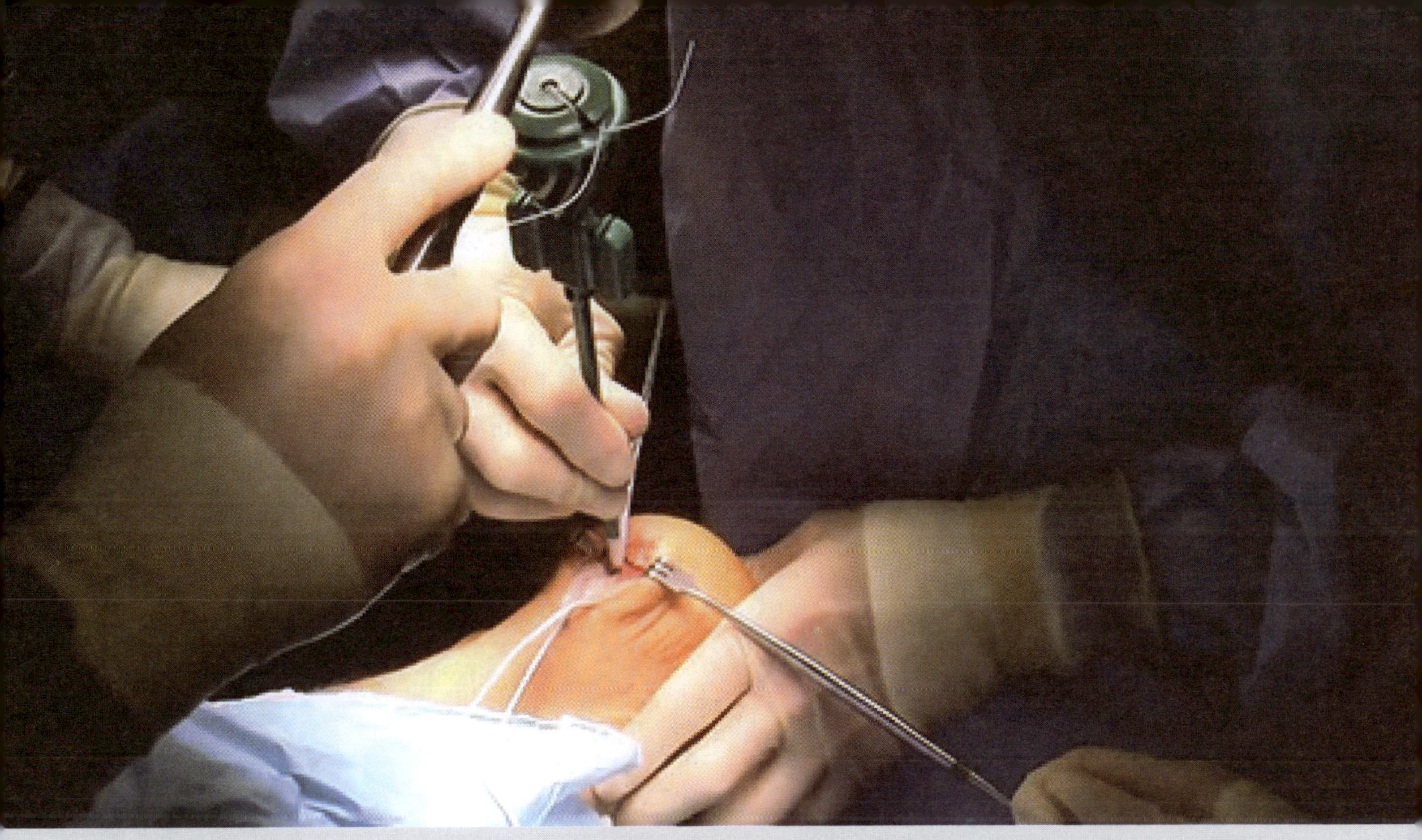

THEORY

1. GENERAL ASPECTS OF SURGERY

NUTRITION

- The best method to assess the nutrition in a surgical patient is serum albumin.
- Malnutrition universal screening tool (MUST) is a clinical tool to assess nutrition based on:
    - BMI
    - Weight loss in 3–6 months
    - Acute disease effect

Differences Between Enteral and Parenteral Nutrition

Enteral nutrition	Parenteral nutrition
Nutrition given via GI tract	**Nutrition given via veins**
Tube feeding • Nasogastric tube (Ryle's tube) • Nasojejunal tube • Percutaneous endoscopic gastrostomy tube • Feeding gastrostomy • Feeding jejunostomy	• Peripheral parenteral • Central parenteral

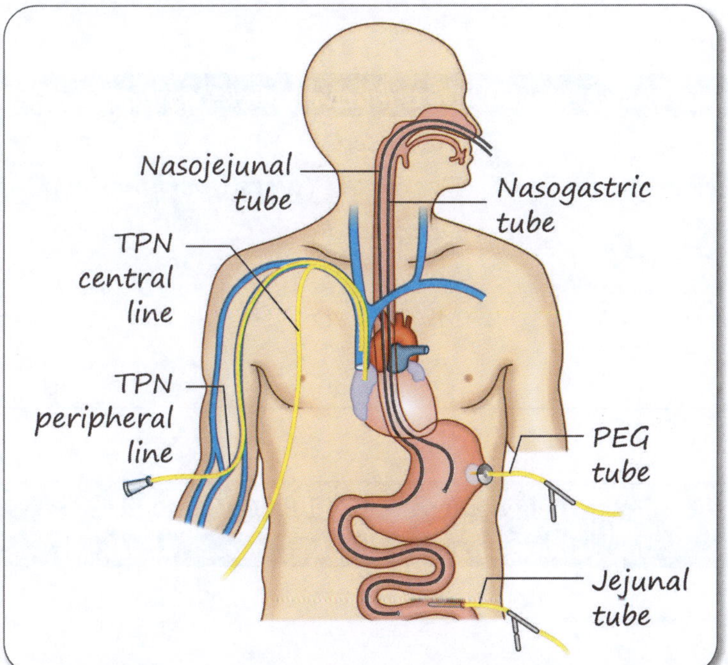

PEG tube

Nasogastric Tube: (Ryle's Tube)

- Ideal length of tube used is calculated by NEX rule (nose to ear to xiphoid process measured).
- Ryles tube is inserted by making the patient sit and keeping the neck flexed.
- Position of Ryles tube in stomach is confirmed by testing the aspirate for pH using litmus paper.

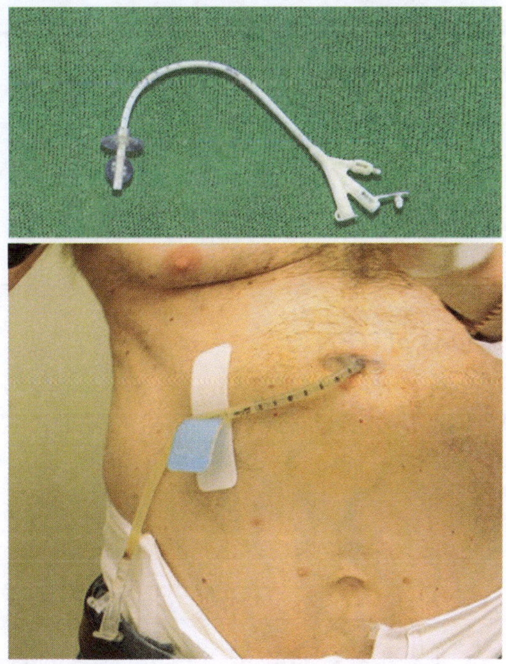

Parenteral Nutrition Types

- **Peripheral PN (<2 weeks)**
    - Peripherally inserted central catheter
    - Hickman lines
- **Central PN (>2 weeks)**
    - IJV, SCV, FV are used

Best Vein to Give Nutrition by Central Vein

- For Elective cases—Subclavian Vein
- For Trauma cases—IJV
- Highest chance of Pneumothorax—SCV
- Most commonly used vein—IJV
- For long-term nutrition—SCV is best
- Risk of thrombosis is highest with Femoral vein route
- Risk of infection is highest with Femoral vein > IJV > SCV > Hickman line

Total Parenteral Nutrition

Components of TPN

- 60% carbohydrates (dextran), 20% protein (amino acids), 20% lipids (fat)
- Fat free TPN—3:1 ratio of only dextrans and amino acids

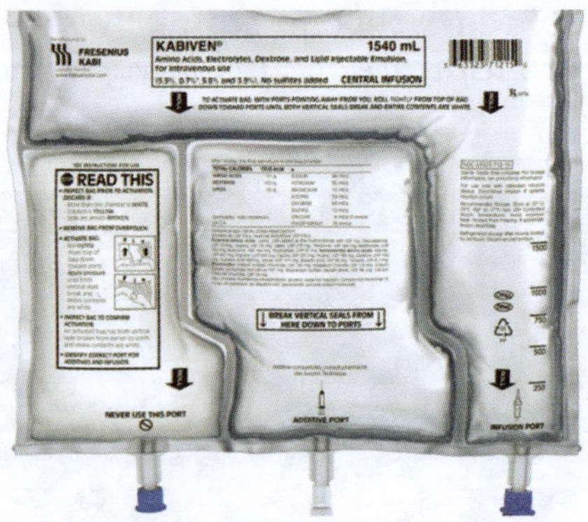

Complications of TPN

- **Catheter related complications are more common:**
    - MC procedure related complication—arterial puncture
    - MC overall complication—catheter related infection
    - Most dangerous complication—tension pneumothorax
- **Refeeding syndrome:**
    - Characterized by severe fluid and electrolyte shifts in malnourished patients undergoing refeeding*
    - It can occur with enteral and parenteral nutrition (MC with TPN)
    - Lab values: **Hypophosphatemia, hypocalcemia, Hypomagnesemia*** and also hypokalemia (Mnemonic—PCM*)
    - Hypokalemia can induce cardiac arrhythmias and congestive cardiac failure and death.

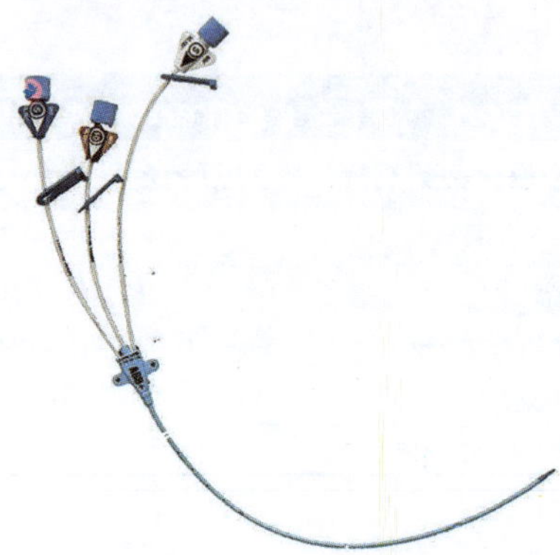

Central vein catheter

SHOCK AND BLOOD TRANSFUSION

Differences between Hypovolemic and Distributive Shock

Features	Hypovolemic shock (hemorrhagic shock)	Distributive shock (septic shock)
Cardiac output	Decreased	Increased
Peripheral vascular resistance	Increased (cold peripheries)	Decreased (warm peripheries)
Oxygen consumption	Increased	Decreased
Venous resistance	Low	Low
Mixed venous oxygen saturation (MVOS) Normal—50–70%	MVOS <50%**	MVOS >70%**

Change in Parameters

Parameters	Hypovolemic shock	Cardiogenic shock	Neurogenic shock	Anaphylactic shock	Septic shock
Pulse rate	↑↑	↑/↓	↓	↑↑	↑
Systolic Blood pressure	↓↓	↓	↓	↓	↑
Cardiac Output	↓↓	↓	↓	↓	↑
Peripheral vascular resistance	↑	↑	↓	↓	↓

Note: *Repeated question
**Multiple times repeated question

Differences between Urine Output, CVP and Serum Lactate

Urine output	CVP	Serum Lactate
• Best clinical parameter • Best clinical method to look for adequacy of resuscitation • Best to look for tissue perfusion.	• Best method to calculate amount of fluid to be given and dose of drug to be given • CVP is not accurate for cardiogenic shock and septic shock.	• Best lab value to monitor tissue perfusion • <2 mmol/L good resuscitation • >5 mmol/L bad resuscitation • Best method to look for muscle and GIT perfusion.

Hemorrhagic Shock

- **Four classes of hemorrhagic shock:** Class 1, 2, 3, 4 based on amount of blood lost.
- Class 1 (<750 mL), Class 2 (750–1500 mL), Class 3 (1500–2000 mL) and Class 4 (>2000 mL)
- Pulse rate and respiratory rate increase; and Pulse pressure decreases from class 2 shock
- BP falls from class 3 shock

Septic Shock

- **SIRS is defined by:**
  Two or more of the following: (Mnemonic—Orthopedics Love THR)
  - L—Leukocyte Count (>12000 or <4000)
  - T—Temperature >38°C or <35°C
  - H—Heart rate >90 beats/min
  - R—Respiratory rate >20/min ($PaCO_2$ <32 mm Hg)
- **Quick Sequential Organ Failure Assessment Score (qSOFA score)**
  (Mnemonic—Royal Challengers Bangalore will be in SOFA)
  - R—Respiratory rate – >22/min – 1 point
  - C—Confused mental status – 1 point
  - B—BP <100 mm Hg – 1 point

  ≥2 point indicates organ dysfunction. Score >2 carries 10% mortality

Blood Products and Complications

Whole blood

- Available as 450 mL pack.
- Contains RBC, WBC, plasma, platelet of which WBC and platelet are nonfunctional**

Packed red cells

- The cells are spun down and concentrated.
- **Each unit is 330 mL***
- Stored at 2°–6°C.

Fresh frozen plasma

- Rich in coagulation factors
- Stored at –40°C to –60°C. (2-year shelf life)*

Cryoprecipitate

- Supernatant precipitate of FFP and is rich in factor VIII* and fibrinogen.
- Stored at –30°C with a 2-year shelf life*

Platelets

- Mostly used in dengue fever cases*
- Platelets are stored on a special agitator at 20°–24°C (Room temperature)
- Half-life only 5 days* as a fresh component
- Useful in patients with thrombocytopenia

Complications of Blood Transfusion

Febrile nonhemolytic transfusion reaction* (most common)—due to WBC present—leukocyte reduction filters remove the WBC*. To avoid this reaction—leukocyte reduction filter is used.

Complications of Massive Transfusion: (>10 Units of Blood/day in Adults)

- Coagulopathy
- Hypocalcemia* (due to binding of ionized calcium by citrate used as anticoagulant)
- Hyperkalemia* (due to RBC lysis)
- Hypokalemia also can happen
- Hypomagnesemia
- Hypothermia
- Dilutional thrombocytopenia
- Decreased oxygen delivery (due to decrease in 2, 3 DPG)
- Metabolic alkalosis (even though the stored blood contains pH - 6.3, because of massive transfusion sodium citrate is metabolized in liver to sodium bicarbonate)
- Rare-metabolic acidosis*

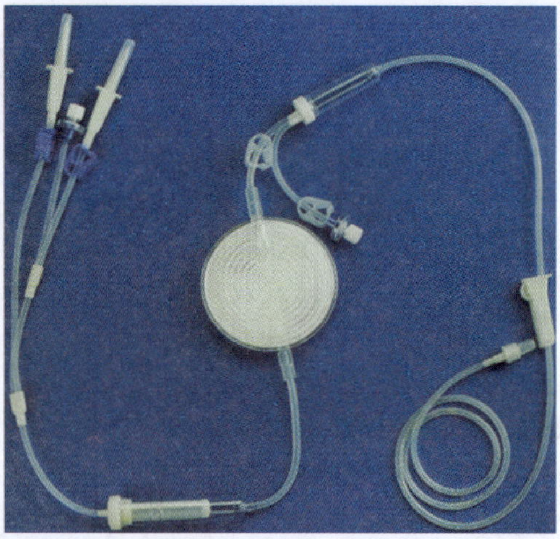

Leukocyte reduction filter

SUTURES AND KNOTS

Sutures

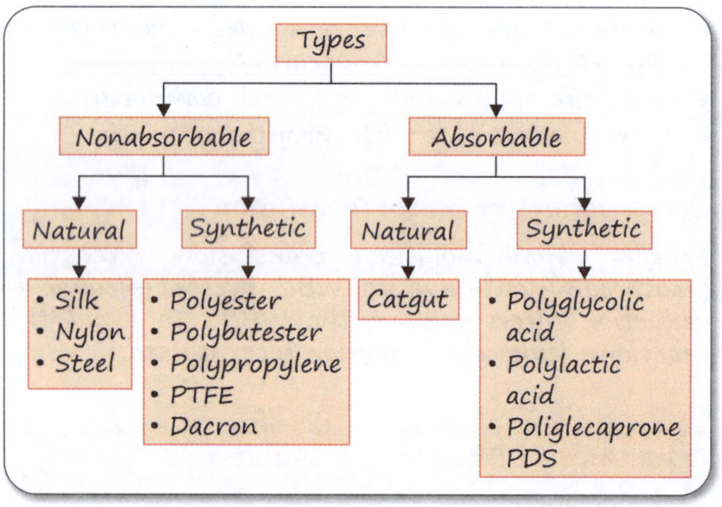

Nonabsorbable Synthetic Suture Materials

Polypropylene

- Blue color
- Monofilament materials
- Coiling back is seen, known as MEMORY*
- Applications of prolene:
  - Hernia repair
  - Hernia mesh
  - Vascular suturing (Aorta, femoral artery)
  - Tendon repair (like Tendo achilles)

Poly Tetra Fluoro Ethylene (PTFE)

Graft materials for Femoral artery, Popliteal artery.

Dacron

Graft material for aorta replacement

Natural Absorbable

Catgut

- Brown in color
- Plain—10 days
- Chromic—90 days
- **Tensile strength:** Plain catgut—7–10 days, Chromic catgut—21–28 days
- Storage solution of Catgut—Isopropyl Alcohol**
- **Applications:**
  - Subcutaneous
  - Muscle approximations
  - Plain catgut—circumcision
- Highest enzymatic reaction*, hence banned in UK
- Absorbed by enzymatic degradation.

Synthetic Absorbable

Polyglycolic acid: (Vicryl)—"Work Horse" material in theater

- Multifilament material (made up of Glycolic acid + Lactic acid copolymers)—as it is multifilament it has good knotting capacity but increased infection.
- Violet color
- Absorption period—60–90 days
- Absorbed by Hydrolysis
- **Types of Vicryl:**
  - Barbed vicryl—No knotting needed, used in facelift sutures, plastic surgery
  - Vicryl plus—Antibiotic coated (trichlosan antibiotic)
  - Vicryl rapide—Absorbed in 10 days
  - White vicryl (MONOCRYL)—Poliglecaprone (Monofilament material)—Suture of choice for Subcuticular sutures in skin (Cosmetic skin closure), complete absorption occurs in 90–120 days.
- **Applications:**
  - Bowel anastomosis (3'0 vicryl)
  - Bile duct anastomosis (4'0 vicryl)
  - Muscle closure
  - Subcutaneous closure
  - Vicryl meshes (Inner side of dual mesh to prevent bowel adhesions)
- Pancreatic duct—Vicryl must not be used (use only prolene or PDS)

Polydioxanone

- Longest absorption period—complete absorption occurs in 180 days.
- Used for Linea alba closures
- Used for tracheobronchial repairs

Blades and Handles

Most important Blades for exam are discussed here:

- **11 Size blade:** For stab incision and for arteriotomy
- **15 Size blade:** For Fine small skin incision
- **20 and 22 Size blades:** For long Incisions like laparotomy and thoracotomy

The handles used to fix the blades are known as Bard Parker (BP) Handles.

- BP handle 3 for holding—10, 11 and 15 size blades
- BP handle 4 for holding—20 and 22 size blades

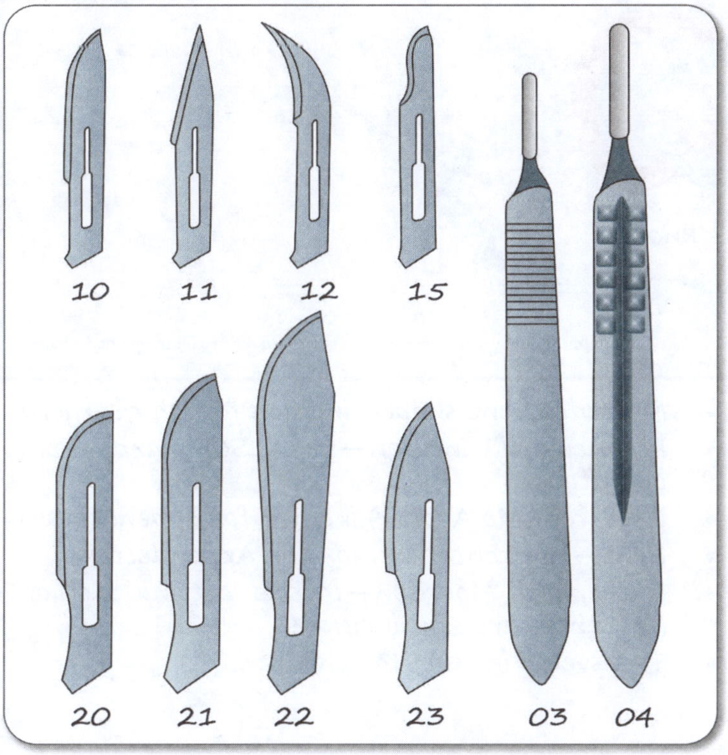

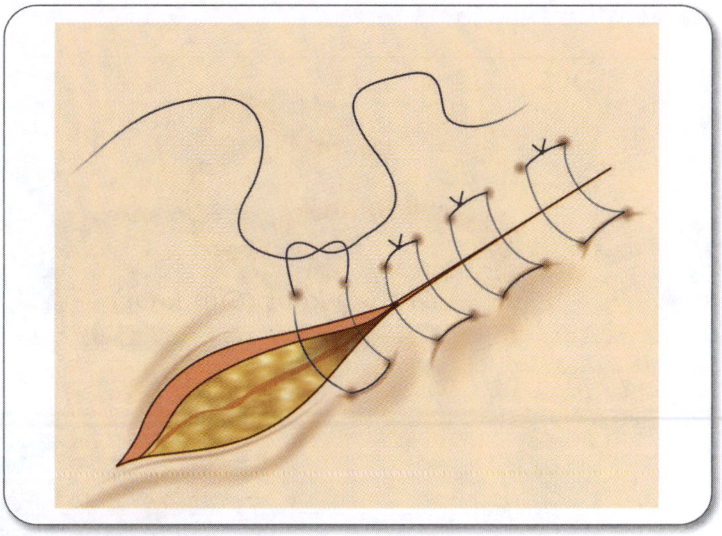

Horizontal mattress

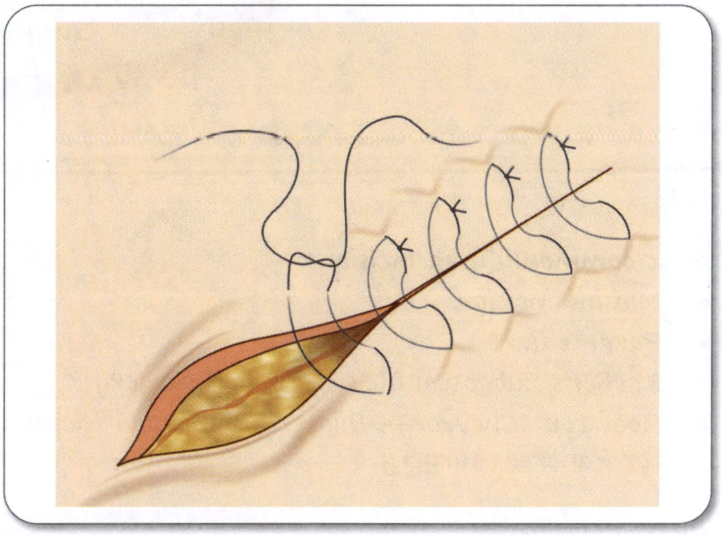

Vertical mattress

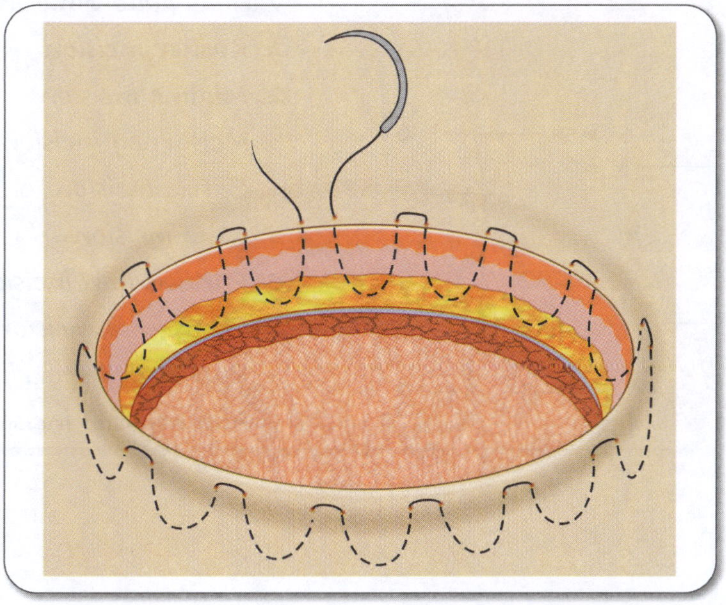

Purse string suture

Remember the Knots

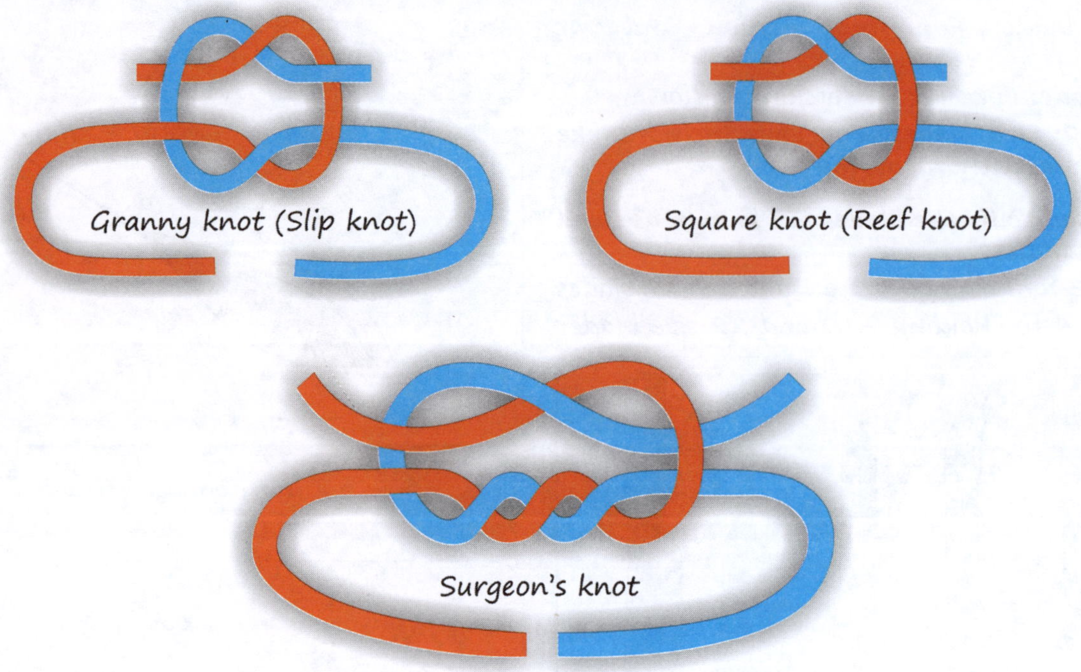

Incisions used on Abdomen

Most commonly used incisions:

- Midline incision
- Paramedian
- Kocher's Subcostal incision for GB surgery
- Roof top (Chevron)—Bilateral Subcostal incision for Pancreas surgery
- Mercedes Benz shaped incision for liver surgery
- Pfannenstiel incision—for LSCS and Pelvic operations
- Grid Iron (Mc Arthur) incision for appendectomy
- Lanz—Horizontal incision for Appendectomy
- Rutherford Morrison—Muscle cutting incision** (all others are skin incisions)
- Transverse incision for children

SKIN SUTURES

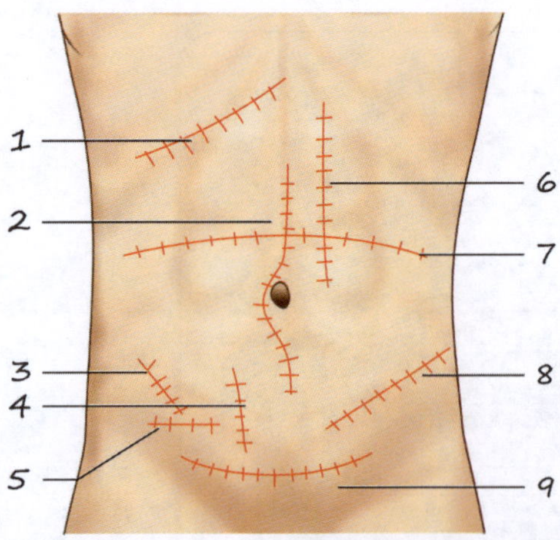

Various abdominal incisions:

1. Kocher incision
2. Midline incision
3. McBurney incision
4. Battle incision
5. Lanz incision
6. Paramedian incision
7. Transverse incision
8. Rutherford Morrison incision
9. Pfannenstiel incision

Removal of Skin Sutures

When to remove the skin sutures?

- Scalp—6–8 days
- 3–5 days—Lids, lips and face
- 8–10 days—Laparotomy, thoracotomy, ear lobe repair
- 10–14 days—Palms and soles, back

Bowel Anastomosis Techniques

- **Kocher's technique of bowel anastomosis**—Two-layer closure of Bowel anastomosis
- Halsted and Matheson method—Single layer extramucosal intermittent anastomosis (sub-mucosa included)
- Most stable layer used for anastomosis—**Submucosa** because it contains high amount of collagen
- Current preferred method for anastomosis is Halsted and Matheson extramucosal method

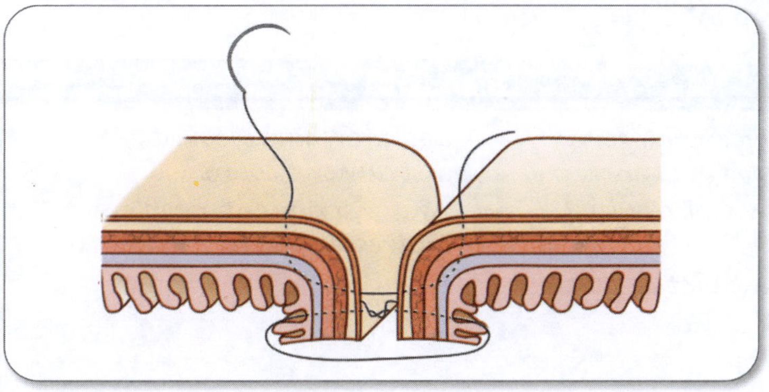

Kocher's technique

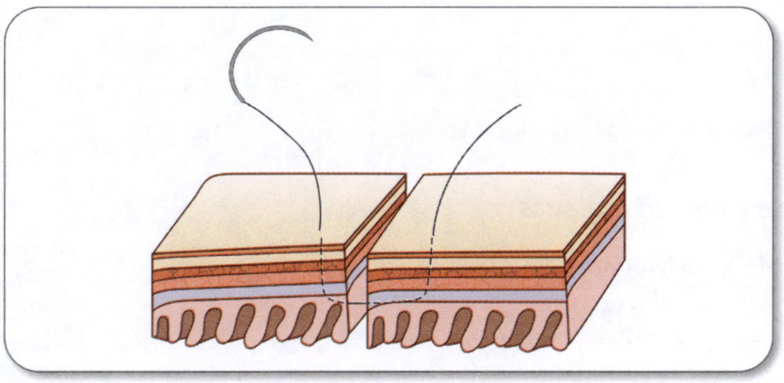

Halsted and Matheson

Cheatle cut: Approximate disproportionate bowel by end to end anastomosis*

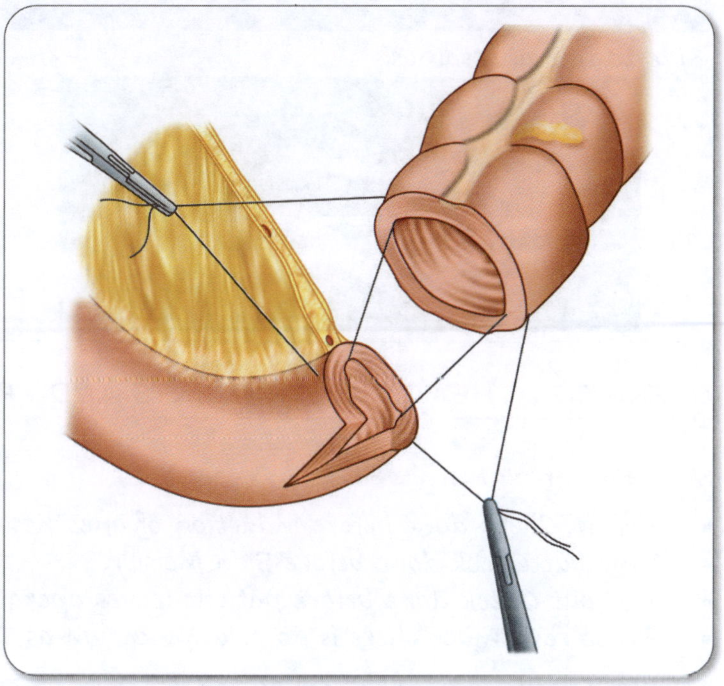

Cheatle cut

Lambert Sutures

- It is a seromuscular suture of the bowel after the inner full thickness or extramucosal anastomosis is being done.
- It gives an additional support to anastomosis.
- It can be intermittent or continuous but the suture runs only the seromuscular layers.

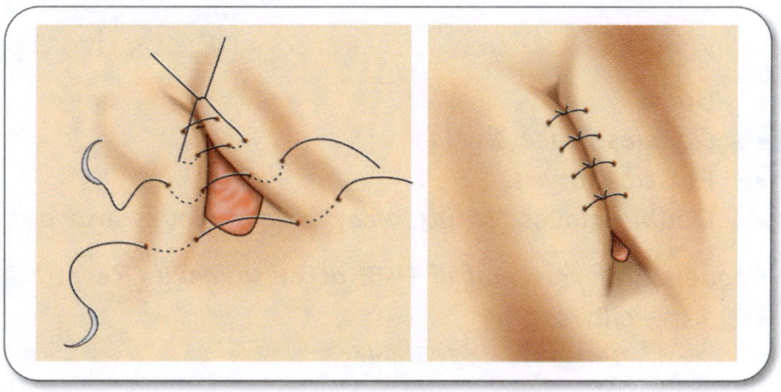

Lambert suture

Stapler Anastomosis of Bowel

Linear stapler (Transverse Linear Cutter—TLC)	Circular stapler (EEA—End to End anastomosis staplers)
Side to side anastomosis 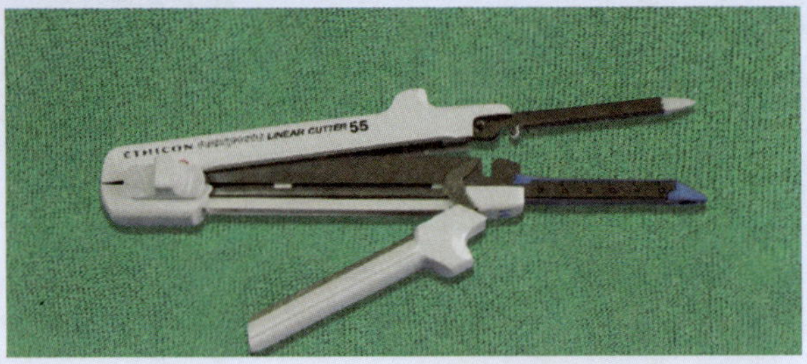	End to End anastomosis 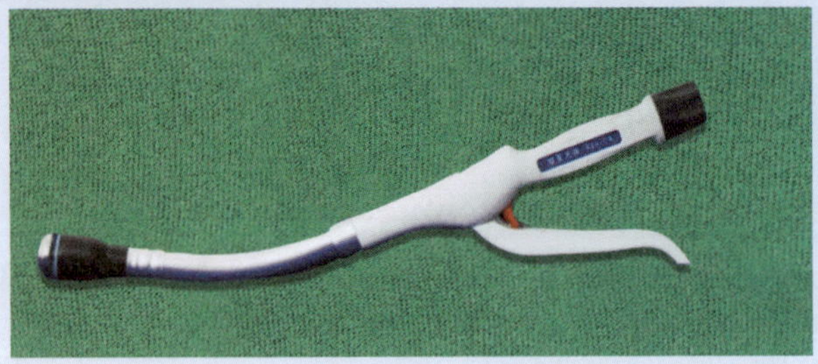

OPERATION THEATER INSTRUMENTS AND PROTOCOLS

Surgical Safety List (WHO UK Process)

- Sign in Check done before induction of anesthesia*
- Time out Check done before Skin incision*
- Sign out Check done before patient leaves operating room**
- Please remember there is no column known as Time in**

Sign in	Time out	Sign out
• Name • Identity • Confirm the disease • Site marked or not • Written consent • H/o drug allergy • Associated diseases	• Discussion between Surgeon and anesthetist. • Anticipated time of surgery and blood loss • Prophylactic antibiotics given or not is noted.	• Look for gauze count, instrument count • Any instrument problem is addressed here.

- Best method to prevent operating wrong limb—surgeon and anesthetist examining each other separately.

Universal Precaution Kit: (Personal Protective Equipment Kit)

- Boots
- Goggles (Face shield)
- Plastic Gowns
- Double gloves (Inside wear bigger gloves and outside your size gloves)

Sequence of removal of PPE after surgery (Recent AIIMS)—Mnemonic- GFPF

- 1st—Gloves
- 2nd—Face shield/Goggles
- 3rd—Plastic Gown/Aprons
- 4th—Facemask/respirator

MC Finger injured during surgery- Nondominant hand index finger*

- Hollow needles have more risk of injury than surgical needles.

Instruments used in operation theater

Allis Tissue Forceps

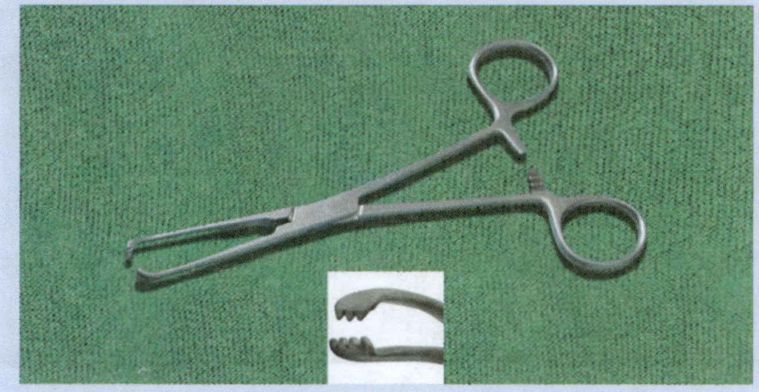

- *Allis forceps for holding the tissues firmly**
- *Used during laparotomy to hold the skin margins.*
- *Used to hold skin flaps during excision of Lipoma, Sebaceous cyst.*
- *It is helpful in creating flaps during thyroid surgeries**

Lane's Tissue Forceps

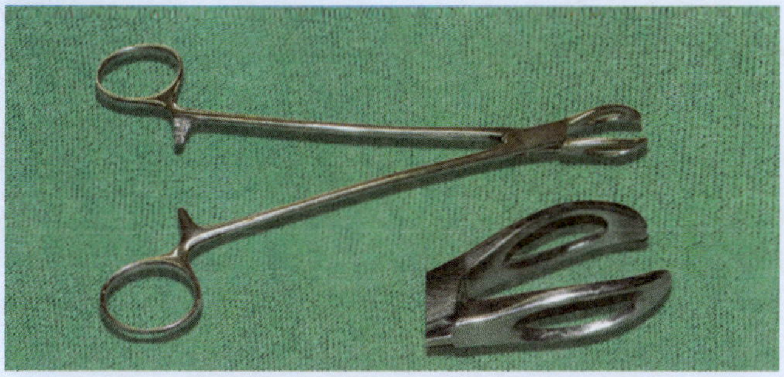

- *Used to hold structures very tight.*
- *It is used to hold submandibular gland and Parotid gland during dissection from adjacent structures.*
- *Helps in holding breast during mastectomy.*
- *Also helpful like a towel clip to hold the suction tubes, draping sheet.*

Babcock's Forceps

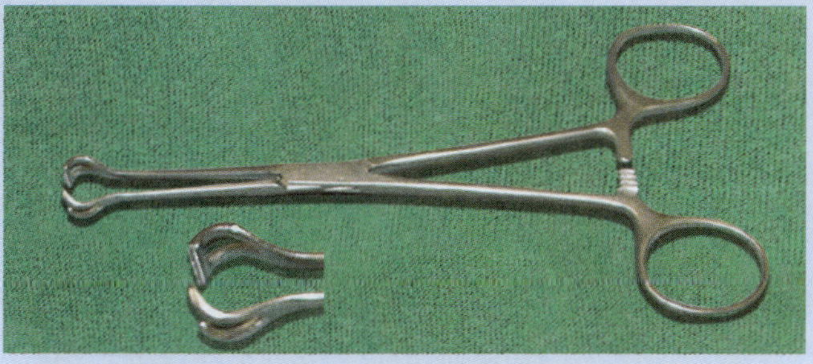

- *Used to hold tissues very softly.*
- *The ideal instrument to hold and grasp the bowel and appendix during surgery**
- *Hold the margins of stomach or small intestine during anastomosis**

Contd...

Instruments used in operation theater

Instruments used in Skin Suturing:

- *Needle Holder*
- *Toothed forceps*
- *Straight scissors*

Curved Scissors not used to cut sutures, only used to cut tissues.

Curved artery forceps—To catch the bleeding vessels

Straight artery Forceps—To hold tissues

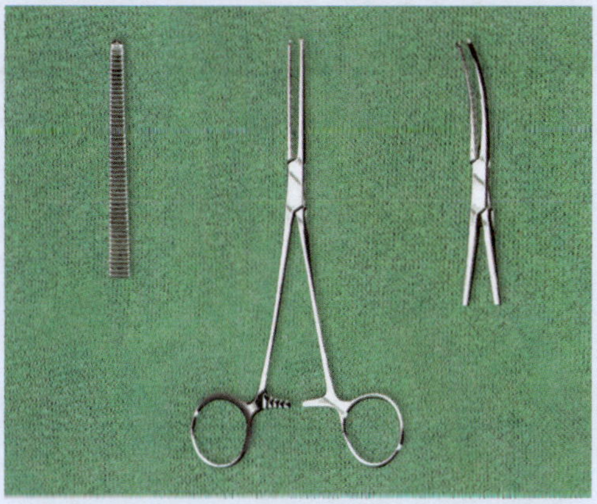

Cheatle Forceps

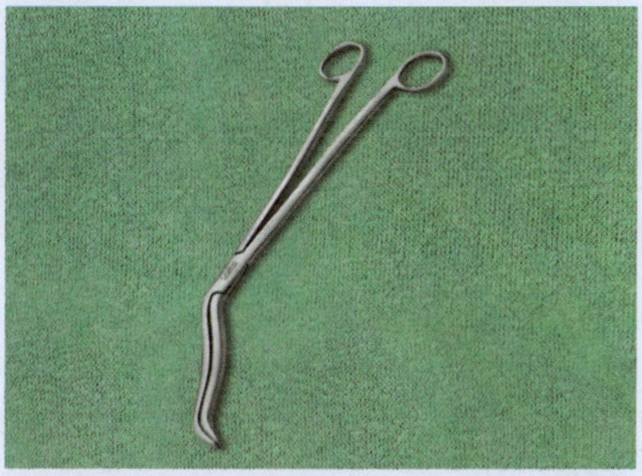

- *It is used to pick instruments and mopping pads/gauzes from bin in a sterile way.*
- *It is kept in a sterile bottle container.*

Langenbeck Retractor

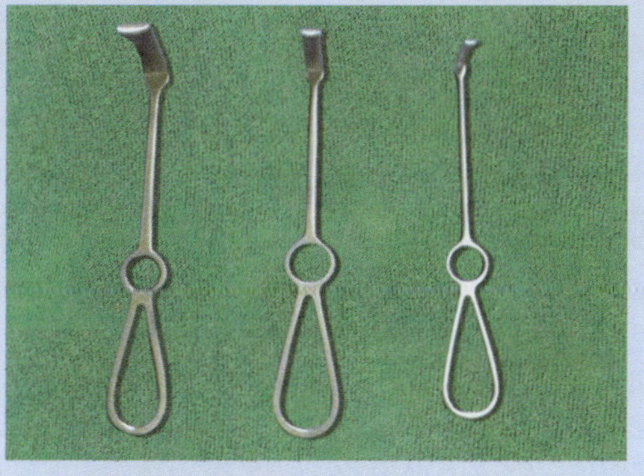

- *Used to retract tissues during hernia surgery, appendectomy, etc.*
- *Available in various sizes.*

Contd...

Instruments used in operation theater

Morris Retractor

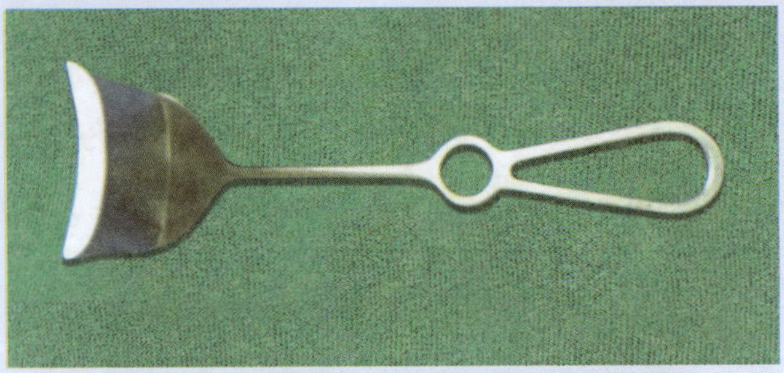

- Used to retract the abdominal wall in a wide manner.
- It is the instrument of choice for retraction in left subcostal region because it avoids the risk of splenic injury*

Czerny Retractor

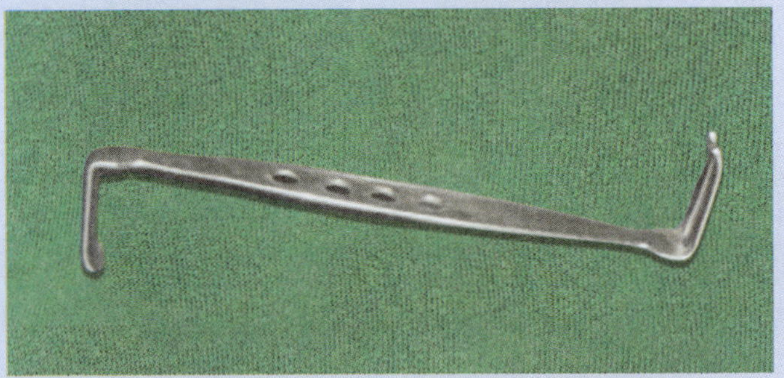

- Serves the same purpose of a Langenbeck retractor, but has another limb with a double hook with space in between.
- Sutures can be made in the tissues between the gap of hooks.

Deaver Retractor

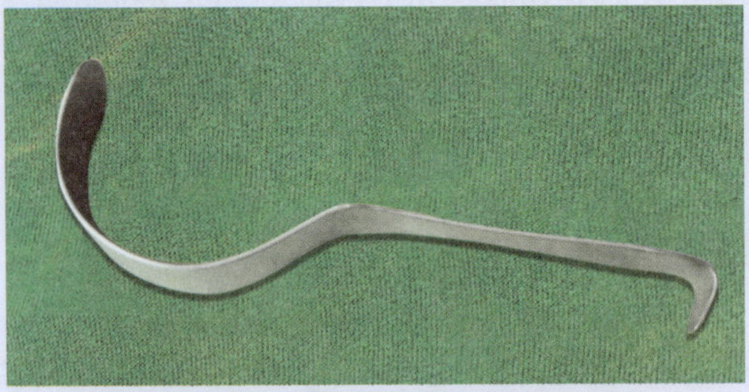

- Used to retract liver without any damage to liver parenchyma.
- Used during Cholecystectomy to retract liver.
- Used in places where a careful retraction without organ damage is needed.

Contd...

Instruments used in operation theater

Doyen's Retractor

To retract the pelvis and bladder at pubic symphysis.

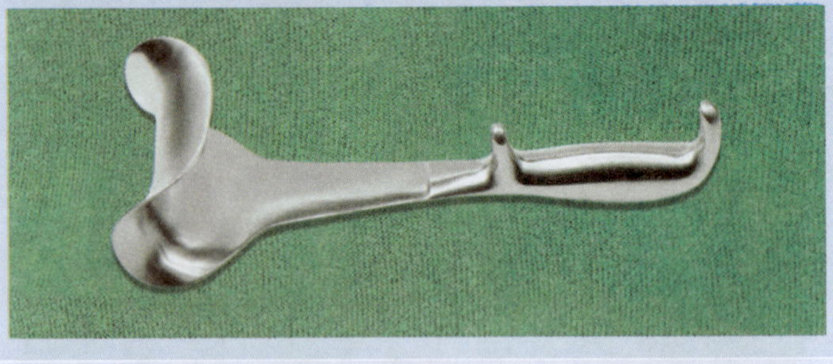

Balfour Abdominal Self-Retaining Retractor

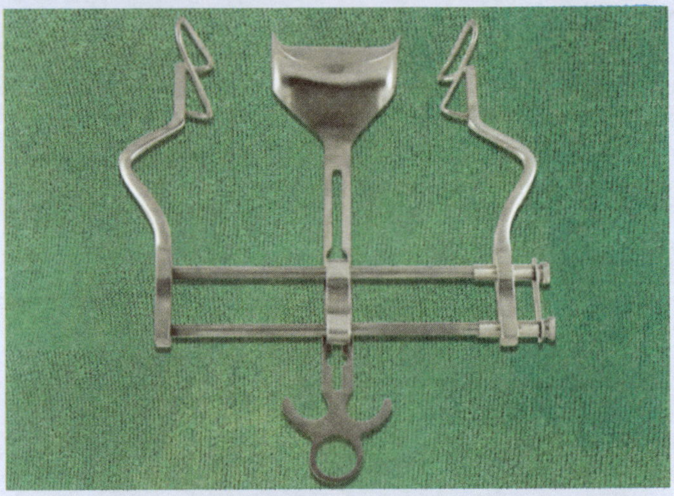

- It is used to retract the lateral abdominal walls.
- The third limb—used to retract the bladder downward.

Joll's Self-Retaining Thyroid Retractor

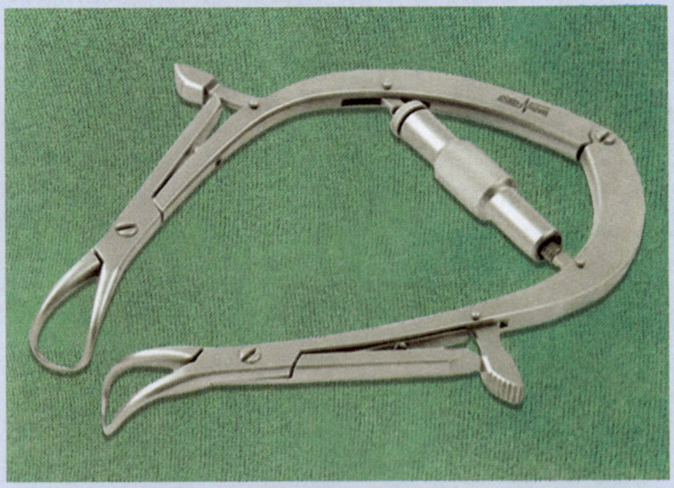

- Used during thyroidectomy* to retract the platysma.
- It is a self-retaining retractor.

Contd...

Instruments used in operation theater

Towel Clips

- Towel clips are used to hold the sterile dressing after drap in position*.
- Some surgeons use this to hold and retract the tongue outside for intraoral surgeries.

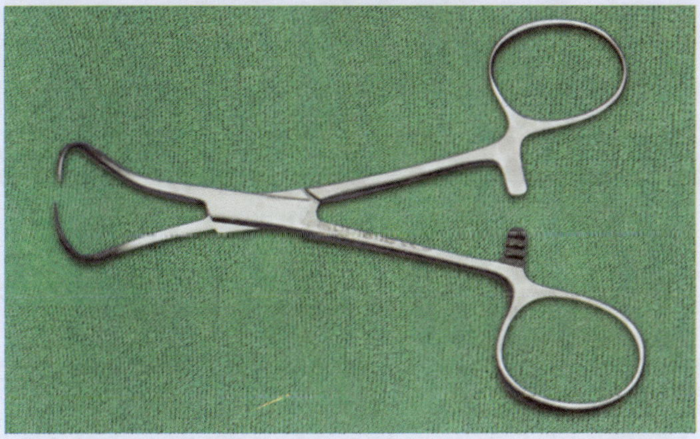

Contd...

Instruments used in operation theater

Blade Handles: (Bard Parker Handles)

- 3 size to load – 11 size blade and 15 size blade
- 4 size to load – 22 Size blade

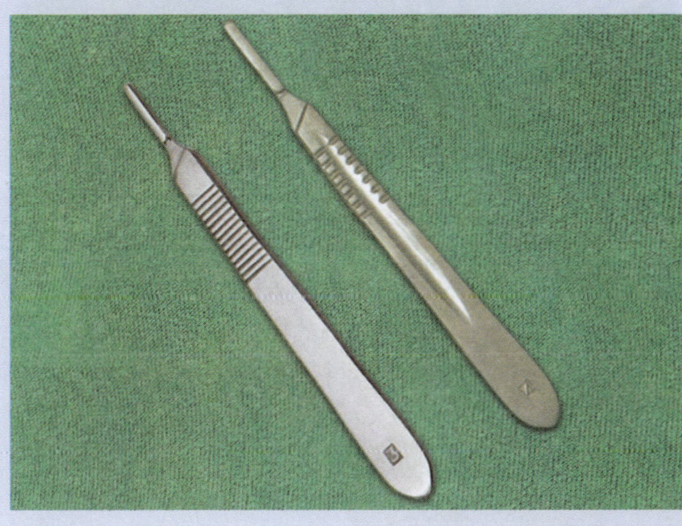

Cannulas

Color codes of Cannulas

Gauge	Color code	Catheter		
		Ext. Dia. "mm"	Length "mm"	Flow rate "mL/min"
G 14	Orange	2.1	45	270
G 16	Gray	1.8	45	200
G 17	White	1.5	45	140
G 18	Green	1.3	45	85
G 20	Pink	1.1	33	55
G 22	Blue	0.9	25	33
G 24	Yellow	0.7	19	18
G 26	Violet	0.6	19	10

- To infuse maximum fluids in dehydration and diarrhea, the ideal cannula is GRAY—16G. **(From the Table note- 200 mL/minute using Gray** and 85 mL/min using Green)**
- In Trauma, we use short and wide bore 2 Cannulas of at least 18 Gauge—2 in numbers as per ATLS guidelines*

Foley Catheter

Materials Used

- Latex rubber
- Silicon

Silicon catheter	Latex rubber catheter
• Less chances of encrustation and calcification and hence, less changing of catheter needed (once in 3 months)	• Increased risk of infection • Hypersensitivity • Irritation of bladder mucosa • Must be changed once in a month

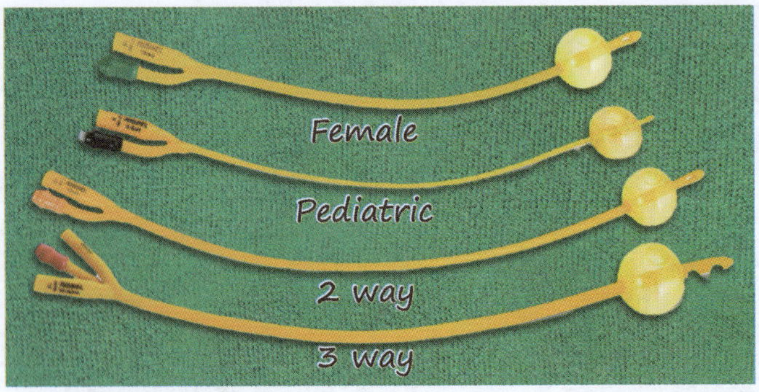

Color Codes for Foley and Size

Color code	Size
Black	8 Fr
Gray	10 Fr
White	12 Fr
Green	14 Fr
Orange	16 Fr
Red	18 Fr
Yellow	20 Fr
Purple	22 Fr
Blue	24 Fr

- MC used is orange (16 Fr)
- Women: 12–14 Fr, Men 16–18 Fr catheter is used,
- Three Way Foley Catheter is used for—**Bladder irrigation**, Commonly used after Prostate Surgery—TURP.
- In case of retention of Foley inside bladder and unable to remove the Foley catheter—we rupture the Foley Bulb using USG guidance.
- 1 mm = 3 French in units (or) 1 French = 0.33 mm
- The size mentioned in Foley catheter is based on **Outer Diameter of the Catheter****
- Balloon is inflated with sterile water only. Saline and air must not be used. Saline may cause blockage with crystals.
- In case of retained Foley how to remove it ideally—USG guided Puncture of Balloon

Energy Devices in Operation Theater

Diathermy

Diathermy is a machine which converts electrical energy into heat energy.

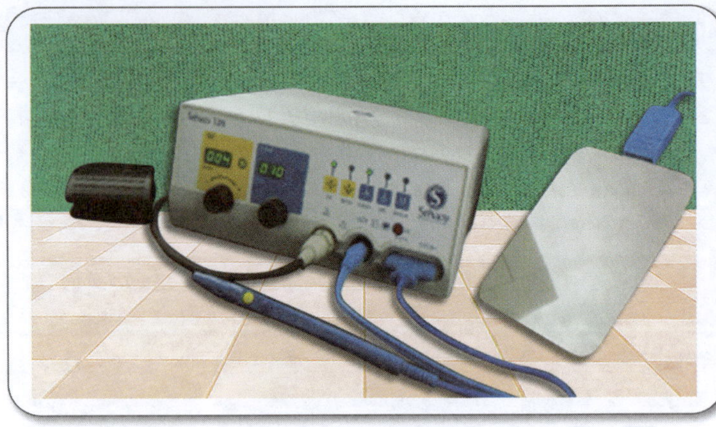

Diathermy machine

- Yellow button in the pencil is for cutting (Continuous Waveforms).
- Blue button in the pencil is for coagulation (Intermittent Waveforms).
- Earth plate prevents electric shock to patient.

Diathermy can be used for three purposes:

1. **Coagulation:** The sealing of blood vessels.
2. **Cutting:** Used to divide tissues during bloodless surgery.
3. **Fulguration:** The destructive coagulation of tissues with charring. It is a blended current which uses both the above forms of diathermy activity.

Monopolar Diathermy

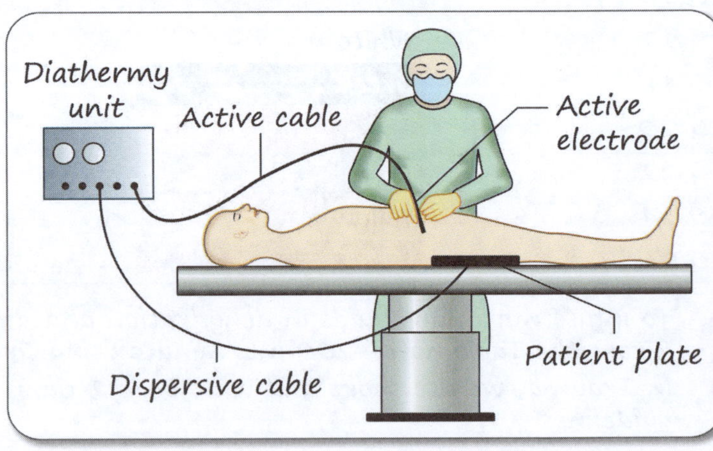

- **Monopolar diathermy:** The electrical energy is passed via the diathermy probe and returned to the machine via the patient earth plate as shown in the image given above.
- MC complication inside OT is diathermy burns**.
- **Pacemaker containing patients** must be carefully watched during monopolar diathermy and earth plate must be far away from pacemaker.

- Contraindications of Monopolar Diathermy:
  - Fingertips
  - Penis (Circumcision)
  - Thyroid and parotid surgery near nerves

Bipolar Diathermy

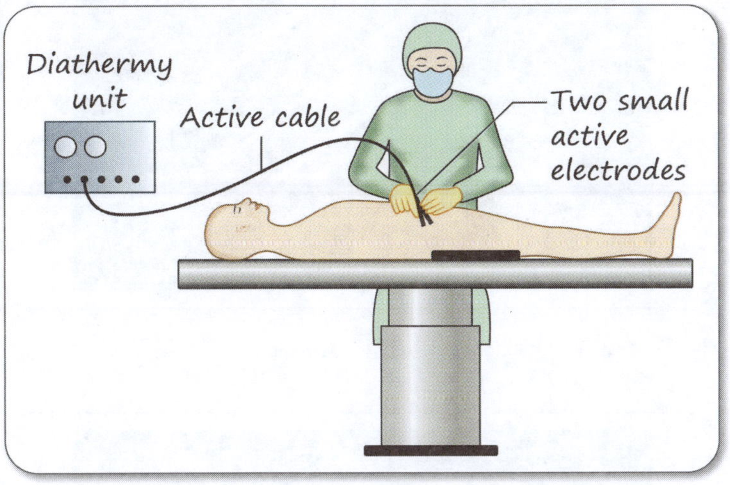

- Bipolar diathermy needs no earth plate.
- The current is passed between the limbs of diathermy probe.
- Safe in surgeries near nerve and circumcision.
- Can be safely used in pacemakers.

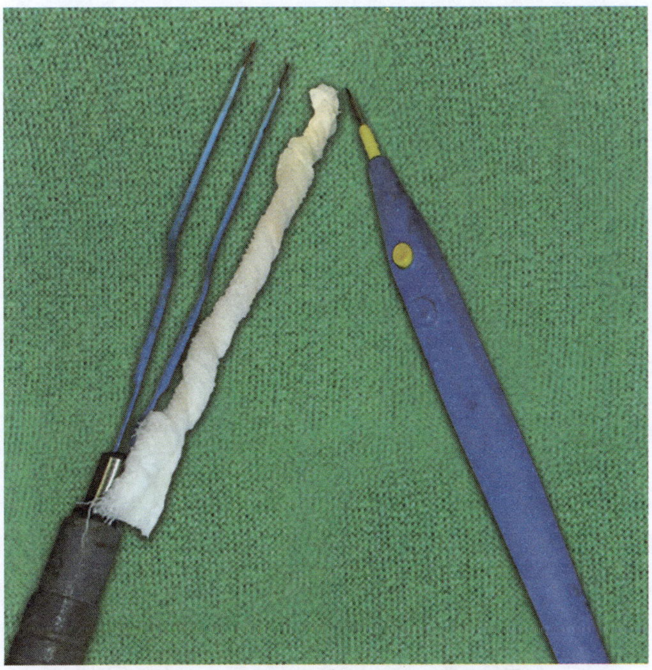

Please note the Bipolar (Left) and Monopolar (Right) Probes

Harmonic Scalpel

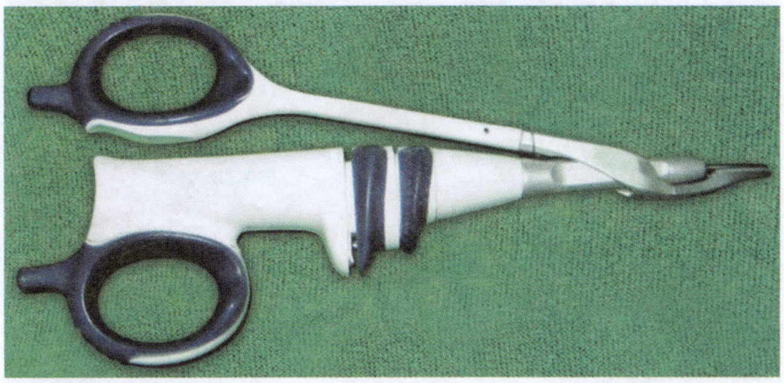

- The harmonic scalpel is an instrument that uses ultrasound technology to cut tissues while simultaneously sealing them and utilizes a hand-held ultrasound transducer and scalpel at frequency of 20,000–50,000 Hz.
- Protein denaturation is caused by vibration** rather than heat.

DRAINS IN SURGERY

Differences between open and closed drains

Open drains	Closed drains
• Include Corrugated Rubber or Plastic Drains	Consist of tubes draining into a bag or Bottle
• Drain fluid collects in a pad or Stoma bag	Abdominal drains, ICD drains, suction drains are examples
• Increased risk of infection seen	Infection risk is less
• Corrugated rubber drain is an open drain	Vacuum suction and Jackson Pratt are all closed drains

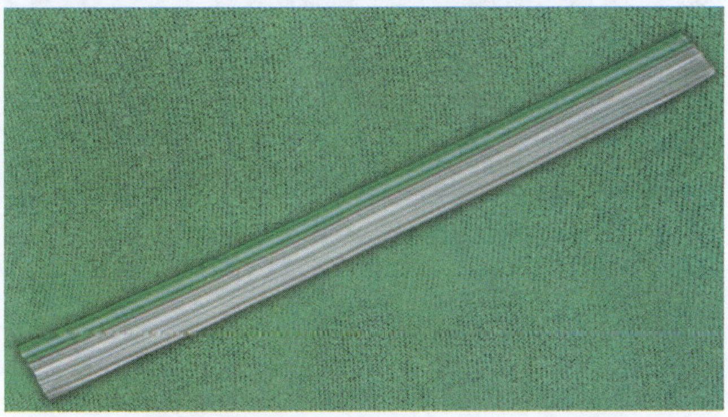

Corrugated rubber open drain

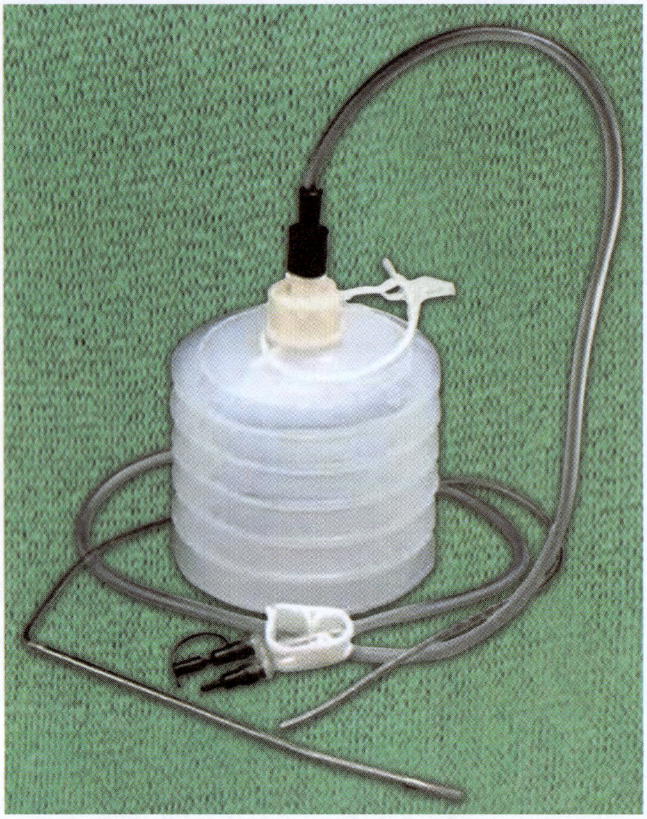

Closed suction drain

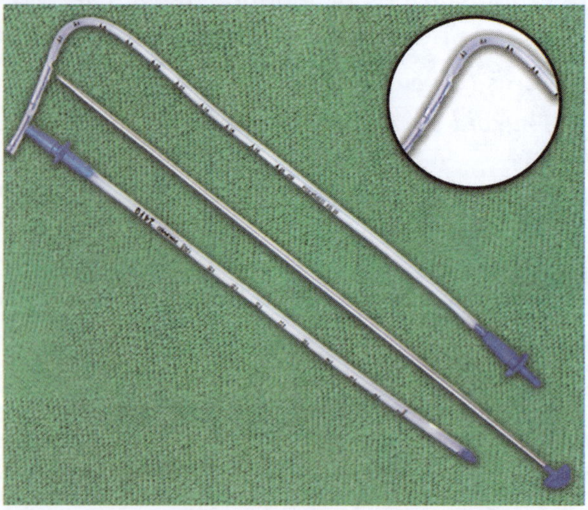

Intercostal drain tube

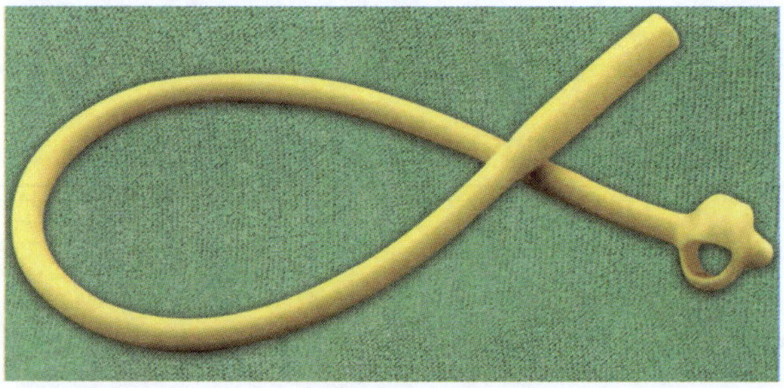

Malecot self-retaining catheter drain

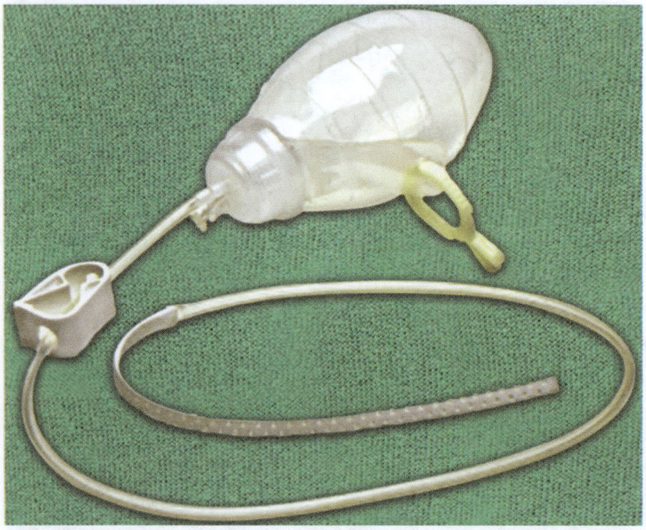

Jackson pratt closed drain

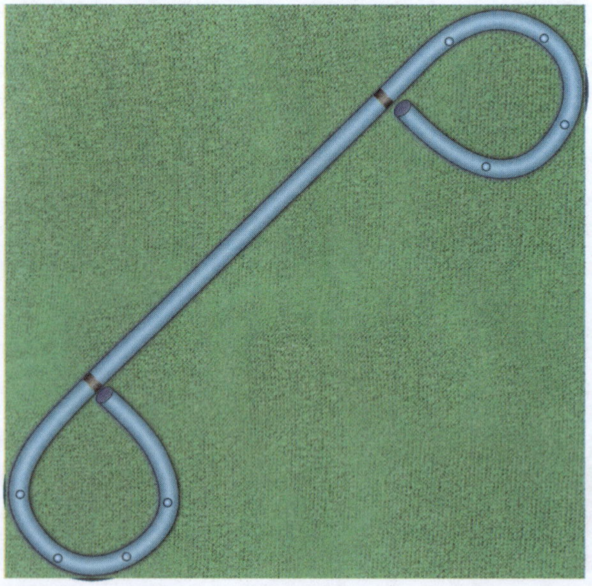

Double pig tail stent (double j stent)—ureter, bile duct

Place of drain	Purpose	Removal after
Thyroid surgery	To identify bleeding	24 hours
Breast surgery	To remove Serous Discharge	5 Days
ICD drain	To drain Collections	Collection <20 mL/day
T Tube Drain	To Drain Bile	10–14th POD
Pelvic drain after Colorectal anastomosis	To identify leakage	7th POD

POSITIONS OF PATIENTS IN OPERATION THEATER

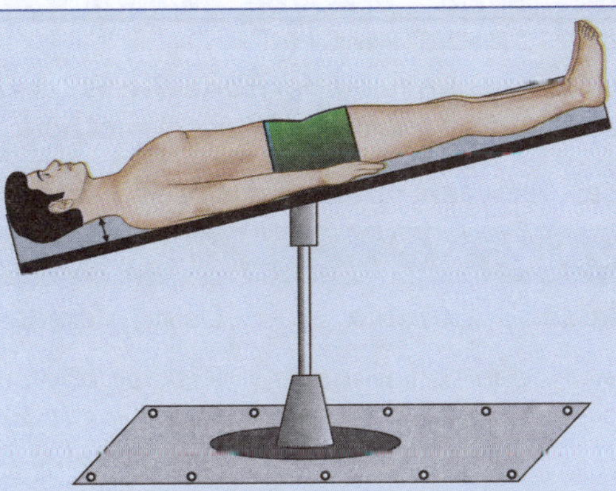

Trendelenburg
Varicose Vein Surgery

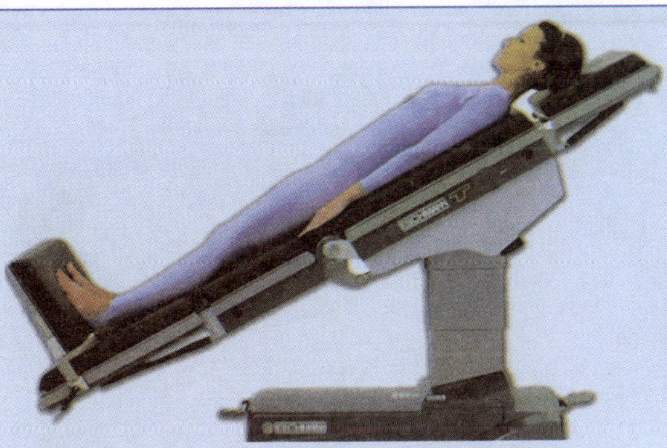

Reverse Trendelenburg:
Thyroid Surgeries

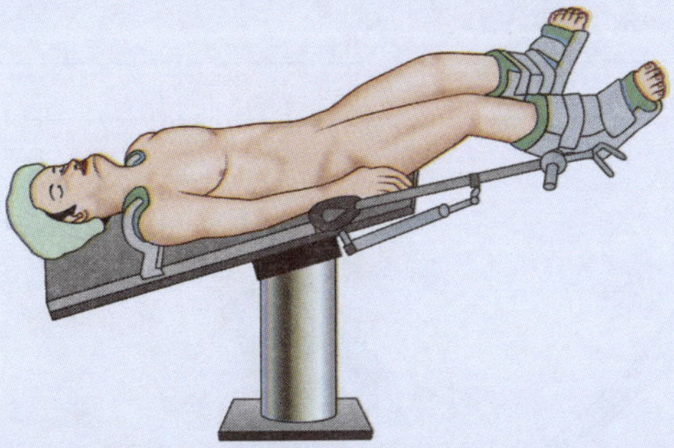

Lloyd-Davies position
- Trendelenburg + Leg Split
- Laparoscopy procedures

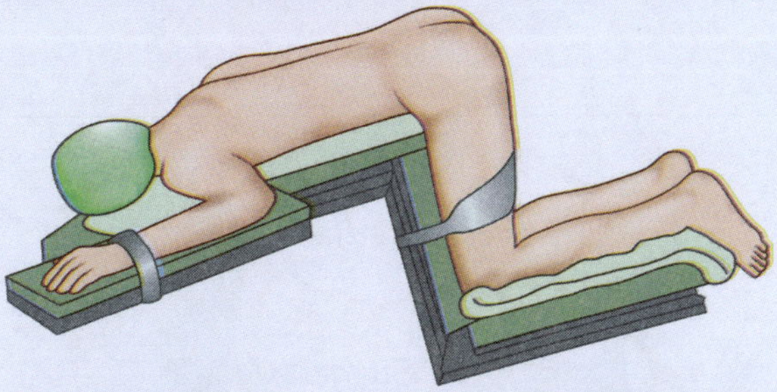

Jack knife position
- Prone Position
- Pilonidal sinus operated
- Positional Asphyxia may happen

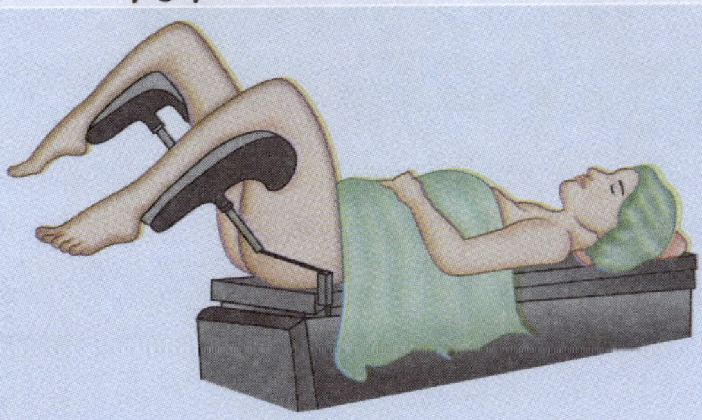

Lithotomy Position
- Gynecology procedures
- Injury to Common Peroneal nerve can happen

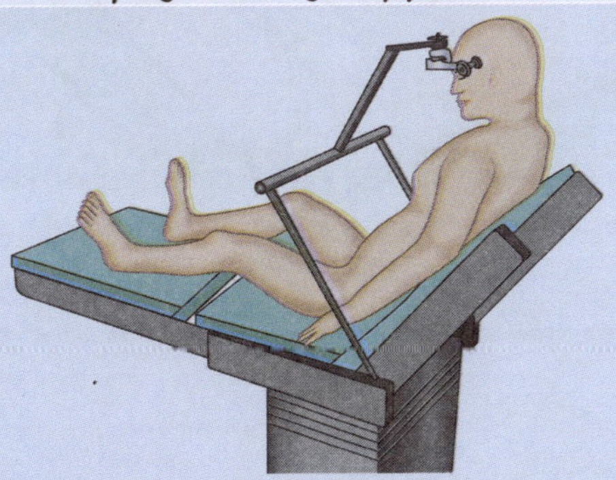

Sitting position:
- Neurosurgery
- Air embolism can happen

DURANT'S POSITION/MANEUVER

A position used in air embolism in which the patient is immediately put in left lateral decubitus with head low position (Trendelenburg) so that gas will remain in the apex of ventricle and may be aspirated under Echo guidance.

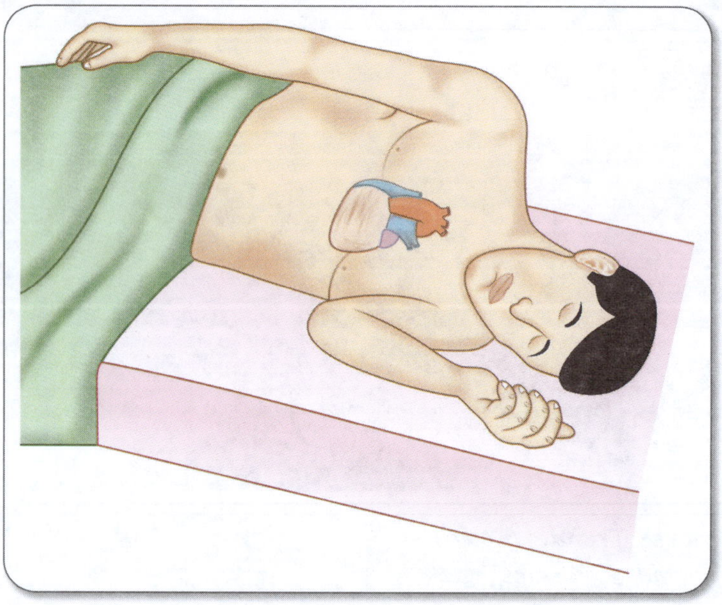

ADVANCES IN SURGERY

Laparoscopic Surgery

- Insufflation of gas in peritoneal cavity and operating via small holes.
- **Gases used:** Carbon Dioxide(MC), Nitrogen, Air
- Carbon dioxide is rapidly absorbable and causes less postoperative pain and less incidence of fat embolism**.
- CO_2 is 200 times more diffusible and rapidly cleared from circulation*.
- Intraperitoneal pressure maintained during surgery- 12-15 mm Hg**
- **Laparoscopy pneumoperitoneum is created by two methods:** Open and Closed method

Differences between open and closed method

Open method	Closed method
Using Hassan's Cannula	Using Veress needle
Risk of major vessel injury is less	Risk of bowel injury is less as it has safety valve at tip.
Trocar penetrates—Skin, Superficial and Deep fascia, Fascia Transversalis, parietal peritoneum.	

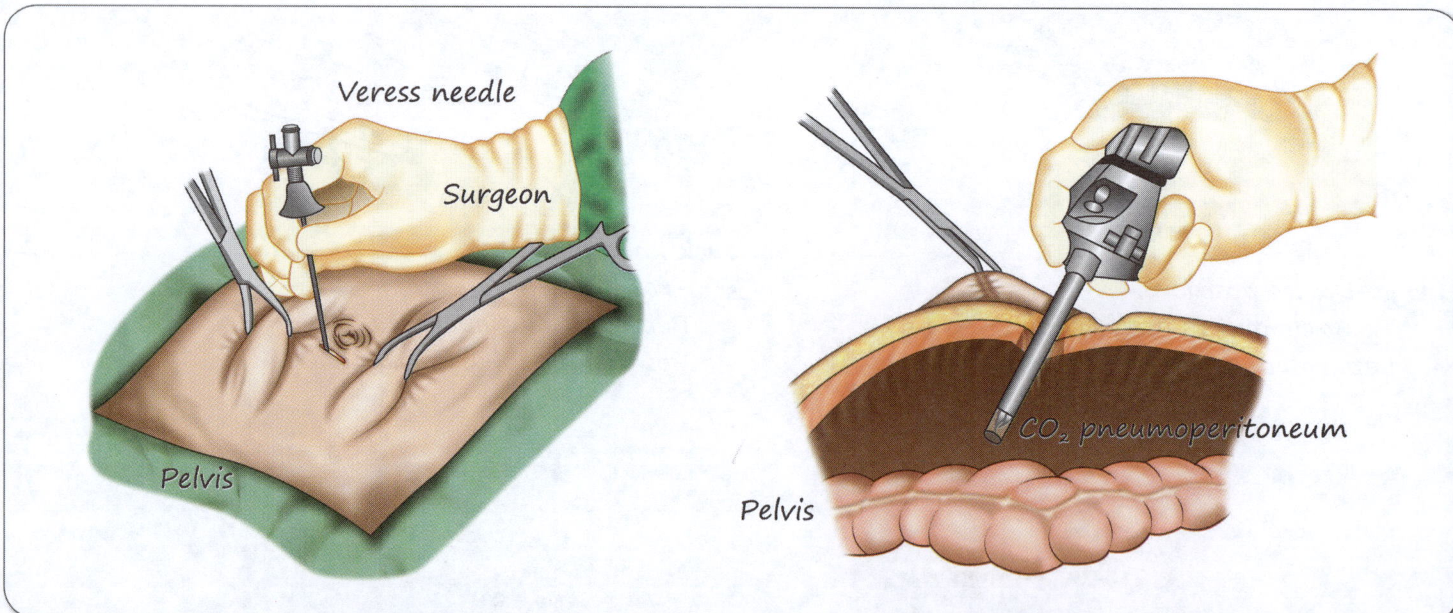

Robotic Surgery

- *da Vinci Robot**

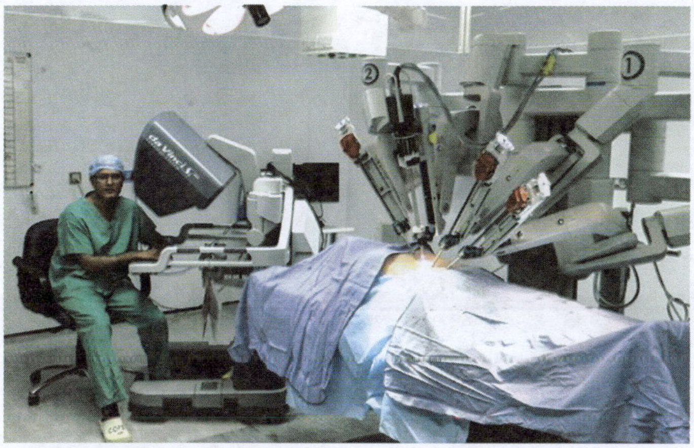

- **Docking—Inserting the limbs of Robot inside**
- **Major Advantages:**
  - Eliminates tremors of the surgeon
  - Multidirectional movement—7 degrees of freedom
  - Tele robotic Surgery can be done

TYPES OF SURGERIES

- **Outpatient surgery:** Not admitted to a ward facility
- **Procedure room surgery:** Surgery not requiring full sterile theater facilities
- **Day or same-day surgery:** Admitted and discharged within the 12-hour day**
- **Overnight stay:** 23-hour admission with early morning discharge
- **Short-stay surgery:** Admission for up to 72 hours

Day Care Surgery

Definitions:

- **Day Surgery**—Patient was admitted in Hospital for 12 hours only**
- **Overnight Stay Surgery**—Patient needs '23 hour stay'
- **Short stay Surgery**—72 hours admission

Criteria for Day Care Surgery

Medical Criteria

- Age—No upper limit
- ASA—Grade 1, 2
- BMI <40 is essential

Social Criteria

- Responsible adult available to take care for 24 hours
- House should be situated at a distance of less than one hour

Surgical Criteria

- Surgery up to two hours only
- Patient must be able to eat and drink self

Anesthesia Points

- Total Intravenous Anesthesia (TIVA) using Propofol is used.
- Short-acting opioids like Fentanyl, Alfenatil is used
- Avoid Long-Acting Morphine to reduce Postoperative Nausea and Vomiting.

Discharge Criteria

- Vital signs stable >1 hour
- Oriented to place, time
- Oral analgesia relieves pain
- Able to dress and walk
- Minimal nausea, vomiting and dizziness
- Oral fluids taken
- Minimal bleed or discharge
- Passed urine
- Adult to take care for next 24 hours
- Knows when to come back
- Emergency contact number given

CAPSULE ENDOSCOPY

- 26 × 11 mm size capsule
- Battery life = 8 hours
- Total images 50000/8 hours
- Dummy capsule which can dissolve in 40 hours is used if you suspect chances of obstruction* or Strictures.

- *Contraindications: Gastroparesis, pseudo obstruction, Strictures, Small bowel obstruction.*
- *Gold standard in Diagnosis of Occult GI bleeding and Crohn's disease***

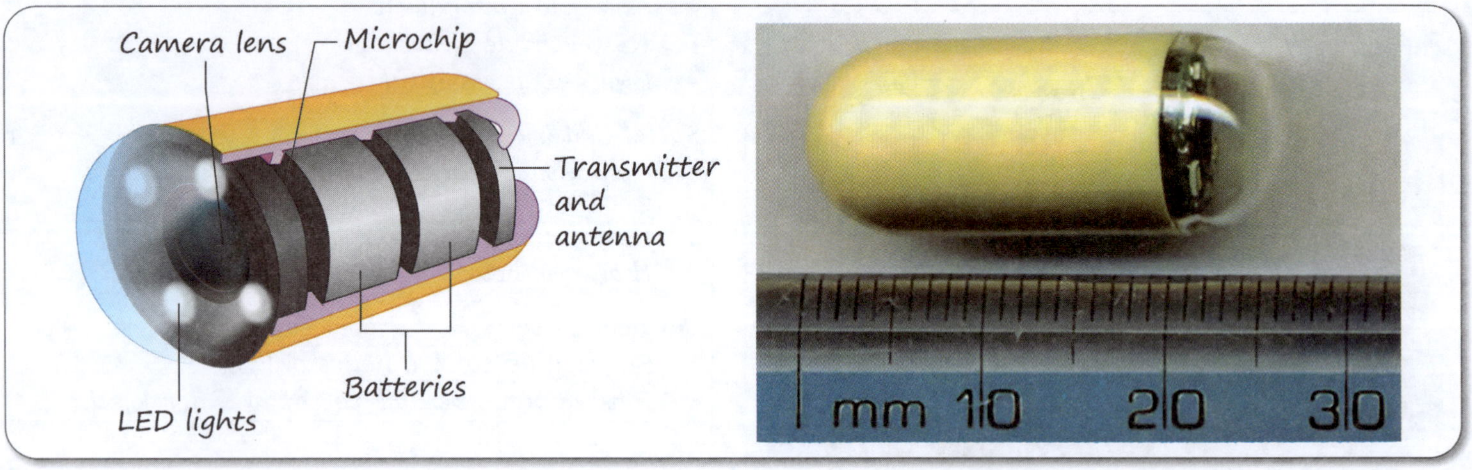

Endoscopy

ERAS PROTOCOLS

- *Early postoperative enteral feeding may decrease the incidence of infectious complications and is a component of most enhanced recovery after surgery (ERAS) protocols.*
- *The ERAS protocol describes the perioperative care pathway with recommendations for patient care at various steps in the perioperative process.*

Points to be taken into consideration for ERAS protocols	
• *Preadmission counseling* • *Avoid mechanical bowel preparation* • *Preoperative carbohydrate loading* • *No NG tubes* • *Small transverse incisions or Laparoscopy surgery* • *Avoid preoperative salt or fluid overload*	• *Short-acting anesthesia drugs* • *Thoracic Epidurals* • *Avoid opiate analgesia* • *Maintain perioperative temperature* • *Prevent postoperative nausea and vomiting* • *Early mobilization* • *Early introduction of oral fluids/ diets/ supplements* • *Early removal of Foley catheter.*

PRACTICE GUIDELINES ESTABLISHED BY THE ASA (AMERICAN SOCIETY OF ANESTHESIOLOGISTS) FOR PREOPERATIVE FASTING

Practice guidelines are methodically developed recommendations that help the health care professional and patient in making decisions about health care.

Some of the recommendations are as follows:

- ***8 hours or more fasting** after intake of fried or fatty foods or meat*
- ***6 hours or more fasting** after ingestion of a light meal, nonhuman milk or infant formula.*
- ***The ASA recommends fasting at least 2 hours from clear liquid intake, including medicines*****. It helps to avoid symptoms of dehydration, hypoglycemia or caffeine withdrawal.*
- *Many fast-track protocols suggest a **"carbohydrate-rich drink 2 hours before surgery"** in order to convert the patient from the "fasted" to the "fed" state causing reduction in postoperative insulin resistance.*

SURGICAL SITE INFECTIONS

Different types of surgeries with examples, infection rate with and without prophylaxis

Type of surgery	Examples of surgeries	Infection rate with prophylaxis	Infection rate without prophylaxis
Clean Surgery: (No viscus opened)	• Heart, Brain, Joint, Transplant surgeries • Herniorrhaphy* • Swelling excision	1%	1%
Clean Contaminated Surgery: (Viscus Opened, Minimal Spillage)	• Wound of Bowel, Biliary and Pancreatic Surgery • Uncomplicated appendicitis* • Gastro Jejunostomy	3%	5-10%
Contaminated surgery	• Appendiceal abscess • Perirectal abscess drainage • Infected laceration • Diverticulitis	6%	10-20%
Dirty Surgery	• Worst wound • Acute cholecystitis with spillage of pus from gallbladder. • Traumatic wound • Bowel obstruction with enterotomy and spillage of content.	7%	Upto 40%

Surgical site infection (SSI) is defined as:

- Wound Infection in <30 days of Surgery
- Wound Infection in <1 year of Implant cases
- Most common SSI pathogens are all gram-positive cocci—*Staphylococcus epidermidis***, *S. aureus* and *Enterococcus***
- For infra inguinal incisions and intra cavitary surgery, gram-negative bacilli such as *Escherichia coli* and *Klebsiella* are potential pathogens.

How to prevent SSI?

- One hour before surgery prophylactic antibiotics (before incision)
- Shaving not advised now (If needed, skin clippers or epilators used to remove the hair just before shifting to OT)
- Avoid hyperglycemia during surgery (Blood sugar <200 mg/dL)
- Avoid hypothermia
- Avoid contamination (Sterile precautions)
- Avoid hypoxia intraop and post op also for 4 hours.
- Avoid hypotension
- Surgery Extending >4 hours (Every 4 hours one more dose is given)—Prophylactic antibiotics not given beyond 24 hours.

Grading Systems for SSI

Southampton Wound grading System: (Mnemonic- EISPA)

Grade	Appearance
0	Normal healing
1	Erythema
2	Inflammation
3	Serosanguinous discharge
Major Complications	
4	Pus
5	Anatomical separation

ASEPSIS Scoring System

	Criteria	Points
A	Additional treatment	0
	• Antibiotics for Wound Infection	10
	• Drainage of Pus under Local anesthesia	5
	• Debridement of Wound under GA	10
S	Serous Discharge	Daily 0-5
E	Erythema	Daily 0-5
P	Purulent Discharge	Daily 0-10
S	Separation of deep tissues	Daily 0-10
I	Isolation of bacteria from Wound	10
S	Stay as inpatient prolonged over 14 days	5

CAUSES OF POSTOPERATIVE FEVER

Day	Cause (Mnemonic—ABCDE)
1	Atelectasis of Lungs
2-3	Hospital Acquired Infection (MC UTI- Bladder infection) Atelectasis- Pneumonia Superficial Venous Thrombophlebitis (Catheters)
4-5	MC-Surgical Site Infection Deep Vein Thrombosis
6	Burst (Exposed) Abdomen in Laparotomy cases Salmon sign—Sudden gush of fluid is the 1st sign**
7 onward	Intra-abdominal Collection (MC in Pelvis/Morrison Pouch)

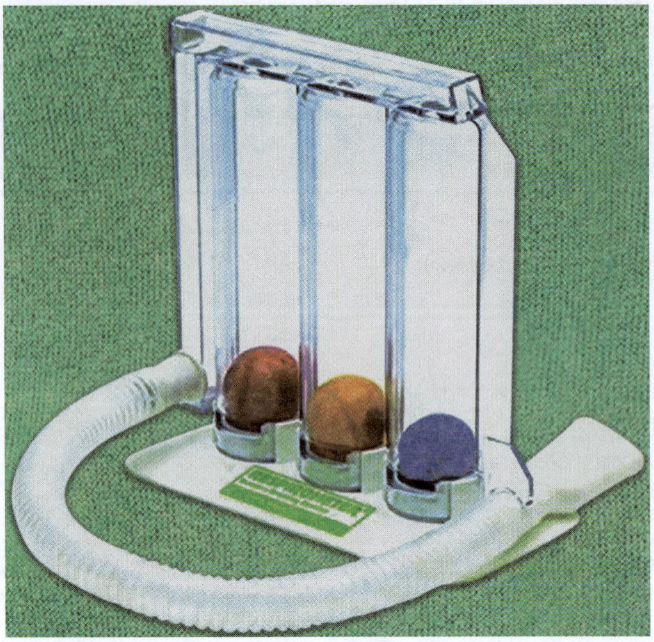

Incentive spirometer for breathing exercises

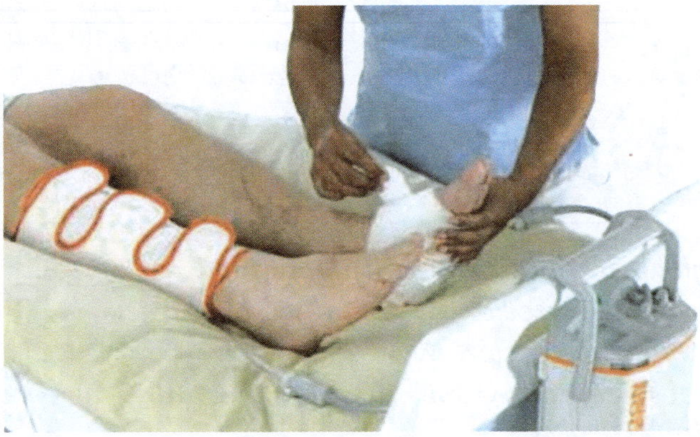

Pneumatic compression device to prevent DVT

SKIN LESIONS

Pressure Sores

- Tissue necrosis with prolonged pressure
- Also known as bed sores, pressure ulcers, decubitus ulcers.
- Incidence—5% in hospitalized patients.
- Pressure sore is MC in Ischium** > Greater Trochanter > Sacrum in the Gluteal region.
- After Gluteal region, the sites in order are- Heel> Lateral malleoli > Occipital region
- Pressure sore occurs if external pressure exceeds 30 mmHg of capillary occlusive pressure.
- **Prevention is the best treatment:**
  - Bedridden patients turned every 2 hours once
  - Wheel chair patients must lift themselves every 10 minutes for 10 seconds.

- **Treatment:**
  - Debridement
  - VAC devices at negative—125 mm Hg Suction pressure**
  - Flaps

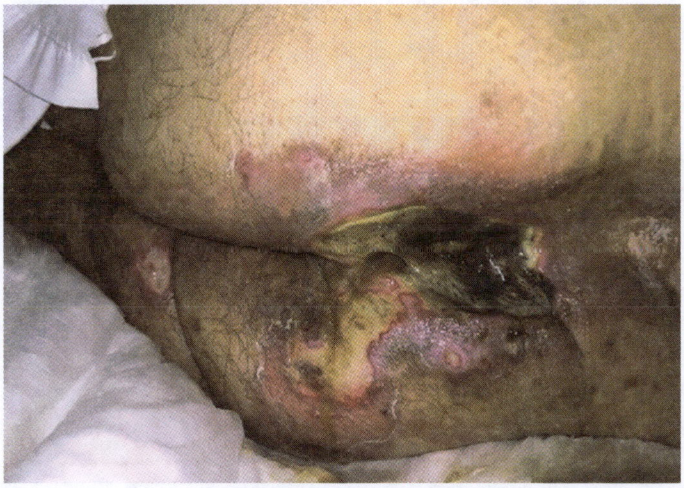

Stage 3 Bedsore

Necrotizing Fasciitis

- Rapid progressive bacterial infection characterized by involvement and necrosis of the subcutaneous tissue and fascia, **with typical sparing of underlying muscle***
- MC site of Infection: **Lower extremity***
- May involve trunk, perineum (Fournier's gangrene), Abdominal wall (Meleney's gangrene), Head and Neck and any other site*
- MC single etiological agent—**Group A beta-Hemolytic Streptococci*** (Usually caused by Polymicrobial organisms)
- Risk factors—Diabetes, immunocompromised, smoking, penetrating trauma, obesity, IV drug abuse, skin infection (abrasions, bites and boils)
- **Pain is the MC presenting symptom*** and pain is disproportionately high.
- Wood hard texture in subcutaneous tissue*
- Systemic features—Fever, hypotension, tachycardia, progression to septic shock, DIC, MODS.
- **Treatment**—Urgent Surgical Debridement+ IV fluids+ Broad spectrum antibiotics+ Supportive treatment.
- Mortality is 100% without debridement*
- Hyperbaric Oxygen Therapy*

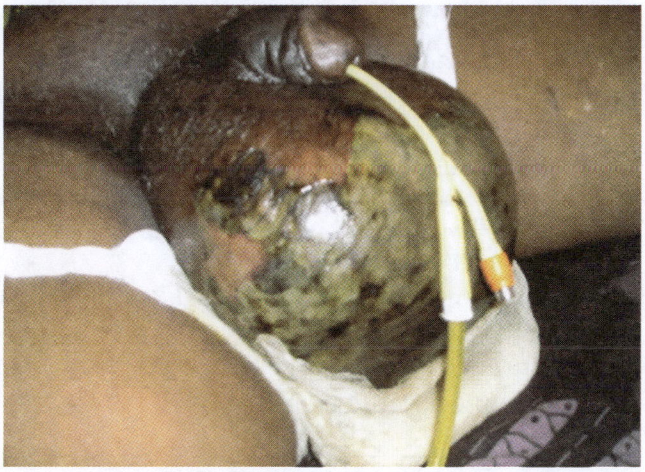

Fournier's gangrene

Hypertrophic Scar Versus Keloid

Differences between hypertrophic scar and keloid

Hypertrophic scar	Keloid
• Proliferation of mature fibroblasts* • No proliferation of blood vessels • Scars crossing Langer's lines • Hypertrophy limited to the scar and does not encroach adjacent tissues • No claw like process • No itching • Equal in male and female • Common in children • Gradually regresses after 6 months • Does not recur after excision **Common site: Flexor surfaces**	• Proliferation of immature fibroblasts* • Proliferation of immature blood vessels • Encroachment of surrounding tissues by claw like process • Itching and blanching • Slightly warm and slightly tender • Most common in people with black or brown skin, has genetic association • Females > males • Common age- 10-30 years • Occasionally malignant change (Marjolin's ulcer) • Recurrence after excision common • Intra keloidal – steroid, hyaluronidase, vitamin A and methotrexate to prevent recurrence. **Common site: Sternum**

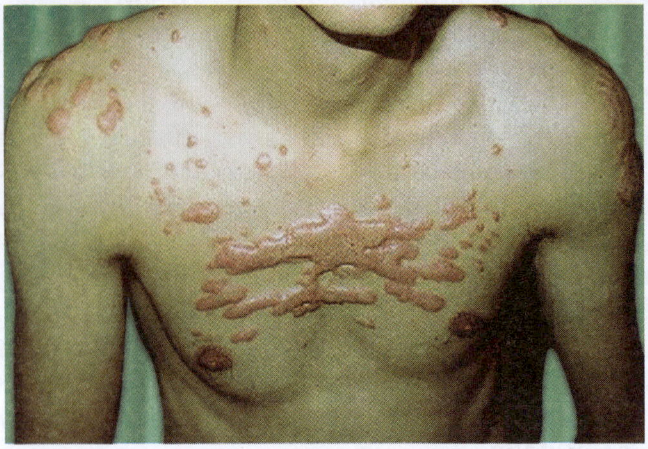

Keloid

Trophic Ulcer

- Trophic ulcer is due to impaired nutrition, blood supply and added neurological deficit.
- Important causes: diabetes, tabes dorsalis, leprosy, peripheral neuritis, etc.
- Also called neurotrophic/neuropathic ulcer.

On examination:

- Painless ulcer
- MC location—pressure points like foot, back (bedsores) etc.
- Punched out
- Base formed by underlying bone

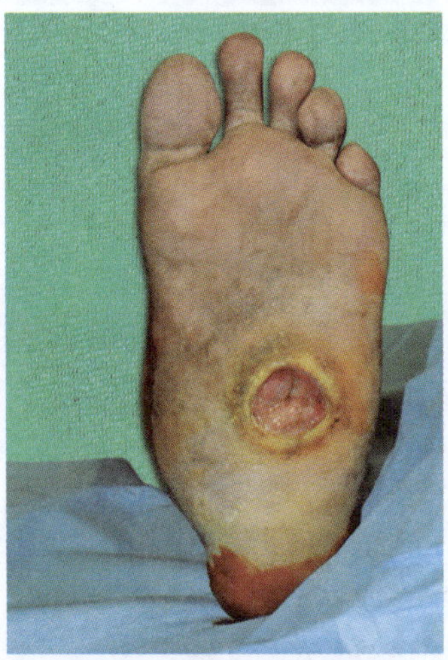

Trophic ulcer foot

Marjolin's Ulcer in a Burns Scar

Venous Ulcer: (Stasis Ulcer/Varicose Ulcer)

- **Site:** Lower 1/3 medial side of leg
- **Size:** Variable
- **Shape:** Oval to circular
- **Margin:** Well defined
- **Edge:** Sloping edge (healing)
- **Floor:** Formed by deep fascia
- **Surrounding:** Pigmentation, Eczema, varicosity (Lipodermatosclerosis)
- **Base:** Extend up to periosteum.
- **Deformity:** Talipes Equinovarus

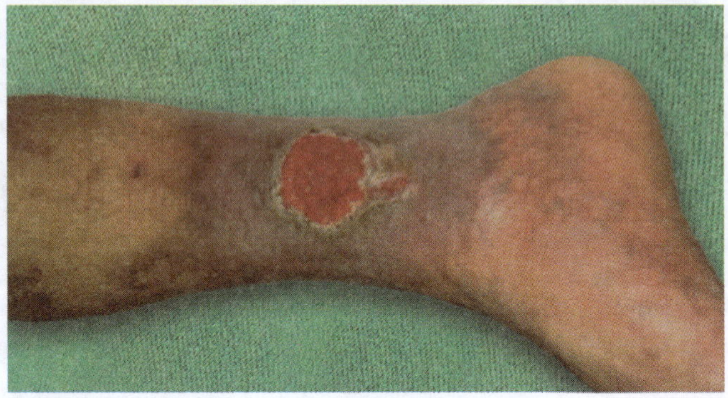

Marjolin's Ulcer

- Ulcers due to burns, keloid or varicose ulcers can get converted to a malignancy known as Marjolin's ulcer
- Marjolin's ulcer is a squamous cell carcinoma.
- No lymph node mets seen.

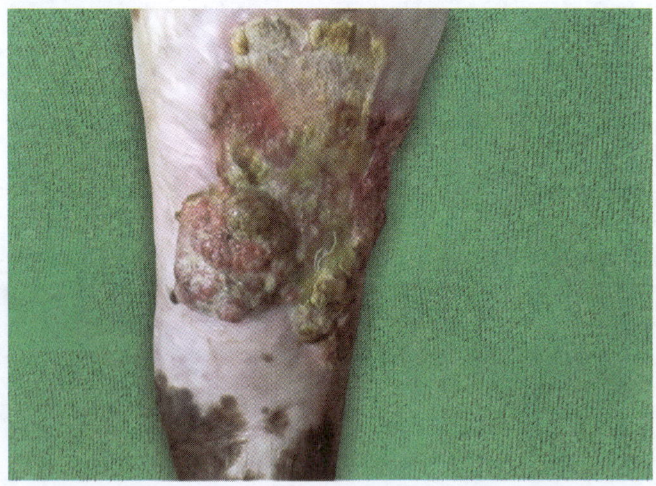

SWELLINGS RELATED TO SKIN

1. Lipoma

- MC benign tumor in the body
- Universal tumor—occurs anywhere in body

Characteristic features:

- Nontender
- Semi fluctuant

- Mobile (slip sign)
- Skin is free

Complications:

- Sarcomatous change
- Saponification
- Calcification
- Submucosal lipoma in intestine causes intussusception and intestinal obstruction

Treatment:

Excision or enucleation

2. Dermoid Cyst

Four types

Sequestration dermoid

- Occurs at line of embryonic fusion
- Epithelium gets sequestrated
- **Clinical features:**
    - Free skin
    - Not transilluminant
    - Fluctuant
    - Indentation of bone

MC sites of sequestration:

- Forehead
- External angular dermoid
- Post auricular
- Root of nose
- Sublingual dermoid
- Anywhere in midline at fusion

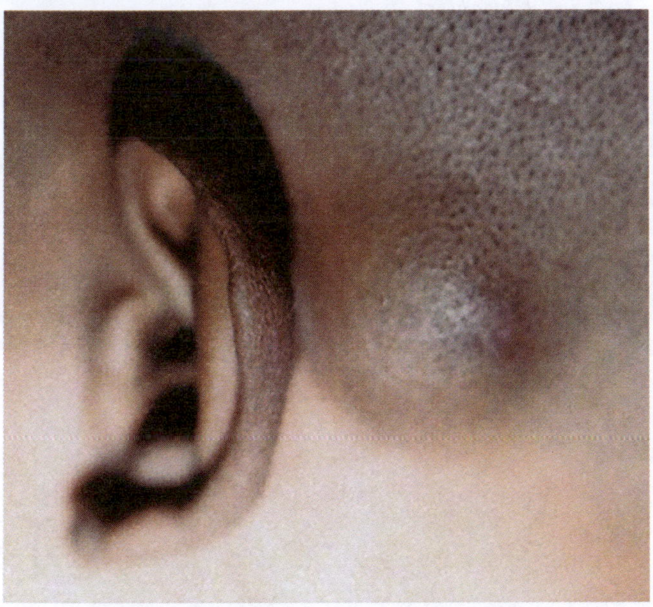

Post auricular dermoid

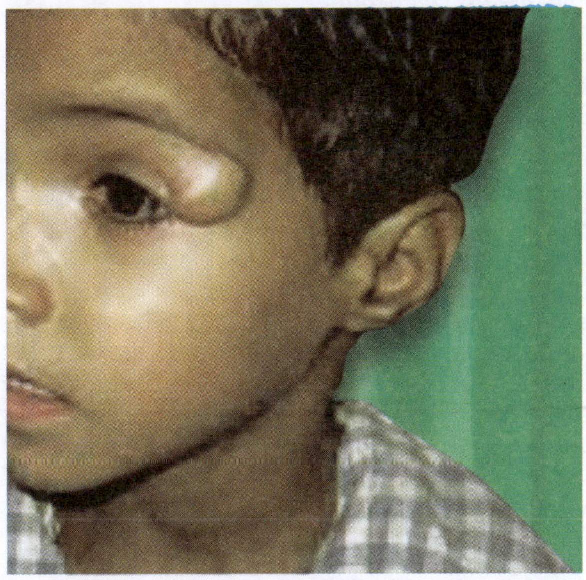

External angular dermoid

Tubulo Dermoid

Arises from embryonic structures

- Thyroglossal cyst
- Post anal dermoid

Implantation Dermoid

- Due to minor pricks or trauma, epithelium get buried into deeper subcutaneous tissue.
- MC site is fingers

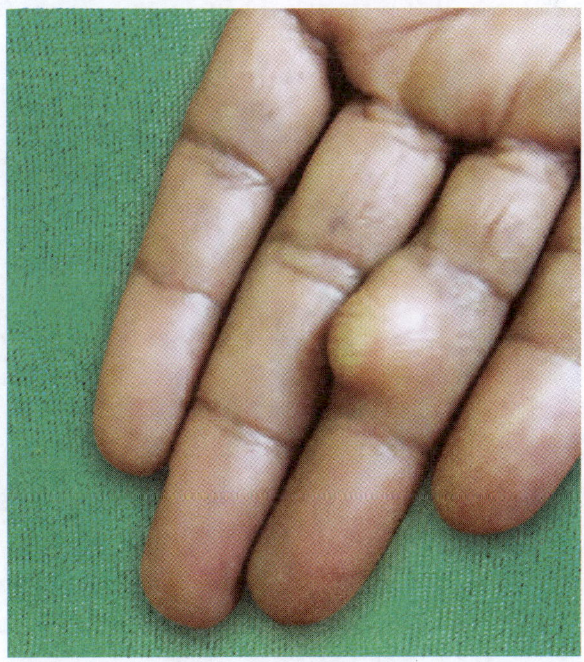

Implantation dermoid

Teratomatous Dermoid

- Arises from all germinal layers ecto, endo and mesoderm
- Occurs in ovary, testis, retroperitoneum and mediastinum.
- Contains hair, teeth, cartilage and muscle
- Can be benign or malignant.

3. Sebaceous Cyst

- Sebaceous cyst is a retention cyst due to blockage of the duct of sebaceous gland causing cystic swelling.
- Not seen in palms and soles

Characteristic features:

- Smooth, soft and nontender, mobile
- Molds on finger indentation
- Punctum – 70% cases (In 30% cases, the cyst opens into hair follicles and hence, punctum not seen)

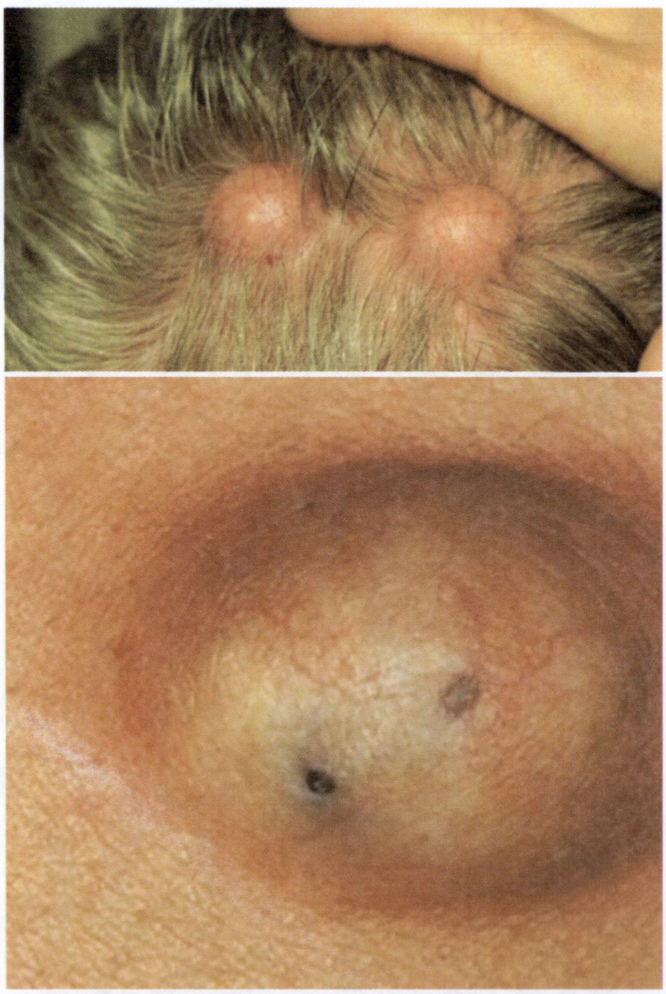

Sebaceous cyst showing punctum

Extra Edge:

- **Cock's peculiar tumor:** Sebaceous cyst surface gets ulcerated leading to painful fungating mass in head.
- **Sebaceous horn:** Hardening of slow discharge sebum via the punctum.
- **Gardner syndrome:** Familial adenomatous polyposis associated with multiple sebaceous cysts.
- **Fordyce disease:** Ectopic sebaceous glands in lip and oral mucosa.
- **Dercum's disease:** Multiple painful lipomas (adiposis dolorosa).

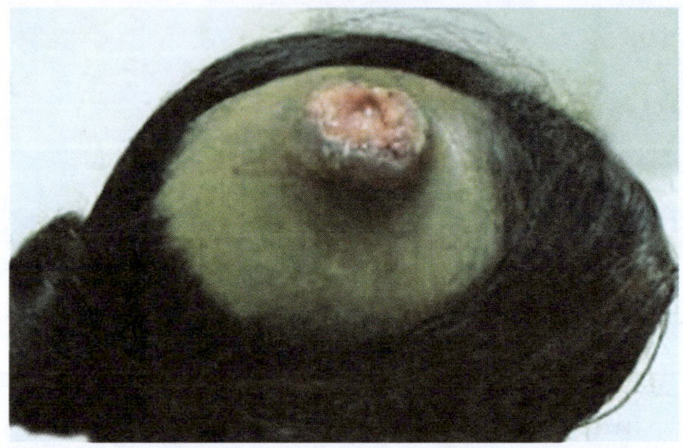

Cock's peculiar tumor

HIDRADENITIS SUPPURATIVA

Chronic fibrous and infective disease of skin bearing apocrine sweat glands.

- Apocrine glands are those which open into hair follicle.
- MC in diabetics
- MC in axilla
- MC due to staphylococci
- Treatment: Excision with grafting.

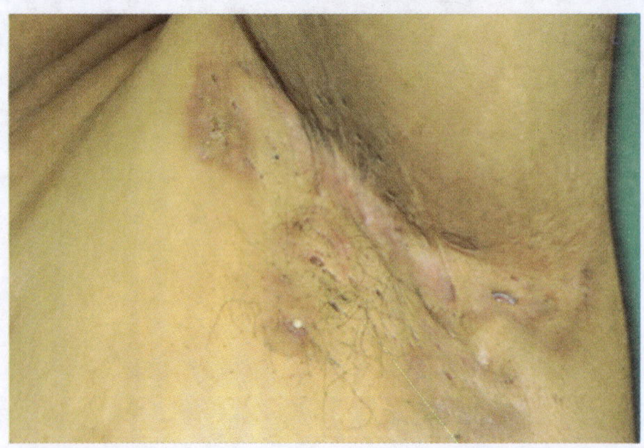

Hidradenitis suppurativa

2. TRAUMA

TRIAGE

Triage, a French word, means *"to sort"*—Sorting out the injuries according to severity

Four color codes are given as follows:

1. **Red:** This represents first priority, i.e., a critical patient (e.g., Tension pneumothorax, pericardial tamponade).
2. **Yellow:** This represents second priority (e.g., Major bone fractures, open pneumothorax).
3. **Green:** This represents minor issues and third priority (e.g., Tibial fractures, wrist bone fractures).
4. **Black:** This represents dead or about to die patients.

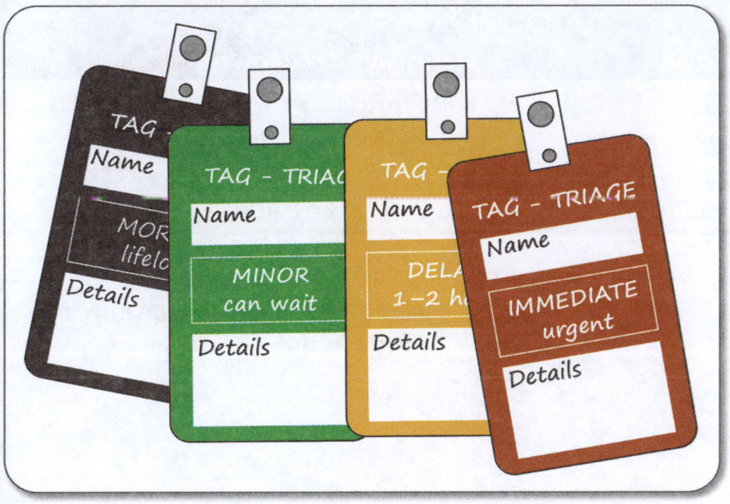

PRIMARY SURVEY: cABCDE

- c – Catastrophic hemorrhage
- A – Airway
- B – Breathing
- C – Circulation
- D – Disability and neurological status
- E – Exposure

MC cause of airway obstruction is falling of tongue backward.

Airway maneuvers to prevent falling of tongue backward are:

- Jaw thrust
- Chin lift
- Guedel airway
- **Definitive airway:** Oropharyngeal, nasopharyngeal airway insertion, tracheostomy intubation.

Orotracheal intubation	Nasotracheal intubation
• MC done method • Contraindicated in maxillofacial injuries (more than one time we must not do)	• Contraindicated in: ○ Base of skull fractures ○ Cribriform plate fractures ○ CSF Rhinorrhea+ ○ Maxillofacial fractures

- Maxillofacial injuries—Tracheostomy intubation advised*

Management of Circulation

- Two large bore, short, peripheral IV catheters. (Minimum two 16 G Cannulas used).
- If peripheral veins are available—IJV central vein is used in trauma.
- Children <6 years—Intraosseous transfusion.
- **Permissive hypotension:** Target systemic pressure 70–90 mm Hg; It must not go very high to prevent rebleeding and must not go very low to prevent cerebral hypoxia.
- CRASH-2 Trial:
  - **Tranexamic acid:** 1 g IV Stat over 10 minutes followed by 1 g for 8 hours.
  - It should be given to all trauma patients suspected to have significant hemorrhage with PR >110/min or BP <90 mm Hg systolic.

Log Roll:

- Not done now as there is a delay in WBCT.
- Done by four people.
- Primarily meant for spine examination.
- Part of primary survey**.
- Along with spine examination, we can also do Anal wink reflex and PR examination.
- During PR—Vermooten sign to look for floating prostate in membranous urethra injury (contraindicated now).
- Log roll is absolutely contraindicated in pelvic fracture patients**.

DAMAGE CONTROL SURGERY (ABBREVIATED LAPAROTOMY)

Indications for Damage Control Surgery (DCS)

Deadly triad**

- Hypothermia
- Acidosis
- Coagulopathy

Others:

- Serum Lactate >5 mmol/L
- ISS >36
- Systolic BP <70 mm Hg
- Transfusion >15 units of blood

Early Trauma Care (ETC)- Definitive management of Trauma Patient

Within 36 hours ETC if none of the above features seen

Serum Lactate – Significance:

- <2 mmol/L—ETC
- 2–5 mmol/L—Management in ICU
- >5 mmol/L—DCS

Damage control surgery is restricted to two goals only:

- Stop any active bleed
- Control any contamination.

Phases of damage control surgery:

- **Phase 1:** Initial exploration
- **Phase 2:** Secondary resuscitation
- **Phase 3:** Definitive operation

Phase 1 Initial exploration	Phase 2 Secondary resuscitation	Phase 3 Definitive treatment
• Control active hemorrhage and contamination* • Midline incision—4 quadrant packing done • GIT perforations closed with sutures or staples* • External drains kept for pancreatic/bile duct injuries • Temporary closure of abdomen using plastic sheet known as OPSITE** • Do Bogota bag method	• Transfer to ICU • Ventilatory support • Correct the deadly triad- hypothermia, acidosis, coagulopathy*	• Planned re-exploration and definite surgery* • Done 48–72 hours after secondary phase* • Complex reconstruction must be avoided* • Abdomen closure done in this phase only**

Stages of Damage Control Surgery as Per Bailey and Love

Stage	Procedure
I	Select the patient
II	Control hemorrhage, contamination
III	ICU resuscitation
IV	Definitive repairs
V	Closure of abdomen

HEAD INJURY

Methods to reduce intracranial pressure:

- Head up position 15°–30°
- Injections to reduce ICP—Mannitol (osmotic diuretics), Diuretics if BP is fine.
- Sedate the patient—Inj Barbiturates (Don't give diazepam as it can cause respiratory depression)
- Seizure prophylaxis—Sodium valproate
- Open skull fractures—prophylactic antibiotics
- Don't give steroids in trauma** (Can be used in malignancy in brain causing increased ICP)
- Lumbar puncture is contraindicated.
- External ventricular drainage is used to remove the CSF**
- Nasal oxygen

Glasgow Coma Scale (GCS)

Eye opening:	Verbal	Motor
• Spontaneous – 4 • To loud voice – 3 • To pain stimuli – 2 • Do not open – 1	• Normal oriented – 5 • Confused – 4 • Inappropriate words – 3 • Sounds only – 2 • No sounds – 1	• Obeys commands – 6 • Localizes to pain – 5 • Withdrawal flexion – 4 • Abnormal flexion – 3 (decorticate) • Extension – 2 (decerebrate) • No motor response – 1

Mnemonic:

- Verbal—One confused word sounds nowhere* (54321)
- Motor—Obey localities with flexion and extension now. (654321)

Essential points about GCS

- **Motor component – most predictive of future neurologic outcome**
- Maximum score = 15
- Minimum score (Dead patient) = 3
- Intubated patient = Mentioned as VNT (Not testable) = Score – 0
- Intubate when score is <8
- At admission when score is <13, take CT scan
- **Score represents the best performance elicited**, e.g., Flexion response to pain in left limb and localizing pain in right limb-take into consideration the best which is in right limb – M5**

Classification of head injury based on GCS:

- **Minor:** GCS 15 with no LOC
- **Mild:** GCS 14 or 15 with LOC
- **Moderate:** GCS 9–13
- **Severe:** GCS 3–8

Base of Skull Fractures

- **Raccoon/Panda eyes:** Bilateral periorbital hematoma (Anterior cranial fossa fractures)
- **Battle's sign:** Bruising over mastoid. Middle cranial fossa fracture
- **CSF otorrhea:** Middle cranial fossa fracture
- **CSF Rhinorrhea:** Anterior cranial fossa fracture
- Hemotympanum or bleeding from ear.

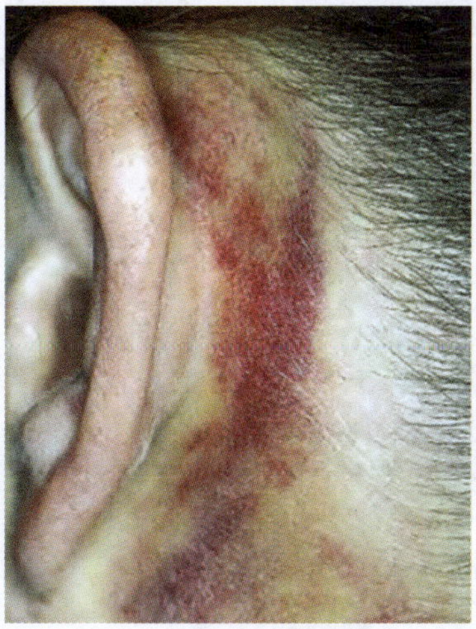

Battle sign*

Indications of NCCT Brain—NICE Guidelines: (National Institute for Health and Clinical Excellence)

Indications of CT in 1 hour:

1. **GCS <13 at any point***
2. GCS <15 at 2 hours
3. Focal neurological deficit
4. Suspected open, depressed or base of skull fracture
5. Post trauma seizure
6. Vomiting > one episode.

Indications of CT within 8 hours:

1. Age >65
2. Coagulopathy (on warfarin, aspirin or Rivaroxaban)
3. Dangerous mechanism of injury
4. Retrograde amnesia (>30 minutes)

EDH	SDH	SAH
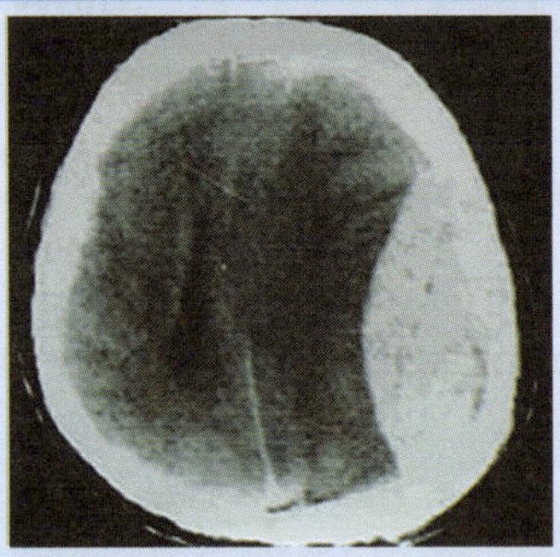	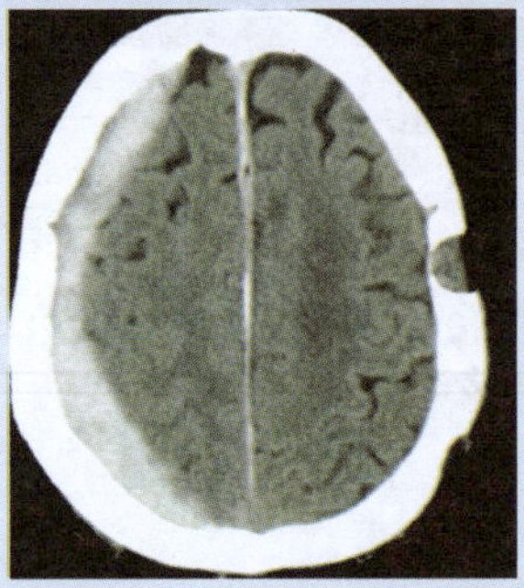	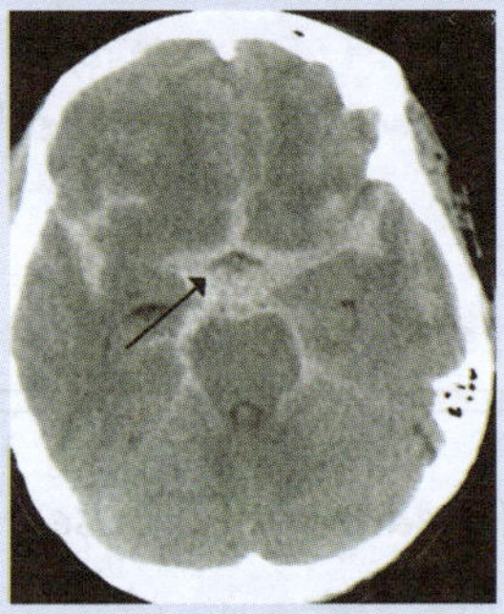
Biconvex appearance	Concavo-Convex appearance	MC type of hemorrhage-Intracerebral hemorrhage due to hypertension in PUTAMEN. The picture shown above is subarachnoid hemorrhage with blood in subarachnoid cisterns
• MC in young male patients • Always associated with skull fracture • Injured vessel—**Middle meningeal artery**** • MC site of injury is **temporal bone at pterion (thinnest part of skull)** which overlies the middle meningeal artery • The hematoma is located between bone and dura mater. • Lucid interval is seen- Period of consciousness before patient becomes unconscious	• Accumulates in space between dura and arachnoid • Associated with bridging vein disruption and brain laceration* • **C/F—Impaired consciousness from the time of impact itself.** • **Acute SDH—Follows trauma** • **Chronic SDH—People on Anticoagulants***	• MC cause of SAH nowadays is trauma • Other cause is sudden rupture of berry aneurysm
Treatment: Burr hole is TOC Mortality – 5%	**Treatment:** **Acute SDH:** Decompressive craniectomy and evacuation **Chronic SDH:** Burr Hole **Mortality:** 40%	

Diffuse Axonal Injury

- High acceleration and deceleration injury
- No surgery done
- Wait and watch
- IOC: MRI

THORACIC INJURIES

Intercostal Tube Placement: (ICD Placement)

- Pass the ICD in upper border of the rib (in lower border, intercostal vessels and nerve are present)
- **Triangle of Safety** – Anteriorly by lateral border of pectoralis major, posteriorly by mid axillary line and inferiorly by an imaginary horizontal line drawn at the level of nipple to meet mid axillary line.

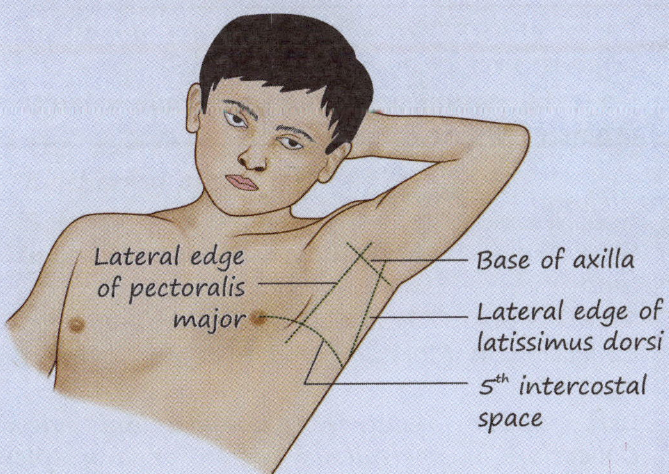

Triangle of safety

- Best space is 5th ICS in midaxillary line.
- 28 Fr, 32 Fr tubes are used. Ensure all holes are inside the chest*
- Underwater drainage device provides **20 cm H_2O suction.****

How to say ICD is functioning well?

- Moving of the air liquid column in ICD tube in correspondence with respiration.

If the column is not moving, this implies:

- ICD is not in position
- ICD is blocked
- ICD is displaced and hole lies outside
- Lung has fully expanded

Indications of thoracotomy in thoracic injury:

- Hemothorax more than 1500 mL (Blunt trauma)
- Hemothorax more than 1000 mL (Penetrating trauma)
- Hourly collection in ICD of >200 mL/hr for 3 hours
- All the dangerous dozen injuries (Except pulmonary contusion, flail Chest)

Pericardial Tamponade

- MC mechanism – **Penetrating trauma****
- Collection of blood inside the pericardial cavity.
- Blood in pericardial cavity will compress the heart.
- **Beck's Triad:** Raised JVP, Low BP and Muffled Heart sounds*
- **X-ray shows Air Bag Appearance**
- **Differential Diagnosis: Tension pneumothorax (tachypnea with absent breath sounds seen)**
- **IOC: eFAST diagnosis**
- **Bailey 28th Edition Update—Needle thoracocentesis is no more advised, directly thoracotomy and repair are needed.**
- **MC complication of needle insertion—Arrhythmias***
- **Definite treatment**—Thoracotomy and repair of myocardial leak.

Tension Pneumothorax

- Mechanisms—Penetrating trauma, Blunt Trauma with rib injuring, Central vein insertion.
- Collection of Air between the parenchyma and pleura.
- Pleura is intact and hence, during every breath, air enters the pleural cavity and compresses the lung which is already compressed.
- This results in **mediastinal shift, absent breath sounds****, low BP and raised JVP. (DD: Pericardial tamponade)
- C/F—Tachypnea and Dyspnea
- **Lifesaving procedure**—5th ICS in midaxillary line in adults and 2nd ICS in children
- **Definite procedure**—ICD insertion.

Hemothorax

- **MC vessel injured—Intercostal artery**
- MC vessel injured in massive hemothorax—Internal Mammary artery bleeding or Internal thoracic vessels.
- 1st line treatment—ICD
- Immediately thoracotomy needed for >1500 mL (Blunt), >1000 mL (penetrating) and >200 mL/hr × 3 hours.

Flail Chest

- **Three or more ribs fractured in two or more places****
- **Even one rib fractured at costochondral junction can cause flail chest.**
- Here, a segment of chest wall does not have continuity with the rest of thoracic cage.

Clinical features:

- On inspiration, **paradoxical movement** of chest occurs (segment moves inside on inspiration and on expiration that flail segment will move outside).
- Due to pain there is hypoxia.
- Underlying pulmonary contusion is the most important prognostic factor*.

Investigation of Choice:

- CT Scan with 3D reconstruction* to display vascular structures is the GOLD STANDARD IOC. It also shows the underlying lung parenchymal injury.

Management:

- Traditionally, the treatment is mechanical ventilation.
- But current treatment is only oxygen administration, adequate analgesia and physiotherapy.
- Mechanical ventilation is reserved for cases that develop respiratory failure, PaO_2 <60% and RR >18/min—Intermittent positive pressure ventilation (IPPV).
- Surgery and internal fixation of ribs are in use again.

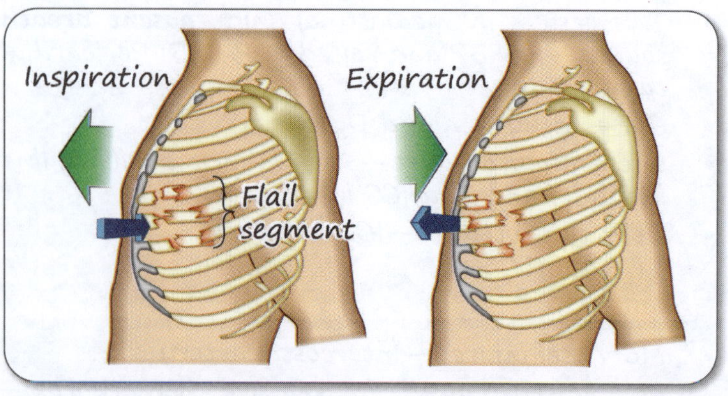

Paradoxical respiration in flail chest

Diagnostic Peritoneal Lavage (DPL)

- Insert a cannula below the umbilicus.
- About 1000 mL of warm ringer lactate is instilled into the abdomen and is then drained out.
- DPL has sensitivity of about 97–98%.
- DPL is especially useful for hypotensive, unstable patients with multiple injuries as a means of excluding intra-abdominal bleeding.

Result: Positive

- >1 lakh red cells/microliter
- >500 white cells/microliter
- Frank aspiration of >10 mL on cannula insertion is also positive*
- >19 IU/L of amylase
- Presence of bile or food particles

Disadvantages

- Invasive
- Nonrepetitive
- So many false positive cases (Nontherapeutic laparotomies happened)

FOCUSED ASSESSMENT WITH SONOGRAPHY FOR TRAUMA (FAST)

- Latest eFAST (extended FAST) is done at 6 regions, previously done by 4 FAST
- Done by casualty doctors or trauma surgeons trained for FAST.

Traditional Four Views

- Subxiphoid **Transverse view**—assess pericardial fluid
- Right upper quadrant **Longitudinal view**—Collection in Morrison pouch or any liver/renal injuries
- Left upper quadrant **Longitudinal view**—Collection in perisplenic region or any splenic injuries
- Suprapubic **Longitudinal and transverse view**—Collection in pelvis; assess bladder and POD
- Added up now two extra areas—right and left thoracic views to rule out pneumothorax (Stratosphere sign) or hemothorax.

Advantages of eFAST

- Repetitive
- Noninvasive
- Bedside investigation
- Short time study

Disadvantages of eFAST

- Detects more than **100 mL blood only**** (Bailey value)
- Does not detect bowel injury
- Not useful for penetrating injury (NEET PG 2020)
- Unreliable for RP collections
- Operator dependent.

IOC for unstable patients: *eFAST*
IOC for stable patients: *CECT abdomen*

Sequence Order Question

Blunt trauma	Penetrating trauma	Gun shot	Seat belt injuries
• Spleen • Liver • Small Intestine	• Liver • Stomach • Small bowel • Diaphragm • Colon	• Small bowel • Colon	• MC injury is mesenteric tear • In GIT—DJ flexure is injured

- Urban bomb blast—Ear drum > Lungs
- Underwater bomb blast—GIT (MC in terminal Ileum)

BLUNT TRAUMA PROTOCOL

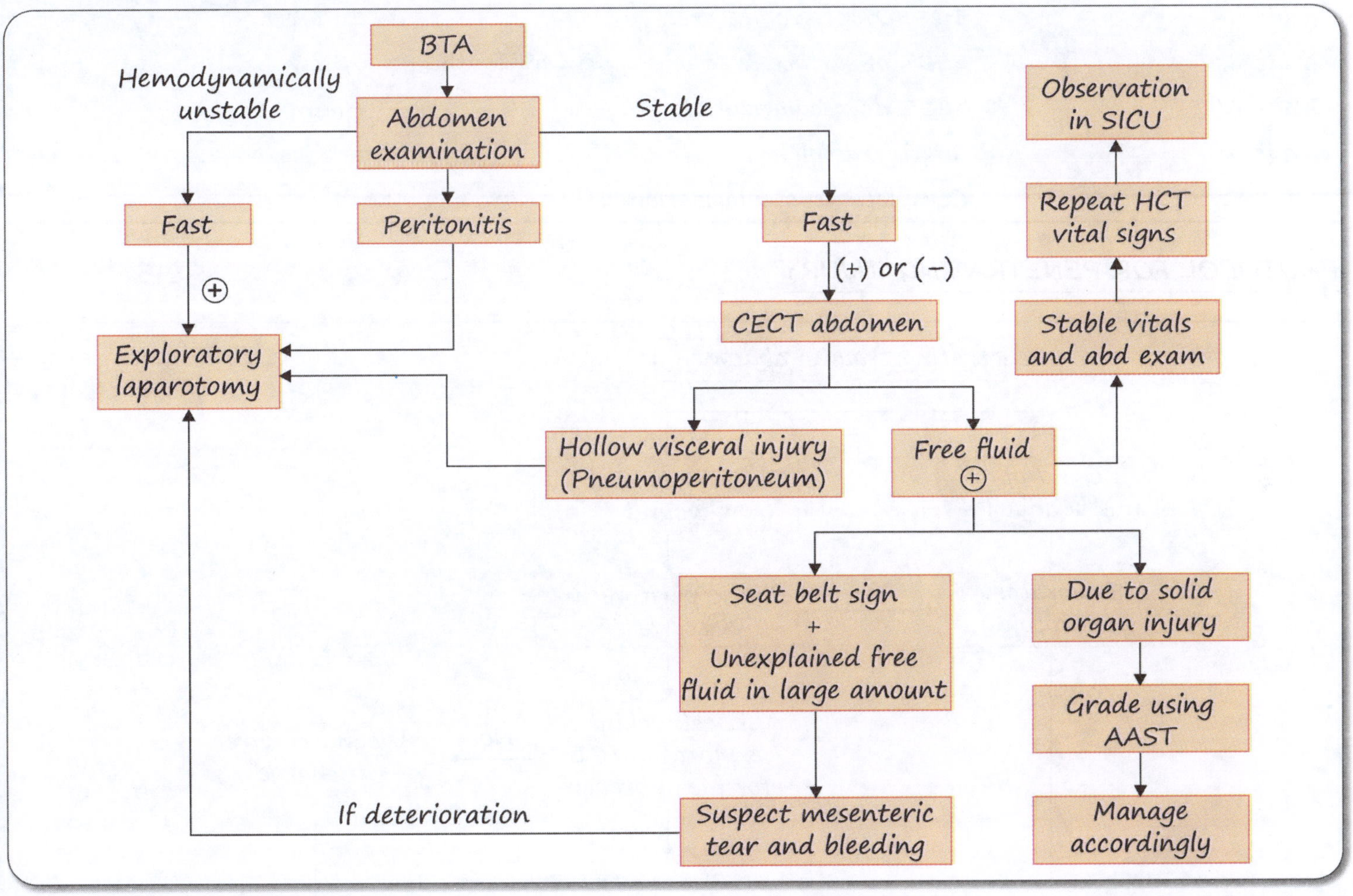

SOLID ORGAN INJURY-AAST GRADING

American Association for the Surgery of Trauma grading scales for solid organ injuries		
	Subcapsular hematoma	**Laceration**
Liver Injury Grade		
Grade I	<10% of surface area	<1 cm in depth
Grade II	10–50% of surface area	1–3 cm
Grade III	>50% of surface area or >10 cm in depth	>3 cm
Grade IV	25–75% of a hepatic lobe	
Grade V	>75% of a hepatic lobe	
Grade VI	Hepatic avulsion	
Splenic Injury Grade		
Grade I	<10% of surface area	<1 cm in depth
Grade II	10–50% of surface area	1–3 cm
Grade III	>50% of surface area or >10 cm in depth	>3 cm
Grade IV	>25% devascularization	Hilum
Grade V	Shattered spleen	
	Complete devascularization	

PROTOCOL FOR PENETRATING INJURY

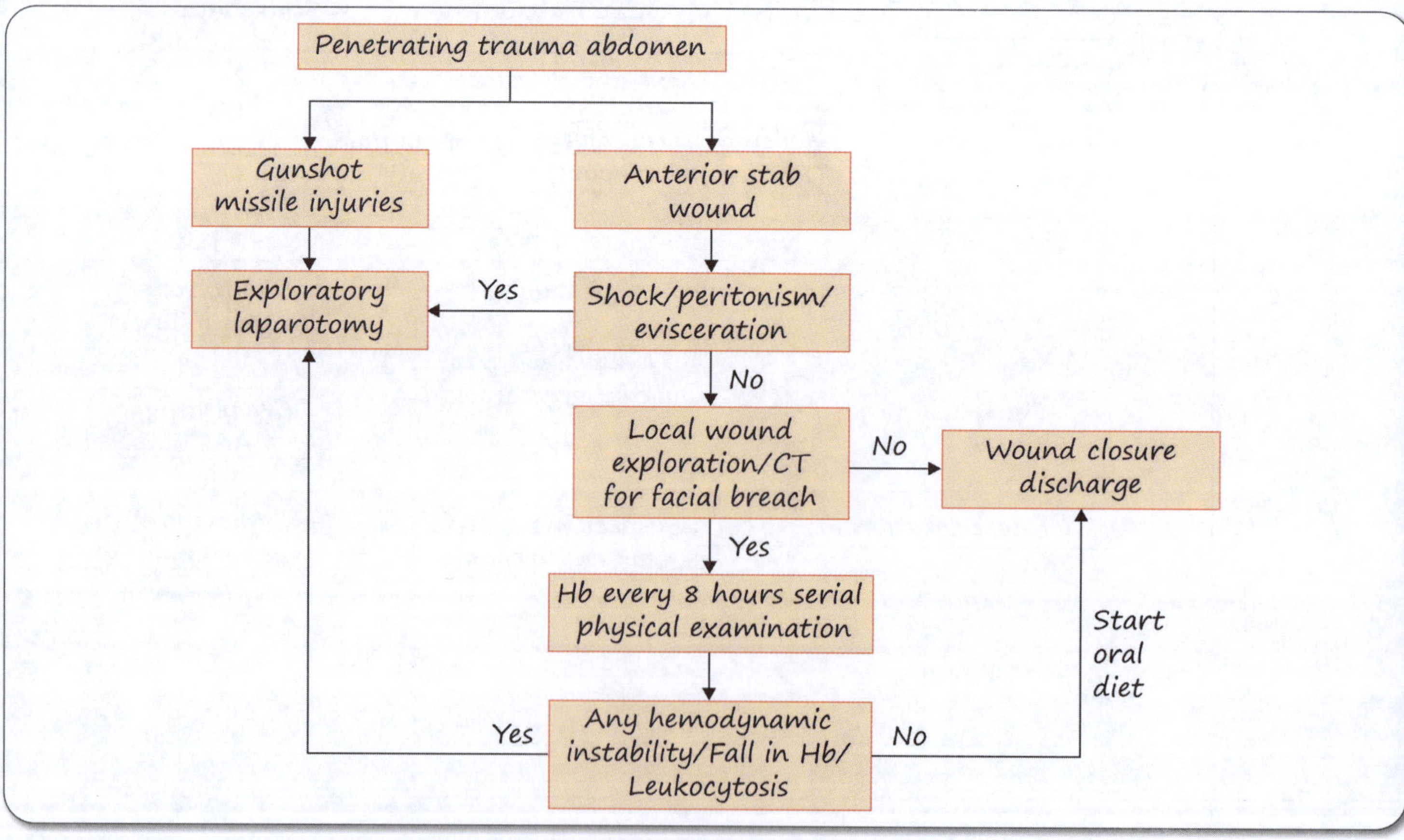

RETROPERITONEAL HEMATOMA

In retroperitoneum, four zones are explained; and management differs based on the hematoma in each zone.

Zones	Contents	Management
Zone I	Central vascular structures such as aorta and IVC	Needs exploration
Zone II	Kidneys and adrenal glands	Observed
Zone III	Retroperitoneum associated with pelvic vasculature	External pelvic compression and fixation
Zone IV	Retrohepatic IVC and hematoma behind portal vein	Observation

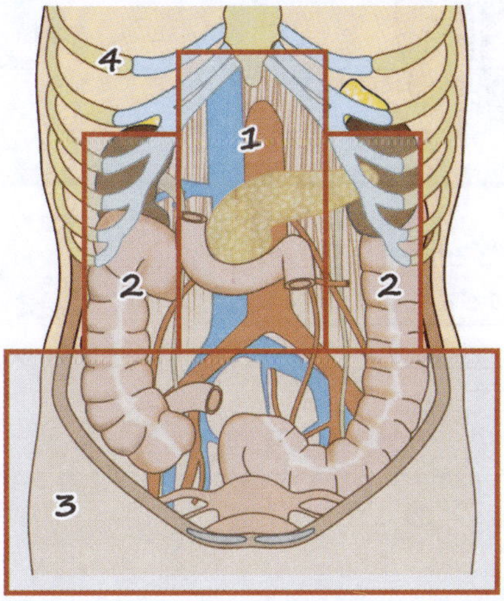

Zones of retroperitoneal hematoma

- **Mattox Maneuver:** Left side medial visceral rotation to reach aorta.
- **Cattell-Braasch Maneuver:** Right side medial visceral rotation to reach IVC.

THERMAL INJURIES

MC cause of death in burns:

- **On the spot (Immediate death):** Asphyxia >Neurogenic shock
- **1–3 days (Early death):** Hypovolemic shock
- **Late death:** Septic shock
- **MC cause of death in burns overall:** Septic shock

If percentage of burns is more than 15% in Adults and 10% in Children, it can develop in hypovolemic shock.

PATHOPHYSIOLOGY OF BURNS

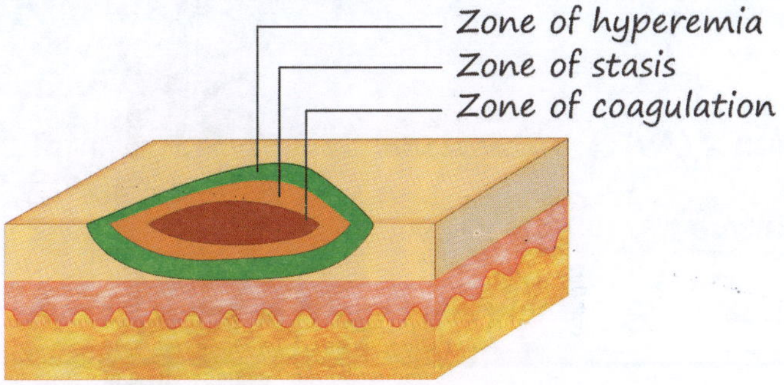

- **Zone of coagulation:** Irreversible damage
- **Zone of stasis:** Can progress or regress
- **Zone of hyperemia:** reversible zone** —Vessels are vasodilated here.

PERCENTAGE OF BURNS CALCULATION

Rule of nine (Alexander Wallace rule)

- Each upper limb—9% TBSA
- Each lower leg—18% TBSA
- Anterior or Posterior Trunk—18% TBSA
- Head and neck—9% TBSA
- Perineum—1% TBSA

Palm rule: Patient's palm = 1%

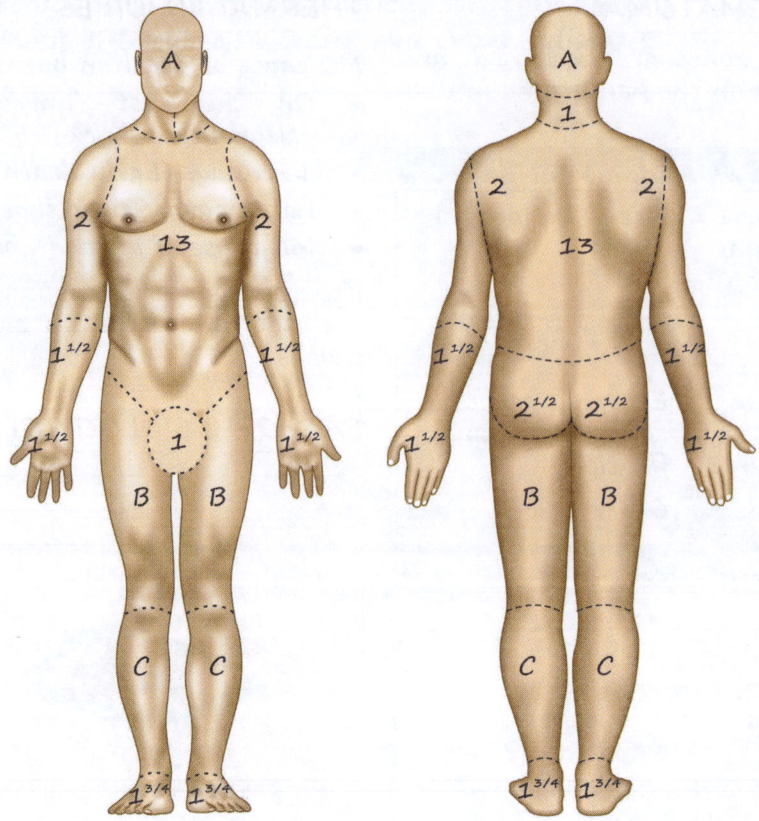

Relative percentage of area affected by growth

Age in years	0	1	5	10	15	Adult
A head	9	8	6	5	4	3
B thigh	2	3	4	4	4	4
C leg	2	2	3	3	3	3

Lund and Browder chart

- Most accurate method for calculating the burns percentage**
- Best method to calculate burns in children.

DEPTH OF BURNS

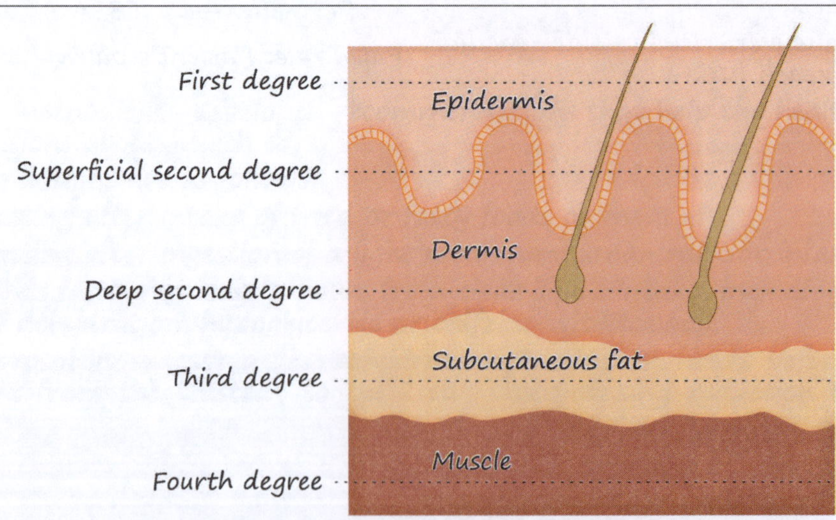

First-degree of burns: Superficial burns:

- Erythema + pain
- Heals without scar in 7 days
- Blanches on pressure

Second-degree superficial (Superficial partial thickness burns)

- Characterized by Blisters.
- Superficial touch (Cotton) – Sensation +
- Pin Prick – Sensation +
- Heals without scar in 3 weeks
- Blanches on pressure

Second-degree deep (Deep partial thickness burns)

- Characterized by Blisters
- Superficial touch (Cotton)—Sensation Absent**
- Pin Prick – Sensation+
- Heals with scar in 5 weeks
- No Blanching on pressure

Third-degree (Full thickness burns)

- Eschar formation seen
- Painless burns.
- Superficial touch (Cotton)—Sensation Absent**
- Pin Prick—Sensation absent**
- Can result in contracture and compartment syndrome

Fourth-degree burns

- Involving deep muscles and tendons**
- Most of them die due to cardiac arrest.

Management

- IV fluid of choice—Ringer lactate*
- Amount of fluid to be infused is calculated by **Parkland formula:**
- **TBSA% × weight (kg) × 4 = volume (mL) needed**
- Half of this volume is given in the first 8 hours, and the second half is given in the subsequent 16 hours.
- **This formula is calculated from time of BURNS** (Not from the admission)**
- In the initial 12 hours, we must give crystalloids only and not colloids as they may have leaking capillaries, which will lead to subcutaneous edema due to the colloids entering the subcutaneous space.
- **>12 hours Colloids like Dextran, hemacel, albumin are given based on "MUIR and BARCLAY Formula".**

Management of Burns Wound

First- and Second-Degree Superficial Burns

- Topical ointments
- MC used—Silver sulfadiazine (Cannot penetrate deeper tissues like Eschar)
- Silver nitrate (Black staining may happen)
- Mafenide Acetate—Can penetrate deeper into eschar (Can cause Metabolic acidosis**)
- Best of all agents—Cerium Bromide (Immunomodulator)—Costly
- SSD+ Cerium Bromide makes the eschar sterile and stimulates cell mediated immunity
- Collagen sheets are available in 2nd degree superficial burns.

Second-Degree Deep Burns

SSG (Thiersch graft is used)—Taken by Humby knife.

Third-Degree Burns

- SSG
- Escharotomy is done to avoid compartment syndrome.

3. HEAD AND NECK DISEASES

ORAL CAVITY AND MALIGNANCY

Conditions Associated with Malignant Transformation

High-risk lesions
- Erythroplakia
- Speckled erythroplakia
- Chronic hyperplastic candidiasis

Medium-risk lesions
- Oral submucous fibrosis
- Syphilitic glossitis
- Sideropenic dysphagia (Paterson—Kelly syndrome)

Low-risk/equivocal-risk lesions
- Oral lichen planus
- Discoid lupus erythematosus
- Discoid keratosis congenita

Leukoplakia

- White patch or plaque involving wide areas of oral mucosa
- 2.4% malignant transformation at 10 years, 4% at 20 years
- Speckled leukoplakia has the highest rate of Malignant transformation**
- Incidence among smokers: 20%; Nonsmokers: 1%
- Can be managed conservatively: Avoid smoking, carbon dioxide laser excision.

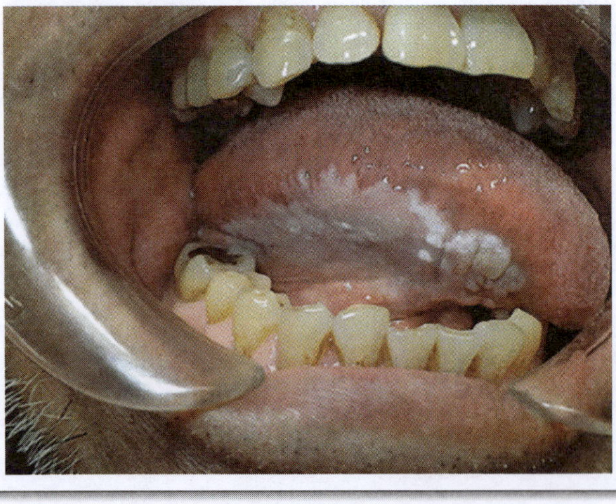

Leukoplakia

Erythroplakia

- Bright red velvety plaques of oral mucosa.
- Has 17 times more malignant potential.

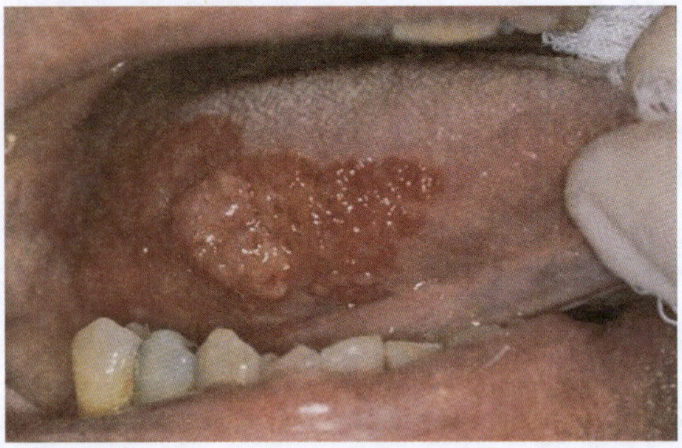

Erythroplakia

Must know:
- MC site of Oral cancer in World/Western countries—Tongue > Lip
- MC site of Oral cancer in India—Buccal Mucosa > tongue
- Histological type commonly seen in Oral cancers—Squamous cell cancer
- MC site of cancer to produce LN mets—Tongue
- Skip Mets are common with—Tongue cancer
- Bilateral LN spread seen in Lower lip, Supraglottis and Soft palate
- IOC for staging Oral and Parotid cancers—MRI
- Staining used to identify areas of Cancer in oral cavity—2% Toluidine blue

TNM Staging of Oral Cancers: (AJCC 8th Edition Update)

Annexure 1: AJCC 8th Edition Oral Cancer Staging

T staging:
- Tis—Carcinoma in situ
- T1—Tumor in greatest dimension <2 cm and DOI <5mm
- T2—Tumor <2 cm and DOI >5 mm but <10 mm or Tumor >2 cm but <4 cm and DOI <10 mm
- T3—Tumor more than 4 cm or any size with DOI >10 mm
- T4 a—Invasion into adjacent structures like cortical bone, inferior alveolar nerve, floor of mouth or skin of nose and chin in lip cancer and skin of face in oral cancer.
- T4 b—Invasion into masticator space, pterygoid plates, carotid sheath or encases internal carotid artery
- **Extrinsic muscle invasion is not considered T4 nowadays**

Contd...

N staging:

- N1—Metastasis in **single node ≤3 cm** in greatest dimension with no Extra nodal Extension (ENE—Negative)
- N2a—Metastasis in **single node** greater than 3 cm but not larger than 6 cm in greatest dimension, **(>3 cm to ≤6 cm)** No Extra nodal Extension (ENE—Negative)
- N2b—Metastasis in Multiple **Ipsilateral** nodes, **none larger than 6 cm**. ENE Negative.
- N2c—Metastasis in Bilateral or **Contralateral** nodes, **none larger than 6 cm**, ENE Negative.
- N3a—Metastasis in a Lymph node larger than 6 cm in greatest dimension, ENE Negative.
- **N3b—Metastasis in any size node with ENE+ve (Newly added point in AJCC)****

M staging:

- M1—Metastasis +

Investigations in Oral Cancers

- Biopsy: Incisional biopsy under local anesthesia* Biopsy must include normal area also*
- MRI is the IOC for oral, oropharyngeal, neck cancers. Ideally it should be performed before biopsy**
  (STIR—Short Tau Inversion Recovery MRI-Contrast enhanced with Gadolinium and Suppression techniques and variation in image sequence acquisition)
- CT is useful in diagnosing Bone invasions**. CT thorax is now mandatory for all Oral cancers to look for mets.
- PET CT is helpful in patients managed by nonsurgical method of oropharyngeal cancer. It also helps in diagnosing recurrence.
- USG guided FNAC of the neck nodes using 21 or 23G needle and there is no risk of dissemination.

Reconstruction of Tongue after Glossectomy

- **RFFF (Radial Forearm Free Flap)**
  - Most commonly used
  - Based on radial artery.
- **PMMC flap (Pectoralis Major Myocutaneous flap)**
  - Based on thoracoacromial artery
  - Cannot do in females—Can lead to Ca breast later.
- **Delto pectoral flap (DP flap)**
  - Can be used in females
  - Based on internal mammary artery.

Carcinoma Hard Palate and Maxillary Alveolus

- Smaller tumors—Transoral Partial Maxillectomy
- Larger tumors—Weber Ferguson Incision is used for a wider excision involving the maxillary floor.

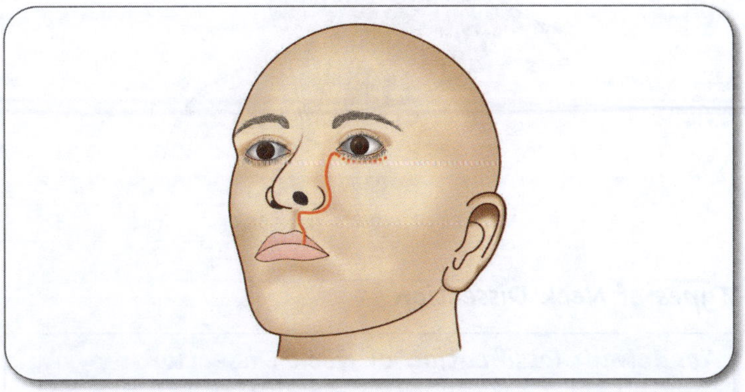

Weber Ferguson Incision for Hard palate tumors

Nodal Dissection in Neck

Level of Nodes

There are 7 levels in neck.

1. Submental and Submandibular nodes	
2. Upper Jugular	Extend from base of skull to hyoid bone
3. Middle Jugular	Extend from hyoid bone to cricoid cartilage
4. Lower Jugular	Extend from cricoid cartilage to suprasternal notch
5. Supraclavicular or Posterior Group	
6. Prelaryngeal/ Pretracheal **(Schwartz says-prelaryngeal as Delphian nodes)**	Extend from hyoid bone to sternal notch
7. Upper mediastinal nodes	

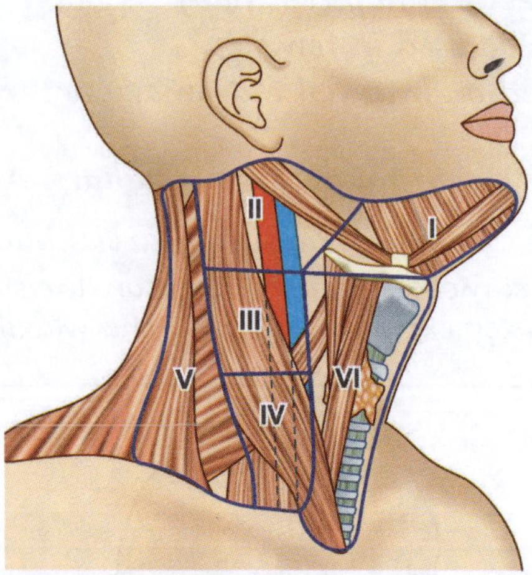

Level of nodes in neck

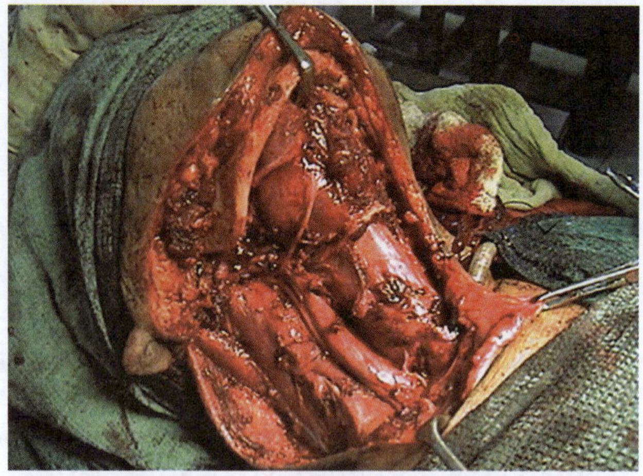
Radical neck node dissection

Types of Neck Dissection

Academy Classification of Neck Dissections

a. Radical neck dissection **by CRILE**.
b. Modified radical neck dissection **by BOCCA**
   - Type I—Preserves spinal accessory nerve
   - Type II—Preserves spinal accessory and internal jugular vein
   - Type III—Preserves spinal accessory nerve, IJV and SCM
c. **Selective Neck Dissection**
   - Supra omohyoid neck dissection Level I, II, III—Lip and oral cavity
   - Lateral neck dissection level II, III, IV—Larynx
   - Posterolateral neck dissection level II, III, IV, V—Thyroid

1. **Classic radical neck dissection (CRILE'S Operation)**
   Structures Removed:
   - Lymph nodes (level I-V), fat, fascia, sternomastoid, strap muscles, internal jugular vein and accessory nerve, submandibular salivary gland; lower part of parotid en bloc.

   Structures preserved:
   - Carotid artery (you can sacrifice branches of external carotid artery), Vagus nerve, Lingual nerve, Hypoglossal nerve, phrenic nerve, cervical branch of facial nerve.
2. **Modified radical neck dissection of Bocca (MRND)****
   - Level 1- 5 nodes are removed**
   - Structures removed are same as Radical neck dissection except for the following are preserved spinal accessory nerve, internal jugular vein and sternocleidomastoid muscle (functional block dissection)**

SALIVARY GLAND

Facial Nerve Trunk Identification During Parotidectomy

- **Conley's pointer (tragal pointer)****
  - Junction of bony and cartilaginous EAC – points downward 1 cm inferior
- Posterior belly of digastric insertion (above this)
- Stylomastoid foramen
- Facial nerve monitors

Nerve Supply of Parotid

1. **Parasympathetic**
   - Salivary nucleus—*Via* glossopharyngeal nerve (crossing Tympanic membrane)—Relay in Otic ganglion—Postganglionic fibers *via* auriculotemporal nerve (branch of trigeminal nerve) supply parotid
   - Leads to increased salivary secretion
   - Serous discharge

2. **Sympathetic supply**
   - Increase blood flow to gland

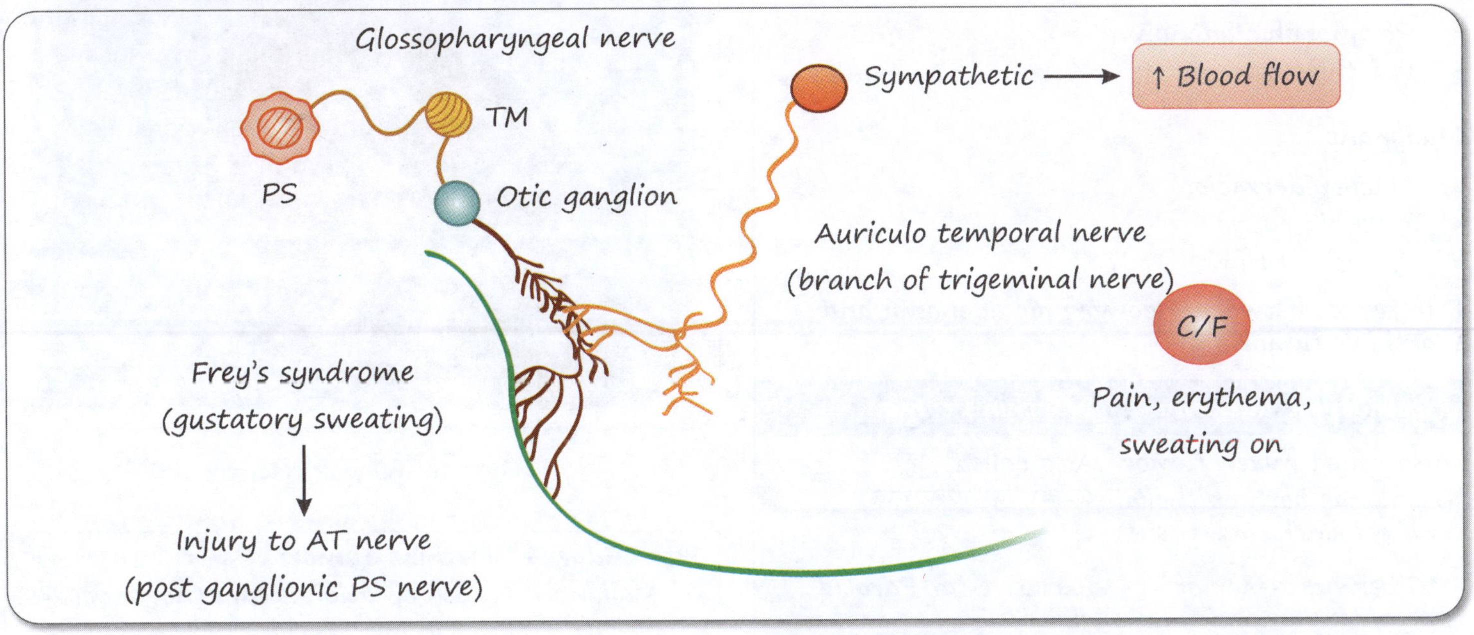

Frey's Syndrome (Gustatory Sweating Syndrome)

- Injury to Auriculotemporal nerve (post ganglionic parasympathetic nerve injury)
- Sympathetic fibers overgrow, join with auriculotemporal nerve and reach skin
- C/F—Pain, erythema and sweating over face on just seeing food
- Presents—2-3 months after parotidectomy operation
- Prevented by interposition of flaps between skin and operative area.
  - Sternomastoid muscle flap
  - Temporalis muscle flap
- **IOC: Starch iodine test**
- **Treatment**—Latest Botox injection at areas of reinnervation appearing as Erythema on Starch Iodine test.

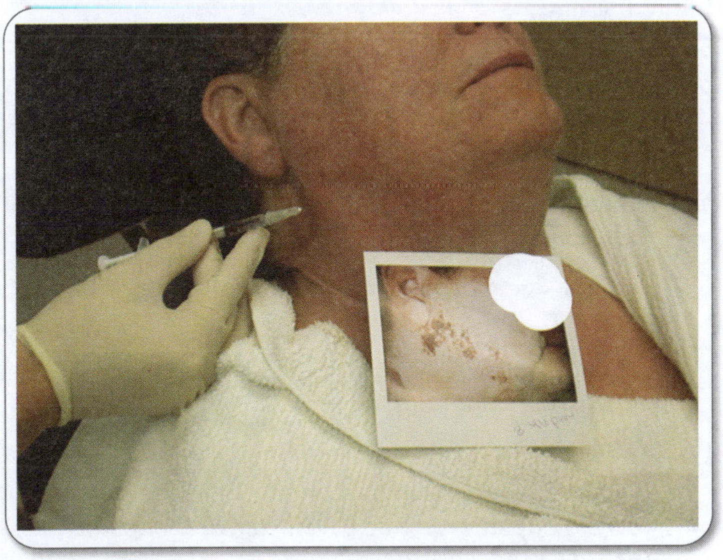

Starch Iodine test

Tumors in Salivary Gland

	Benign	Malignant
Parotid	80%	20%
Submandibular	50%	50%
Minor Glands	10%	90%

As the gland becomes smaller, malignancy increases.

Types of Epithelial Tumors

Benign

- Pleomorphic adenoma
- Warthin's tumor

Malignant

- Mucoepidermoid
- Adenoid cystic
- Acinic cell tumor

Differences between Pleomorphic adenoma and Warthin's tumor

Pleomorphic adenoma	Warthin's tumor
Also called mixed tumor (As it has both epithelial and mesenchymal tissue)	Also called adenolymphoma
MC benign tumor of parotid, submandibular gland and minor salivary glands	**Exclusive for Parotid gland****
Seen in tail of parotid	**Lower pole of parotid****
Three classical features 1. Lift the ear lobule 2. Curtain sign positive 3. Obliteration of retromandibular groove	–
Bi digitally palpable +	–
Tonsil pushed medially (if deep lobe is enlarged)	–
Pathology: • Rarely capsule+ – not well defined capsule • Pseudopod extension into normal gland	Well defined capsule
Only Parotidectomy is TOC	Enucleation or parotidectomy
C/F: All salivary gland tumors are most common in females.	Old male (5th–7th decade)

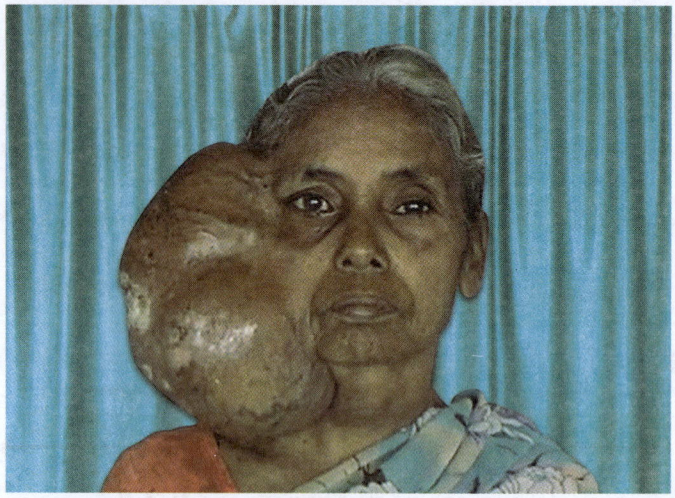

Huge Pleomorphic adenoma

Extra Edge – Warthins Tumor:

- Malignant transformation is rare (never occurs)
- Occurs exclusively in Parotid.
- MC site is lower pole* (Pleomorphic adenoma at Tail of Parotid)
- Multicentric/bilateral occurrence is more common
- MC occurs in lower pole (at angle of mandible)
- MC in smokers
- MC in males (5th to 7th decade)
- Hot spot in technetium 99m scan

Differences between mucoepidermoid cancer and adenoid cystic cancer

Mucoepidermoid cancer	Adenoid cystic cancer also known as cylindroma
High or low grade variants	High or low grade variants
MC malignant tumor of parotid	• MC malignant tumor of submandibular gland • Perineural infiltration + • Base of skull extension
30% LN enlargement (Increased LN mets)	No LN mets

Surgical Aspects

Sistrunk Incision—Lazy S Shaped Incision done for Parotidectomy

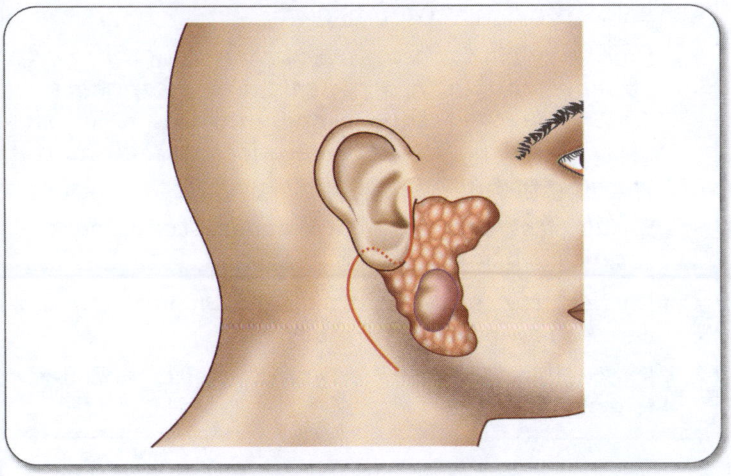

Sistrunk incision for parotidectomy

- **Simple parotidectomy:**
    - Only superficial lobe removed
    - Deep lobe and facial nerve preserved
    - Done in benign tumors
- **Total conservative parotidectomy:**
    - Superficial + deep lobe removed
    - Facial nerve is preserved
    - Done in deep lobe benign tumors
- **Radical parotidectomy:**
    - Superficial + deep lobe + facial nerve removed
    - Done in malignant
        - Mucoepidermoid
        - Adenoid cystic tumor

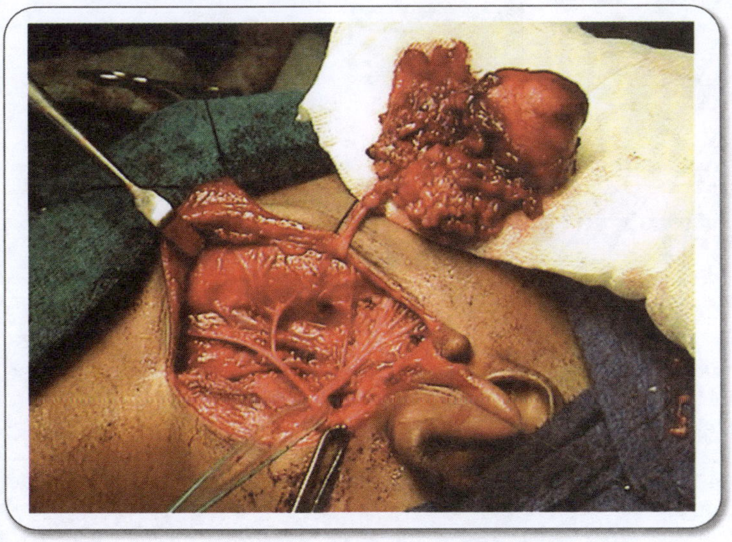

Total conservative parotidectomy

Postop Complications

Nerve Injuries

- MC nerve injured—**Any branch of facial nerve**
    - Bell's phenomenon
    - Deviation of mouth
    - Loss of nasolabial fold
- MC cutaneous nerve injured—**Greater auricular nerve****
    - Paresthesia in shaving area
- Auriculotemporal nerve (postganglionic parasympathetic injury)—**Frey's syndrome**

Extra mile

Parotid surgery:

- While doing parotid surgery—if a branch is adherent the tumor, it must be resected.
- The resected nerve can be reconstructed using Greater auricular nerve.
- All nerve branches compromised can be reconstructed except the Buccal branch**

High Yield Facts:

Ranula

- Mucous extravasation** cyst arising from sublingual gland
- Latin word Rana means—Frog's Belly**
- Develop on floor of mouth.
- Surgical management: Excision of cyst and affected gland.
- Incision and drainage result in Recurrence.

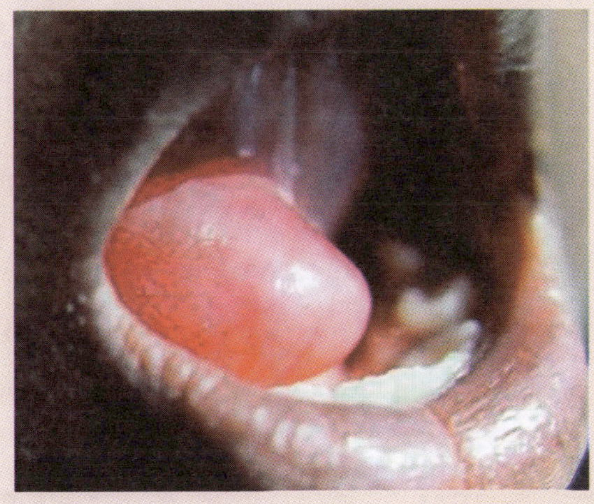

Ranula

Plunging ranula:

- Mucous retention cyst** that can arise from both sublingual salivary glands.
- Mucous collects around the gland and penetrates the mylohyoid diaphragm to enter the neck.

Stafne Bone Cyst

- Most common site of ectopic salivary tissue*
- Located below inferior dental neurovascular bundle (at angle of mandible – radiolucent area)
- No treatment needed

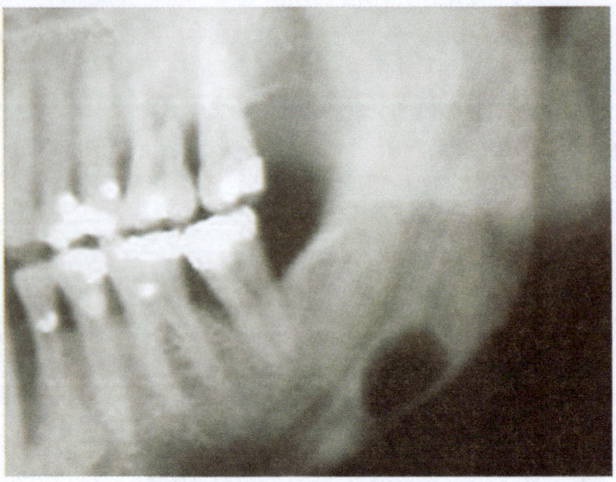

Stafne bone cyst

Obstruction of Submandibular Duct

- MC cause of obstruction is stone (sialolithiasis), 2nd MC cause is Stricture**
- 80% stones are radiopaque.
- Painful swelling occurs in Submandibular region – appears rapidly after meals and disappears in 1–2 hours*—Meal-time Syndrome** (if the obstruction by stone is complete usually at the opening of Submandibular duct)
- Small, less than 4 mm, mobile stones can be retrieved using a Dormia basket**
- Larger stones can be broken by Lithotripsy and can be removed with a basket**
- Recently – Pneumatic Intraductal Lithotripter is used.

SWELLINGS IN THE NECK

Anatomy of Triangles of Neck

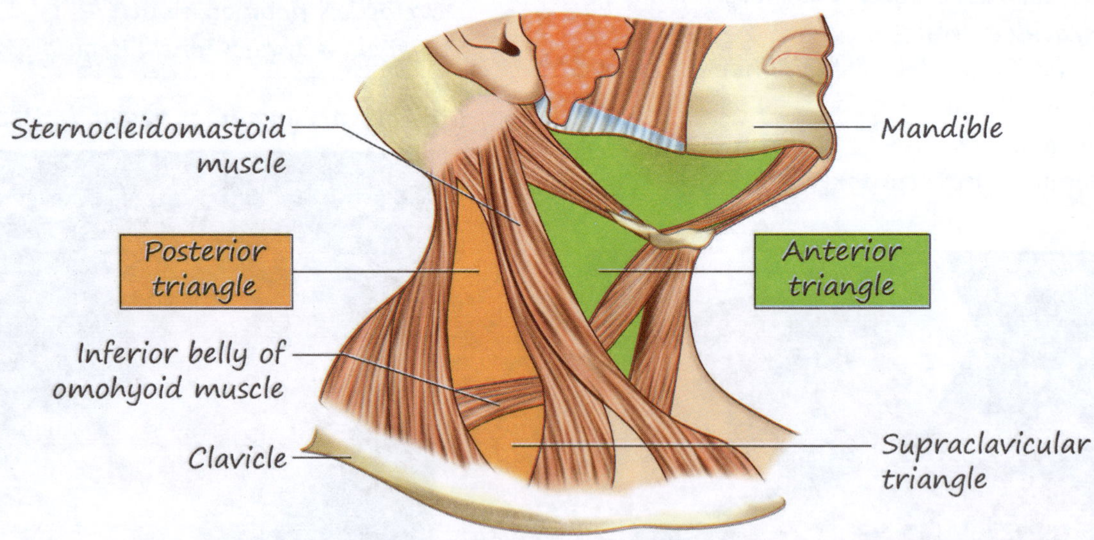

Neck triangles

The triangles you must know are as follows:

- Anterior triangle:
  - Carotid triangle
  - Digastric triangle
  - Submental triangle
  - Muscular triangle (More in midline)
- Posterior triangle:
  - Supraclavicular triangle
  - Suboccipital triangle

Differences between carotid triangle and posterior triangle

	Carotid triangle	Posterior triangle
Solid type	Carotid body tumor	Cervical rib
Liquid type	Branchial cyst	Cystic hygroma
Air filled swelling	Laryngocele	Pharyngeal pouch (Zenker's diverticulum)

Carotid Body Tumor (Potato Tumor/ Paragangliomas/Chemodectoma)

Pathology

- Histologically—Non chromaffin paraganglioma
- Associated with pheochromocytoma**
- Usually unilateral; MC in 5th decade, MC in women
- 10% have family history
- MC in high altitudes and due to Hypoxia*
- Incidence is 0.5%

Must know:
Carotid body tumors arise from chemoreceptor cells (not baroreceptor cells) of carotid body and are stimulated by decreased arterial oxygen tension, e.g., Cyanotic heart disease, chronic hypoxia in high altitude inhabitants**.

Clinical Features

- 75% cases present with neck mass (Slow growing firm mass)
- Mobile side to side—But not vertically (FONTAINE SIGN)**
- Pulsatile but not expansible*
- Malignancy seen in 5–10% cases
- Rarely metastasize

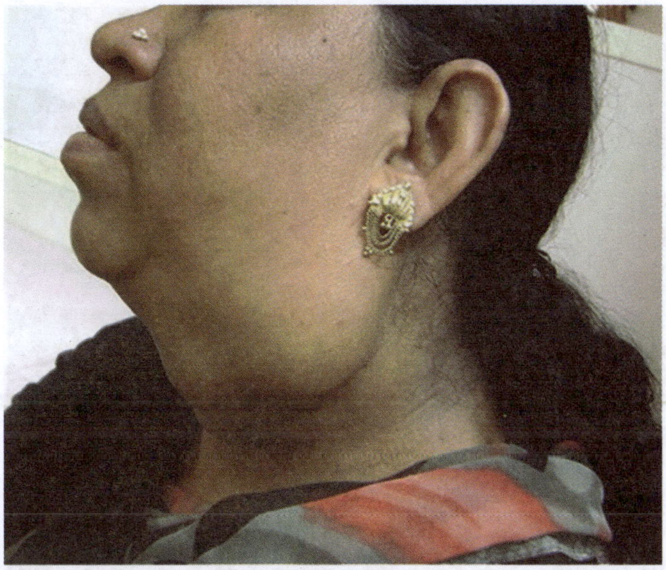

Carotid body tumor

Investigations

- Duplex scan
- CT contrast/MR angiogram

Lyre Sign**

- Angiogram finding—Splaying of internal and external carotids due to tumor in between
- Biopsy and FNAC are absolutely contraindicated

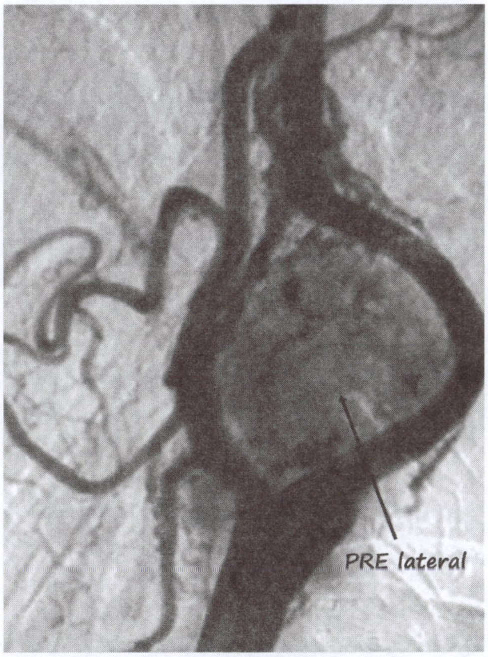

Conventional angiogram shows Lyre sign

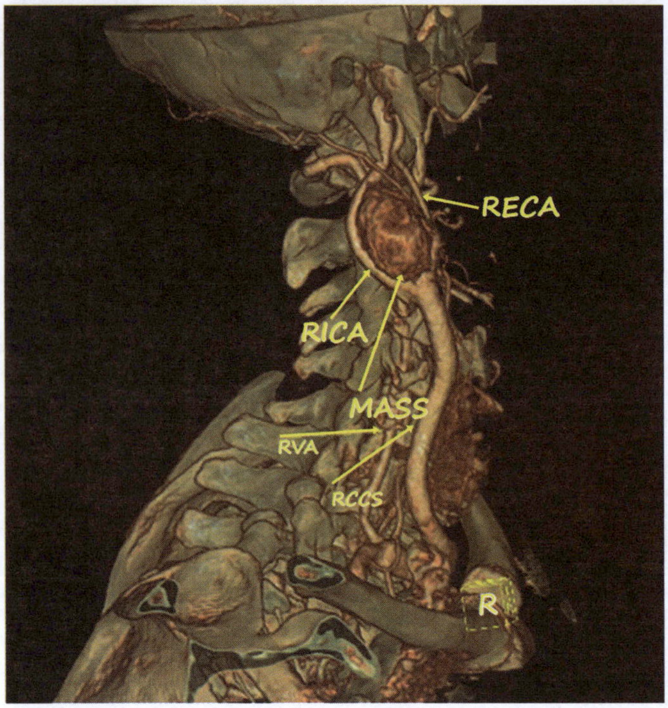

MR angiogram reconstructed showing Lyre sign

Treatment

Shamblin classification of Types and Management

Types	Pattern	Surgical procedure
Type 1	Localized (25%)	Excision
Type 2	Adherent partially (50%)	Subadvential dissection (temporary intraluminal shunt may be used)
Type 3	Adherent completely surround Internal Carotid Artery (25%) cases	En bloc removal of tumor and ICA en bloc great saphenous vein grafting

Thoracic Outlet Syndrome

Applied Anatomy

Subclavian artery leaves the thoracic cage by passing over the first rib between scalenus anterior anteriorly and scalenus medius posteriorly along with brachial plexus

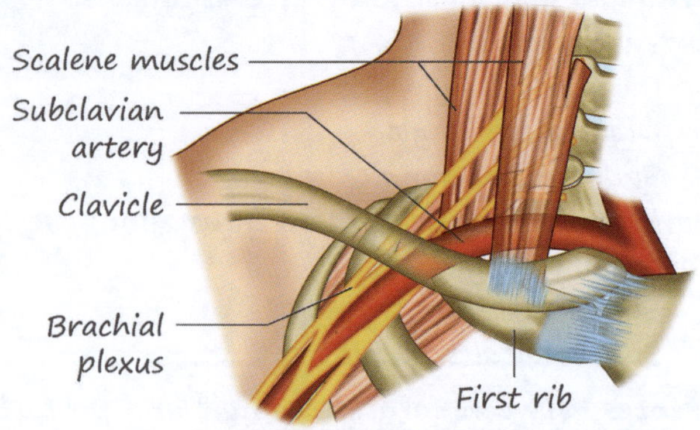

Thoracic outlet anatomy

Causes of Thoracic Outlet Syndrome

Congenital	Acquired
Osseous • **Cervical rib (Most common cause)**** • Long C_7 transverse process • Abnormal 1st rib	• Fracture clavicle, callus and pseudo arthrosis • Fracture 1st rib • Exostosis/tumors
Soft tissue: • Anomalous scalene insertion • Scalene muscle hypertrophy • Congenital bands and ligaments **Postural:** • Heavy breast • Sagging shoulders	• Scalene muscle injury • Previous surgery/scar • Soft tissue tumors • Direct brachial plexus injury

Must know:

Neurogenic symptoms	Vascular symptoms
MC nerve compressed is lower trunk of Brachial Plexus C8T1 (Ulnar nerve)	Intermittent occlusion of Subclavian artery resulting in Poststenotic aneurysm and distal emboli.
Clinical features: • Pain, paresthesia, along ulnar nerve distribution • Hallmark – pain in arm, shoulder, forearms	**Clinical features:** • Claudication • Ischemic ulcers • Gangrenous tips • Cold hands, color changes

Clinical Features

- MC in 20–40 years
- 70% are females
- O/E—Pulsatile supraclavicular mass – due to Poststenotic aneurysm*
- Tinel's sign over brachial plexus
- Hard and fixed lump in lower part of posterior triangle** – Cervical rib.

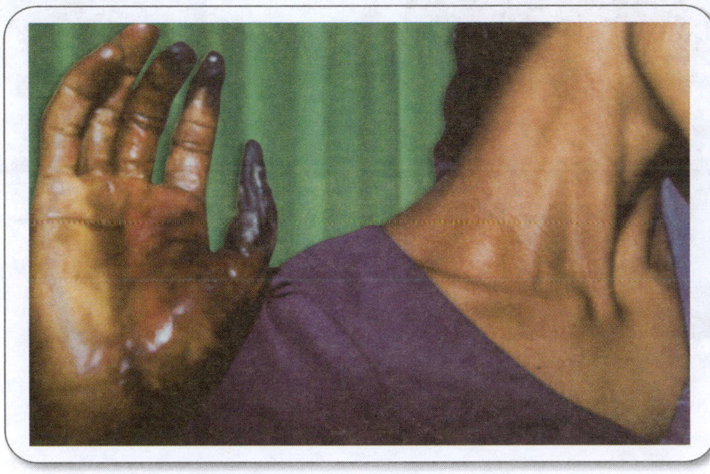

Cervical rib and gangrene of fingers due to TOS

Investigations

Adson test	Roos test**	Halstead test	Wright test
• Extend arm • Turn to same side • Take a deep breath • Radial artery dynamicity decreases (not pulse rate)	• Abduct arm • Flex elbow • Open and close fist for 5 minutes • Claudication pain develops • Patient puts hand down	• Standing in military position • Turning to opposite side just opposite to Adson test • Check for pain and color changes in limb and for radial pulse	Hyperabduction of arm causes pain and decreases in radial pulse dynamicity

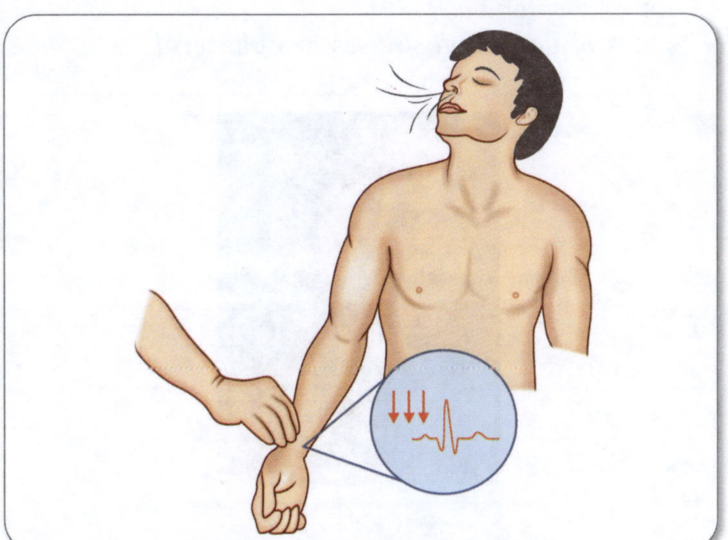

Adson test

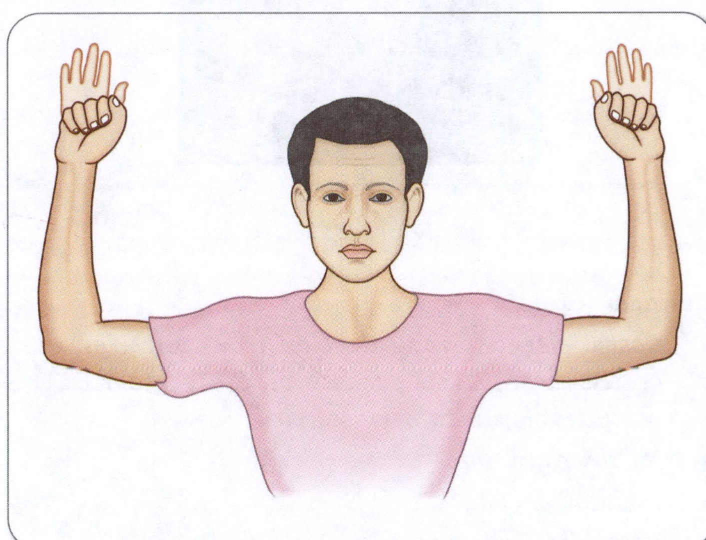

Roos' test (abduction with exercise)

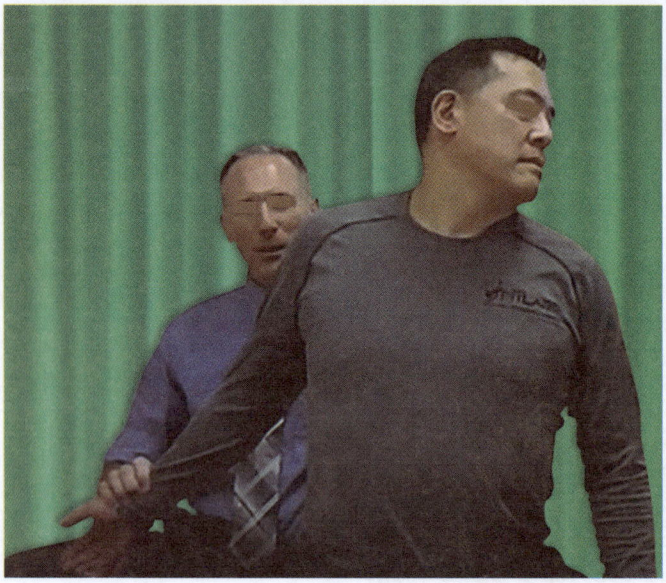

Halstead maneuver

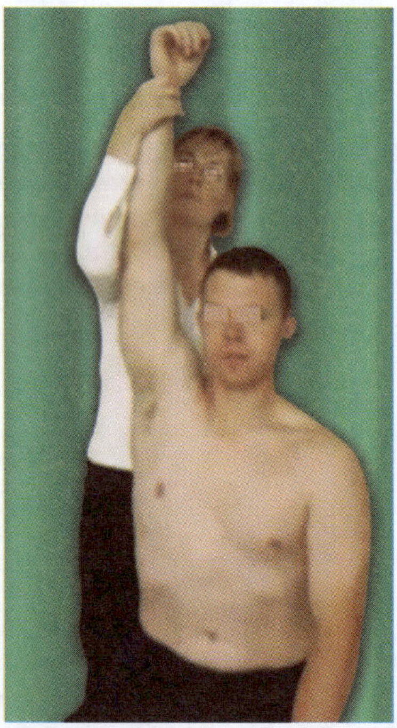

Wright hyperabduction test

Cervical Ribs:

- Costal element may develop from anterior part of the transverse process of C7 vertebra. This may develop into cervical rib.
- MC in right side
- Incidence: 0.45%
- 50% bilateral cases

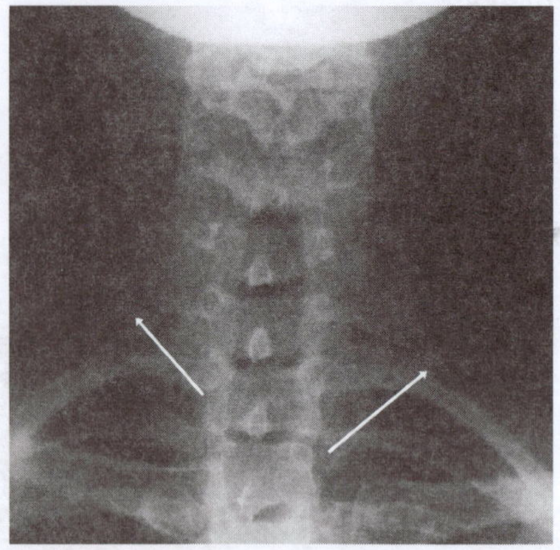

Bilateral cervical ribs

Surgical Treatment

- Excision of cervical rib (extra periosteal excision)
- Scalenotomy

Branchial Cyst

- Cystic swelling arising from the persistent cervical sinus which is formed due to fusion of 2nd branchial arch with 6th branchial arch.
- MC in young age (20–25 years)

Embryology

- 2nd branchial remnants are most common*
- 1st branchial remnants are MC located in front or back of ear. (fistula seen between parotid and external auditory canal)
- 2nd branchial remnant is what discussed in detail below.
- 3rd branchial remnant is located at suprasternal or clavicular region*
- 15% of branchial sinuses are bilateral

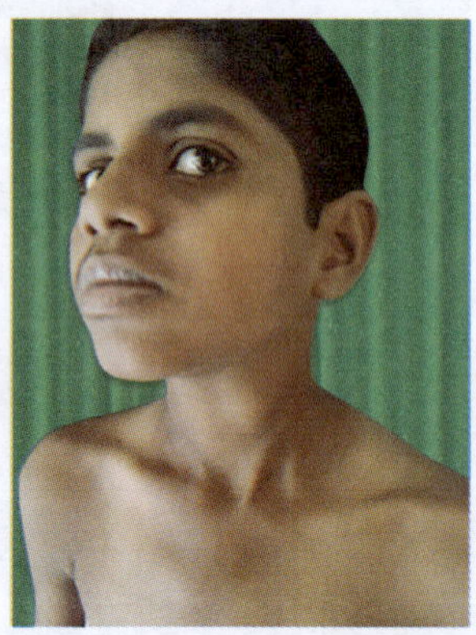

Congenital branchial cyst

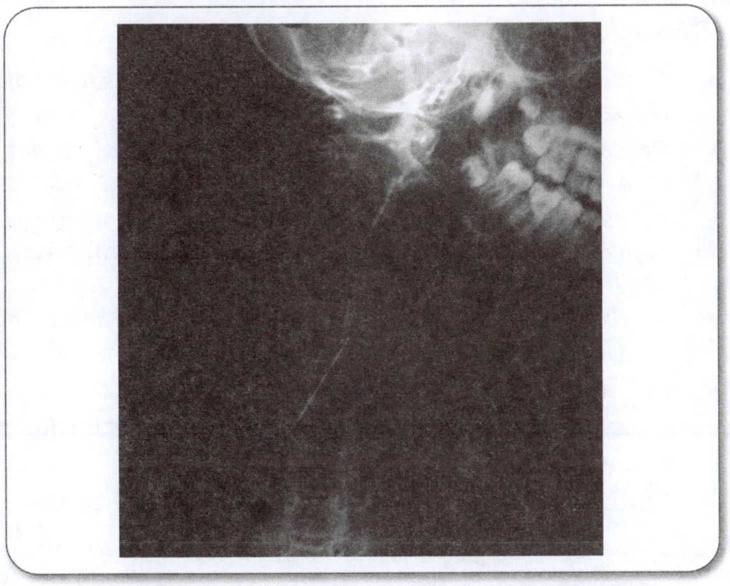

Fistulogram of 2nd branchial remnant

Differences between branchial cyst and branchial sinus/fistula

Branchial cyst	Branchial sinus/fistula
Swelling + in upper 1/3rd of Sternocleidomastoid muscle anteriorly	Opening seen in the neck anterior to SCM Congenital – Lower 1/3rd Acquired – Upper 1/3rd
Transillumination negative Thick content (contains cholesterol crystals- also seen in Hydrocele)	–
Lined by squamous epithelium**	Ciliated columnar epithelium**
Persistence of 2nd pouch	Congenital branchial sinus/fistula Inner opening - in tonsillar fossa Anterior to the posterior pillar**
Complications: • Recurrent infection • Acquired branchial sinus due to inadvertent incision or infection and rupture of cyst • Branchiogenic carcinoma - Can have squamous or columnar epithelium	Fistula passes through Bifurcation of common carotid Pierces superior constrictor of pharynx Tonsillar fossa
Treatment: Complete excision of cyst	Multiple stepladder incision – follows fistula and removes it completely • Hypoglossal nerve, glossopharyngeal nerve and spinal accessory nerve lie deep to the cyst and are at danger during surgery. • Medially it can extend up to the pharyngeal wall.

Contd...

Branchial Sinus

Failure of fusion of the second branchial arch with sixth branchial arch and persistence of cervical sinus results in this condition. In most cases, the internal opening is not found, so this is better called a sinus rather than a fistula.

- **Congenital:** Persistent cervical sinus
- Acquired

External Opening

- **Congenital:** Typically located in lower 1/3rd of neck at the anterior border of sternocleidomastoid.
- **Acquired:** Typically located at upper 1/3rd to middle 1/3rd junction.

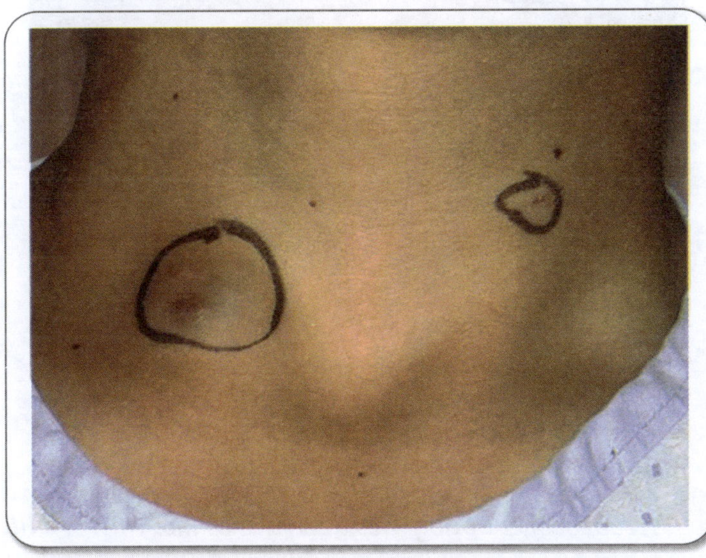

Bilateral congenital branchial fistula

Internal Opening

Behind the tonsil and anterior to posterior pillar of the fauces in the lateral wall of the pharynx lies the interior opening.

Treatment

Excision of fistulous tract.

Cystic Hygroma

- Sequestration of a portion of jugular lymph sac from lymphatic system accounts for the appearance of these swellings in the neck.
- It is a swelling in the **posterior triangle** of neck in the lower third.
- **Earliest swelling** one can see in the neck.
- Cystic hygroma is **present in neonate** or in early infancy.
- It may also be present at birth as obstructed labor.
- Swelling is **brilliantly translucent** and **partly compressible, cough impulse is also positive.**
- Cysts are **filled with clear lymph** and lined with a single layer of epithelium.

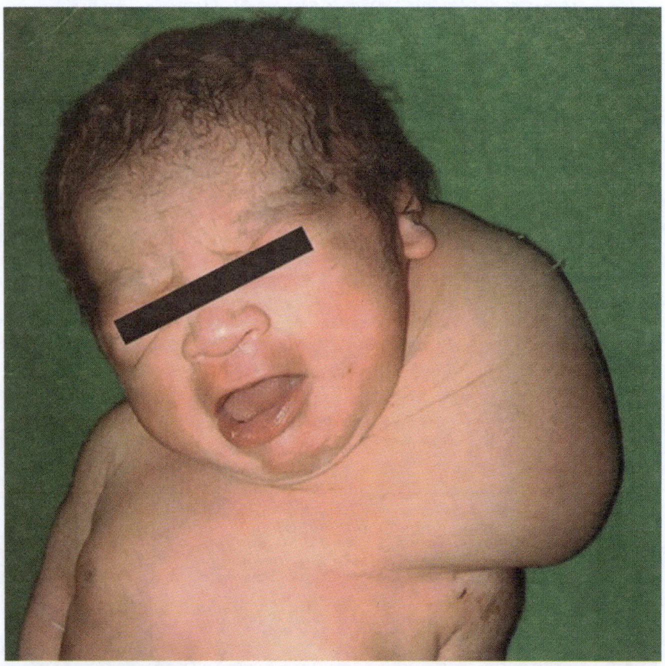

Cystic hygroma

- Recently sclerosants like BLEOMYCIN and streptococcal pyogenes derivatives like PICIBANIL (OK432) injected into the lesions.

Thyroglossal Cyst

- Cystic swelling developing in the remnant of thyroglossal duct or tract.
- Present in any part from thyroglossal tract foramen cecum to isthmus.
- MC sites—subhyoid, region of thyroid cartilage, suprahyoid, in floor of mouth, beneath foramen cecum.
- Midline swelling shifted to left at level of thyroid cartilage.
- MC age—15–30 years.
- Cyst can be moved sideways but not vertically.
- Moves with deglutition and protrusion of tongue
- Lined by pseudostratified columnar epithelium.

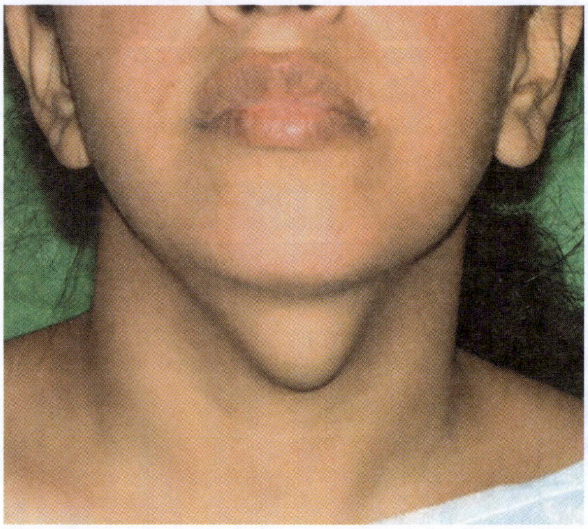

Thyroglossal cyst

Complications

- Infection
- Fistula
- Papillary carcinoma can develop.
- Thyroglossal cyst is congenital but fistula is always acquired** due to improper drainage or surgery inadequate.

Sistrunk Operation

- Excision of tract along with excision of central part of hyoid bone.
- Sistrunk operation is also named for filarial leg surgery**.

4. THYROID DISORDERS

NERVE ANATOMY

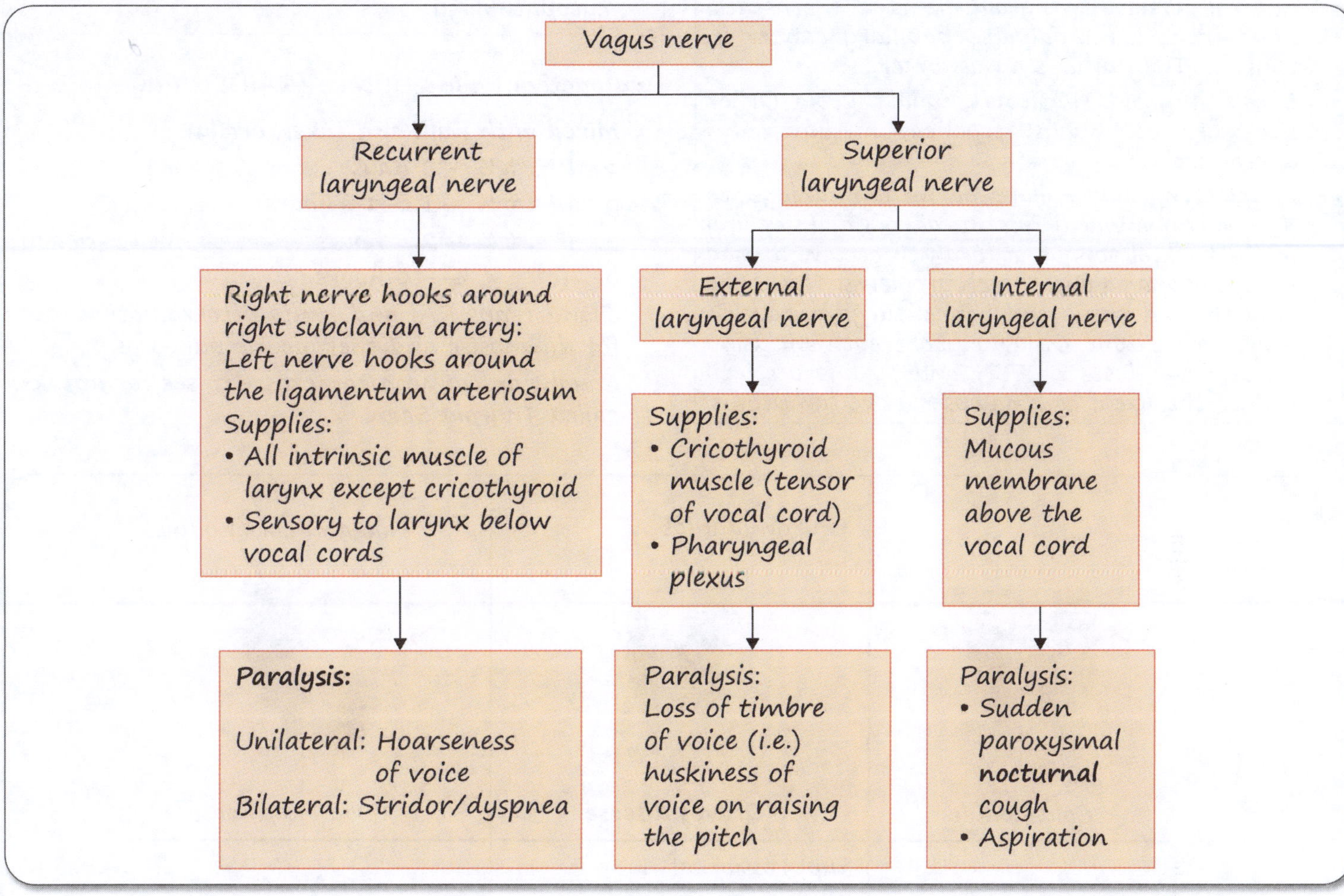

Most common nerve injured: External Laryngeal Nerve**

DISEASES AND INVESTIGATIONS IN THYROID

Deficiency of iodine: MC cause of hypothyroidism in the world.

Hypothyroidism

- Free T3—N/decreased
- Free T4—N/decreased
- **TSH—Increased**

Hyperthyroidism

- **TSH—Decreased**
- FT3—N/increased
- FT4—N/increased

- Most sensitive IOC for hypo/hyperthyroidism-TSH value.
- Subclinical cases—Free T3 is most sensitive.
- Congenital thyroid peroxidase deficiency—**Pendred syndrome**
  - Sensory neural hearing loss
  - Congenital hypothyroidism
- **Hashimoto thyroiditis:** Inhibitory antibody against.
  - TPO—Most common
  - Thyroglobulin
  - TSH-R
- **Graves' disease:**
  - Stimulatory antibody to TPO, TG and TSH-R which results in increased T3 and T4 production.

Must know:

- **Delphic nodes:** They are pretracheal nodes and prelaryngeal nodes (Bailey mentions Pretracheal nodes as Delphic Nodes).
- **Lateral aberrant thyroid:** It is a metastatic node from a nonpalpable papillary cancer in thyroid. The name is a misnomer.
- **Ectopic thyroid:** MC site is Lingual thyroid. Other sites are esophagus, trachea, mediastinum, aortic arch.
- **Lingual thyroid:** Failure of median anlage to descend downward. Presents as rounded swelling in the back of tongue at foramen cecum. It may cause dysphagia and speech problems. This is the only thyroid tissue and hence, surgical excision must not be done. Only medical treatment using suppressive doses of TSH and RAI is used to reduce the size if causing obstructive symptoms.

Extra edge of FNAC of thyroid disease

- Appropriate FNAC specimen must contain- 6 Follicular cell groups containing 10 cells each**.
- Bethesda criteria is used for reporting thyroid cytopathology.

Radioactive Iodine Uptake (RAIU) Study

- **Mixed with milk and taken orally)**
  - **I^{131}: t ½ - 8 days**
  - **I^{123}: t ½ - 12–14 hours**
  - **I^{132}: t ½ - 2.5 hours**
  - **Tc^{99m}: t ½ - 6 hours**
- Gland traps RAI and emits beta radiation, used for diagnostic and therapeutic purposes.
- Caught on Gamma cameras - to see for uptake - called **Thyroid Scan.**

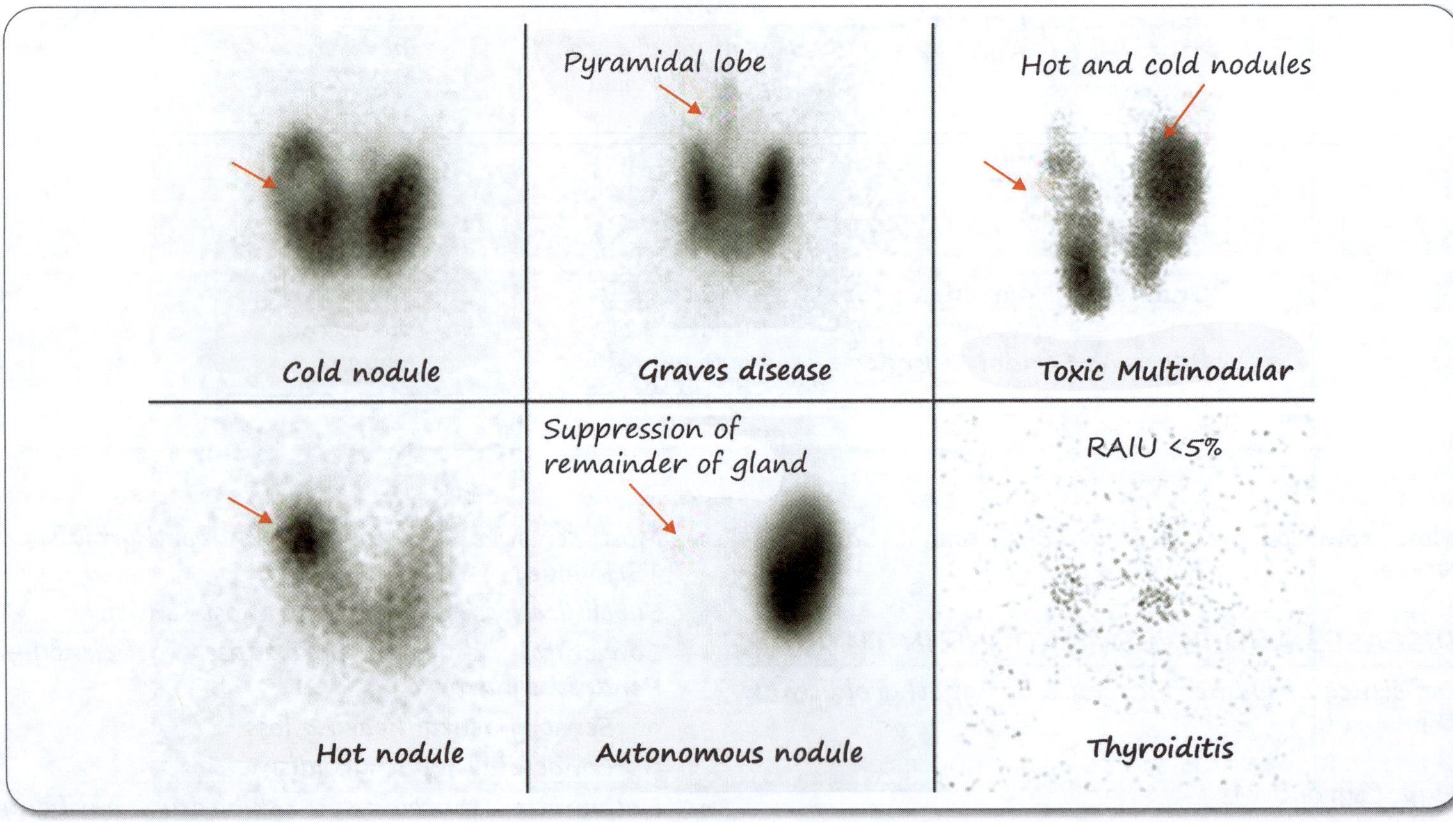

Images of RAI uptake study

Hypothyroidism	Hyperthyroidism
Obese	Slim
Less intake	Increased intake
Cold intolerance	Heat intolerance
Constipation	Diarrhea (increased bowel movement)
Menorrhagia – amenorrhea (anemia)	Oligomenorrhea

Contd...

Tendon reflex – decreased Pseudo myotonic reflex/hung-up ankle reflex-delayed ankle jerk	Tendon reflex – increased Fine tremors
• Loss of eyebrows • Macroglossia • Mask like faces • Depression	**Eye signs—exophthalmos (early)** • **Pretibial myxedema**—Deposition of mucopolysaccharides in front of tibia • **Acropachy**—subperiosteal bone resorption of fingers - look like clubbing **Both are late features**
Names of Hypothyroidism: • Cretinism (pediatrics) • Myxedema (adults) **Most common causes** • Iodine deficiency: India • Hashimoto's disease: Western/world	**Causes:** • Graves' disease (1' toxicosis) • Plummer's disease (2' toxicosis) due to MNG >SNT (for exams) **TYPES OF TOXICOSIS:** **Primary** Swelling and toxic features appear together. E.g., Graves' disease. **Secondary** Swelling is long standing, toxic features appear later. E.g., MNG, toxic nodular goiter.

Graves' Disease

- Most common cause of hyperthyroidism.
- Autoimmune disease: HLAB8, HLADR3, HLADQ1
- Diffuse enlargement, soft consistency, highly vascular.
  - **Palpation:** Thrill in superior pole
  - **Auscultation:**
    - Arterial bruit
    - Venous hum + (due to increased sympathetic activity causing hyperdynamic circulation)

Pretibial Myxedema

Name is misnomer. Pretibial myxedema is not seen in myxedema, it is seen in Graves' disease.

- Glycosaminoglycans deposited in front of leg*
- Symmetrical in both legs below knee
- Usually associated with true exophthalmos, hyperthyroidism, high levels of TSH receptor Ab.

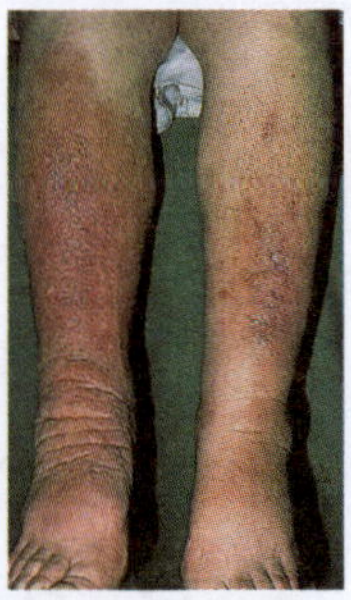

Pretibial myxedema in Graves' disease

Clinical Tests in Thyroid

- Thyroid is always examined from behind.
- Short neck—**PIZZILLO'S METHOD**. (hand behind neck and hyperextension of neck)
- Retrosternal goiter—**Pemberton sign** (to look for svc compression—lift both arm with arm touching ears—look for facial congestion)
- **Lahey's test**: 4 finger examination (push on one side and palpate with four fingers)
- **Crile's test**—for doubtful nodule (using only thumb—ask patient to swallow - feel for nodule)
- **Berry's sign**—nonpalpable carotid artery against vertebrae (d/t engulfment of the tumor)

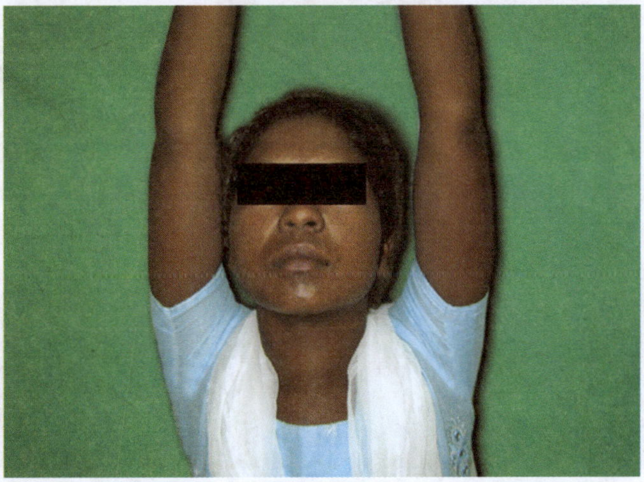

Pemberton sign

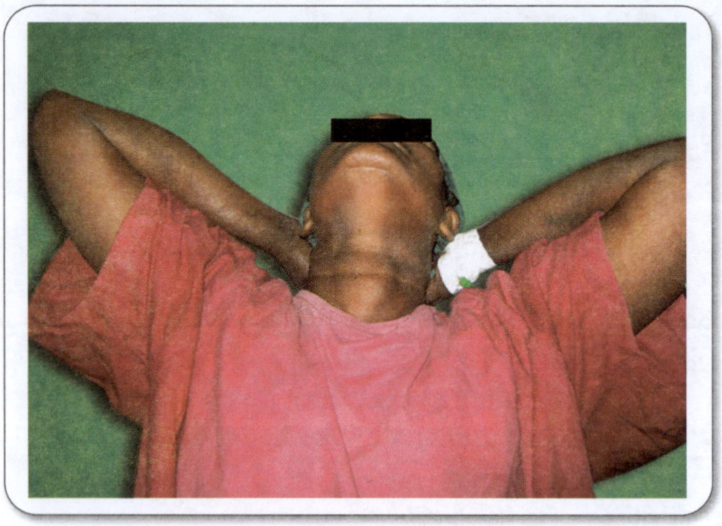

Pizzillo's test

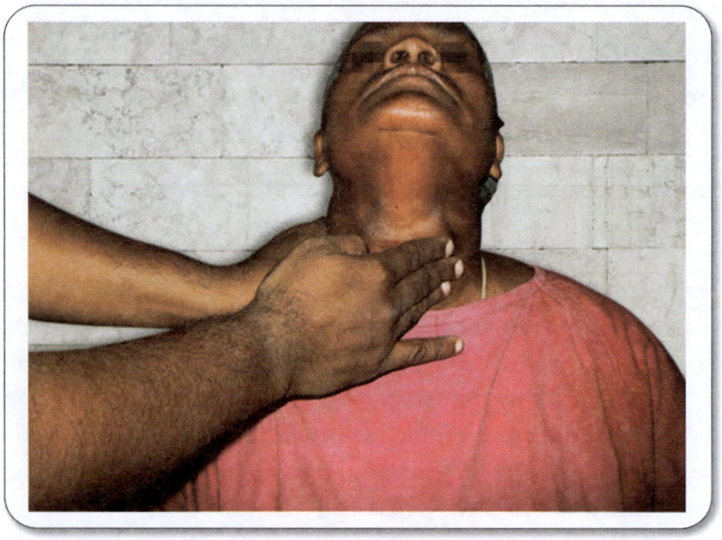

Lahey's test

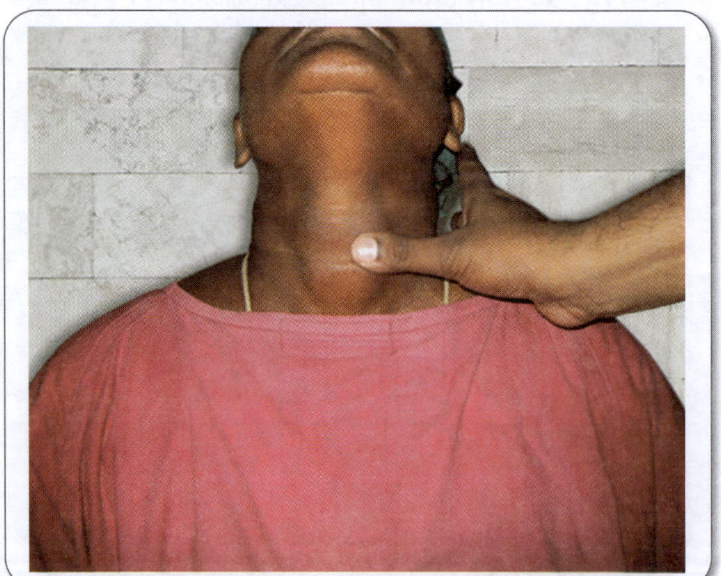

Crile's test

Eye signs in Graves' disease:

Mild exophthalmos – due to only sympathetic activity

- Von Graefe's lid lag sign - ask patient to follow vertical movement - lid lags behind
- Dalrymple's sign/lid retraction sign - visible upper sclera
- Stellwag's sign - starring look

Moderate – due to retro-orbital accumulation of glycosaminoglycans

- Joffroy's sign- absence of forehead wrinkle on looking up
- Ask patient to look at the ceiling of the room – as patient has eyes protruded, no wrinkle happens to see up

Severe – due to intraocular accumulation and paralysis of muscle

Mobius sign - Inability to converge (paralysis of intraocular muscle)

Other signs:

Naffziger's sign - Eyes seen through supraorbital ridge – normally eyes not seen.

Diagnosis

- T3, T4 increased, TSH decreased
- RAIU increased
- Autoimmune antibodies increased: Anti TG, Anti TPO – 75% cases
- **LATS - Long-Acting Thyroid Stimulator** is elevated in 90% cases. Also Known as Thyroid stimulating Antibody or TSH-R stimulating Ab
- FNAC is **not beneficial**.
    - Hemorrhagic aspirate.
    - Therefore, not advised in Graves' disease.

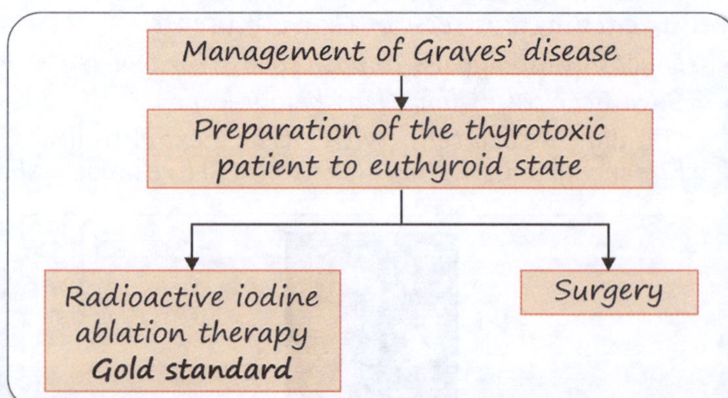

Preparation of the thyrotoxic patient to euthyroid state

If not done properly—thyroid storm can happen (MC cause is inadequate preparation for Surgery)

Anti-thyroid drugs	Quick preparation	Lugol's iodine
Inhibit • Trapping of iodine • Oxidation of iodine • Peripheral conversion T4 to T3	• Decrease sympathetic overactivity of the gland. • Early preparation is possible	**Mechanism:** • Decrease vascularity of the gland • Makes the gland firm
Carbimazole – leads to reversible agranulocytosis	**Beta blockers** • Propranolol (Short acting) – 40 mg TDS • Nadolol (Long acting) 160 mg - OD	5% iodine + 10% KI 10 drops TDS
Methimazole – 10-30 mg TDS		
Propylthiouracil - used in pregnancy – does not cross the placental barrier		
Take for 3 months to become euthyroid.		**LAST 10 DAYS BEFORE SURGERY**
Last dose of carbimazole is given a night before surgery	Note: Continue beta blocker 7 days post operation including Intraoperative period**	

After patient is prepared, RAI Ablative therapy is given

Contraindications for RAI therapy:

- Severe ophthalmopathy
- Pregnancy and lactation
- Children
- Nodules +
- Smoking females

Surgery is indicated in above cases where RAI is contraindicated.

Thyroiditis

- MC in females between 30 and 40 years
- Inflammation of thyroid gland

Hashimoto	Riedel (fibrosis)	De Quervain
MC type		
Also known as chronic lymphocytic/ autoimmune thyroiditis	Associated with • Invasive fibrosing thyroiditis • Dupuytren's contracture • Retroperitoneal fibrosis	• Also known as post viral or subacute (after a few weeks of viral infection) • Associated with HLAB35
Abs: (inhibitory) • TPO-MC • TG • TSH-R		
FNAC: • Hurthle cells/Ashkenazy cells (Abundant cytoplasm with varying size of nucleus) • Lymphocytes +	**FNAC:** cannot be done - woody hard - mimics cancer Do Tru - cut biopsy	

Contd...

C/F: • Pain + • Thyrotoxicosis (d/t increased release not production) • Burn out leading to hypothyroidism • When patient presents- painless enlarged thyroid with hypothyroidism.	ALWAYS HYPOTHYROID** - produce compressive symptoms	• Predominantly hyperthyroid with pain for a long period • Later become hypothyroid **DD: Graves'- increased RAIU** **De Quervain-** • Decreased RAIU • Increased ESR
Complications: • Hypothyroidism • Compressive symptoms • Premalignant - lymphoma and papillary Carcinoma can happen**		

Retrosternal Goiter

Types:

Primary Mediastinal:	**Secondary Mediastinal: (Retrosternal Goiter)**
• Arising from ectopic thyroid gland present inside chest • Blood supply from thoracic vessels • Sternotomy is required	• Typical retrosternal extension – 99% patients • Blood supply from superior and inferior thyroid artery. • Approach through neck incision- put finger and hook it. • Pemberton sign+ - (hands on ear- flushing of face).

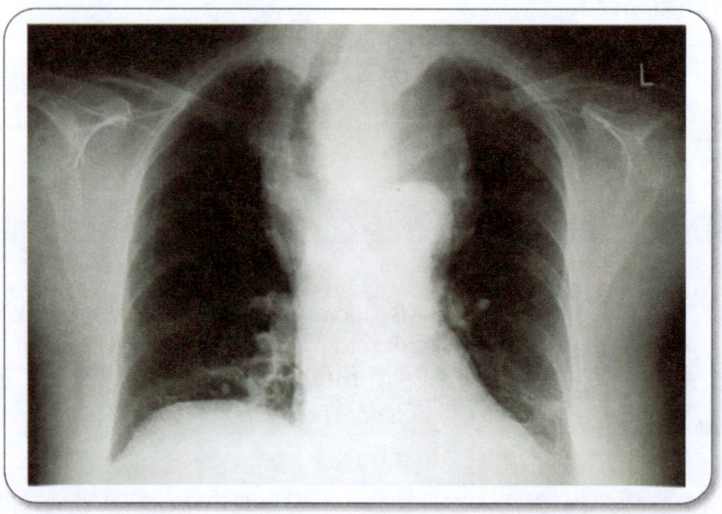

X-ray shows retrosternal extension of goiter

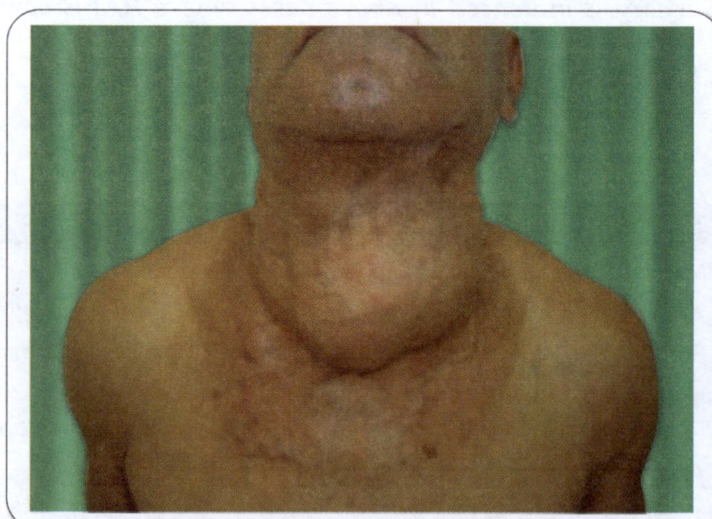

Retrosternal goiter

Management:

- Investigation of choice: (COMPULSORY) CECT THORAX/NECK
- Retrosternal goiter is removed by neck incision

THYROID MALIGNANCIES

Dunhill Classification

Differentiated	Medullary	Undifferentiated
Papillary Ca – 80%	2.5%	Anaplastic – 5%
Follicular Ca – 10%		Lymphoma (NHL) – 2.5%
Hurthle cell Ca		

Sequence-Based Question: Papillary > follicular > anaplastic > medullary = lymphoma

Papillary carcinoma	Follicular carcinoma
MC thyroid cancer	MC in iodine deficiency areas
Pathology • Multifocal- one lobe many foci • Multicentric – B/L • May or may not have capsule	• Single • Well-defined capsule
Spread: **Lymph node mets** • "Lateral aberrant thyroid" • Metastatic node from an occult papillary Ca. **Distant mets:** Lungs	**Hematogenous** **MC site:** Skull - pulsatile osteolytic secondaries **Distant mets:** Skull
FNAC: (3p) 1. Psammoma bodies (concentric calcification) 2. Pale empty orphan annie-eye nucleus 3. Papillary projections	• Inconclusive (can't define benign/ malignant) • Capsular invasion cannot be detected with FNAC

Contd...

Papillary carcinoma	Follicular carcinoma
Predisposing factors: • Irradiation • Hashimoto's • Thyroglossal cyst	Long standing multinodular goiter
Prognosis: **Excellent:** 95% 10 years survival	Good prognosis
Treatment: Total thyroidectomy + modified radical neck dissection (if nodes +ve)	**Management:** • If >4 cm – do total thyroidectomy directly • If Thy 3 (<4 cm) ↓ Hemithyroidectomy ↓ cut and send for HPE (not frozen- miss malignancy) ↓ result in 2-3 days **Based on result:** ○ **if benign:** discharge patient ○ **if malignant:** on day 3- do completion total thyroidectomy.

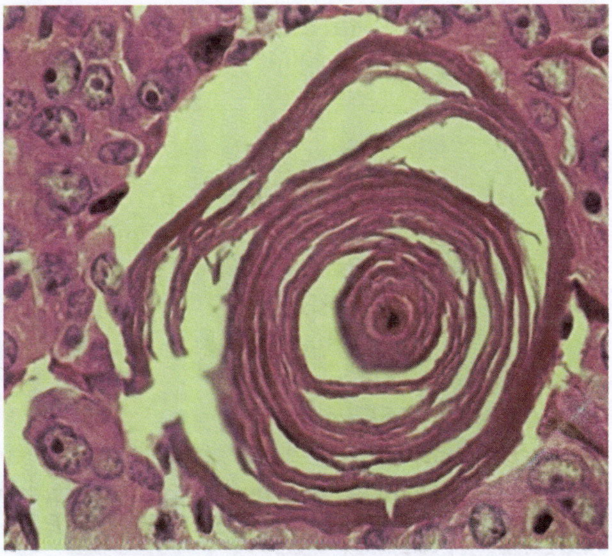

FNAC shows Psammoma bodies in papillary cancer

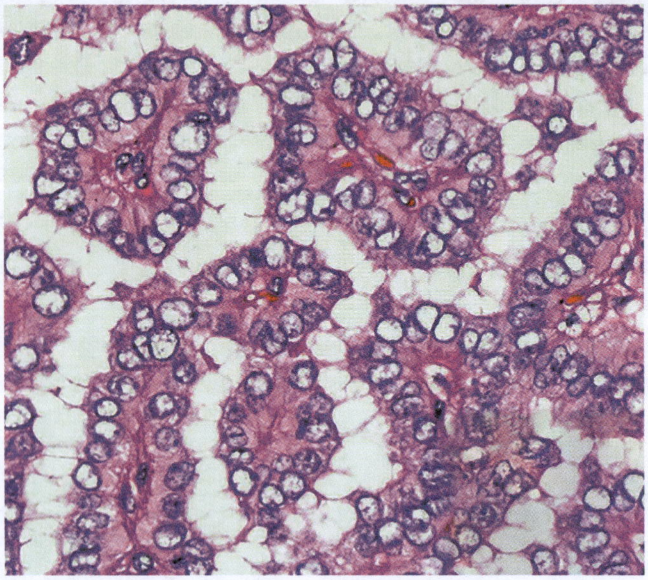

Orphan annie-eye nuclei in papillary cancer

Medullary Ca of thyroid

- Incidence—2.5%
- Parafollicular c cells—(ULTIMOBRANCHIAL BODY)
- RET oncogene mutation: MEN2A, MEN 2B

Sporadic	Familial
80% - M/C TYPE	20%
Unilateral	Bilateral—multicentric and multifocal
	MEN2A, MEN2B, Familial medullary carcinoma thyroid syndrome

Properties:

- **Neuroendocrine tumor (secretory)**
  - Calcitonin—tumor marker for follow-up (**>0.08 ng/mL is significant**)
  - CEA—for prognosis
  - ACTH—Cushing syndrome
  - Serotonin—diarrhea
  - PGE_2 and PGF_2 alpha
  - Histaminidase
- **Rule out pheochromocytoma**—24 hour urinary VMA INCREASED. IF PRESENT – OPERATE Pheochromocytoma first.
- FNAC shows - amyloid stroma

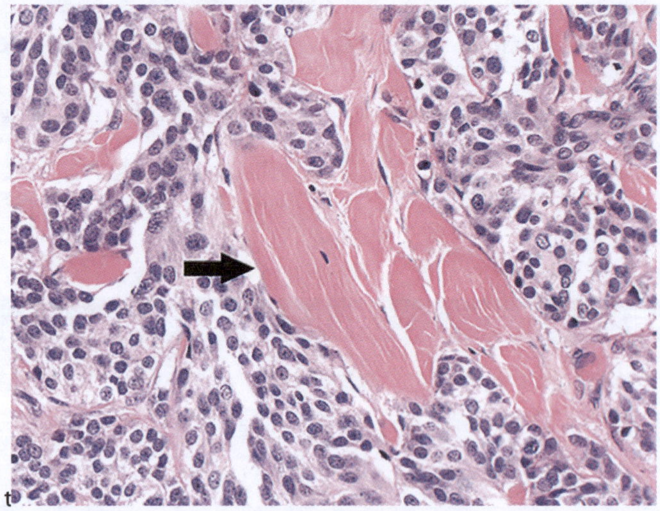

FNAC showing (arrow) amyloid stroma in medullary cancer

- **Treatment:** Total thyroidectomy + central neck node dissection (irrespective of node –/+) + mRND (if node +)
- MC site of distant metastasis – Liver (like other neuroendocrine)
- **Prophylactic thyroidectomy**:
  - MEN2A: <5 years
  - MEN2B: <1 year

THYROID SURGERY

- Lobectomy/hemithyroidectomy – remove isthmus + one lobe
- Subtotal thyroidectomy – leave behind 8 g in each TE groove
- Near total thyroidectomy/Hartley—Dunhill procedure – 2-4 g is left behind on one side
- Total thyroidectomy – nothing is left behind

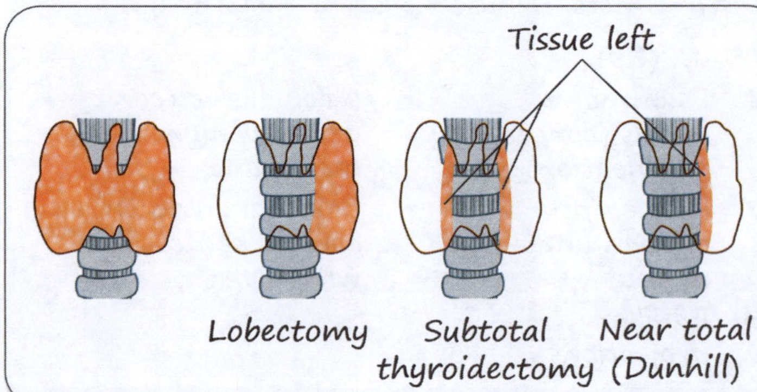

Postoperative Complications

- **Stridor – B/L RLN injury/neuropraxia**-reintubate -wait for 48–72 hours by giving steroids and anti-inflammatory drugs:
  - If stridor disappears—extubate
  - If persistent stridor—extubate and do tracheostomy
  - Permanent B/L RLN injury—do lateralization of cord/Arytenoidectomy
- **Life-threatening complications in postoperative:**
  - Hematoma—due to slippage of ligature of superior thyroid artery
  - Management—remove suture in bed side-then prepare OT
  - Nowadays we don't get it as we have drain-
  - If bleed is seen in drain—shift patient to OT and capture the bleed.
- **Nerve injuries**
  - U/L RLN—Hoarseness of voice
  - B/L RLN—Stridor
  - ELN (MC) Huskiness of voice (timbre is lost)
  - ILN—Paroxysmal nocturnal cough/aspiration
- **Laryngomalacia**—After removal of thyroid—the larynx collapses
- **Postoperative Hypocalcemia**

Hypocalcemia

- 2–5 days post op
- Due to loss of blood supply to parathyroid gland
- Manifestations: **subclinical or overt**

Subclinical	Overt
• On measuring BP-Carpopedal spasm – trousseau sign • On tapping face-Chvostek sign	• Tetany-opisthotonus • Laryngismus stridulous
Management – oral Calcium	IV Calcium gluconate

- No need to monitor serum calcium for looking hypocalcemia
- Normal Serum calcium - 8–12 mg/dL.
- For a preoperative patient with 12 mg/dL—postoperative value of 8 is also hypocalcemic though in normal range. So, serum calcium is not reliable.
- For transient—oral calcium
- For severe—IV calcium
- **Permanent (<10% cases where all 4 parathyroid glands are removed)—oral calcium + vitamin D3 for lifetime**

CANCER OF BREAST

- This is the most common cancer in females in World and even in India as per latest statistics.

Triple assessment of breast**
- Clinical examination
- Radiological imaging
- Pathological examination

The positive predictive value of diagnosis using this combination exceeds—99.9%**

CLINICAL EXAMINATION

Position:
- Sitting
- Sitting and leaning forward—to look for chest wall fixity (ribs)
- Arm on hip with alternate contraction and relaxation—to look for pectoralis major fixity
- Arms raised above head—to look for Nipple retraction and Peau d'orange
- Semirecumbent position—Best position—fat gets dispersed and tumor is well elicited.

cTNM (8th Edition of the AJCC) Staging

- **cTNM:** Clinical TNM staging
- **pTNM:** Pathological TNM staging
- **yTNM:** Post-neoadjuvant chemotherapy (CT)/ radiotherapy (RT) staging
- **Tis:** Tumor in situ—ductal Ca in situ, Paget's disease
  (Lobular Ca in situ is removed in 8th Edition as it is a physiological precursor for Ca breast)

T staging:
- T1: <2 cm
- T2: 2–5 cm
- T3: >5 cm
- T4:
  - **Chest wall fixity**—involvement of intercostal muscles, serratus anterior, ribs
  - **Skin involvement:**
    - Peau d'orange (subdermal lymphatics infiltrated)
    - Ulcer in skin
    - Satellite nodules +, on skin
  - **Both a + b**
  - **Inflammatory breast cancer** (worst prognosis)

Things not included in skin involvement are as follows:
- Fixity
- Tethering
- Nipple retraction
- Dimpling
- Puckering

N staging:
- **N1:** Mobile axillary nodes
- **N2:**
  - Fixed axillary nodes
  - Internal mammary nodes (by CECT—but comes in cTNM)
- **N3:**
  - Infraclavicular node(apical)
  - Both axillary and internal mammary
  - Supraclavicular nodes

Contralateral nodes: Always metastatic (e.g. opposite supraclavicular nodes)

M1: metastatic

Most common (MC) site: Lumbar vertebrae (via Batson plexus)

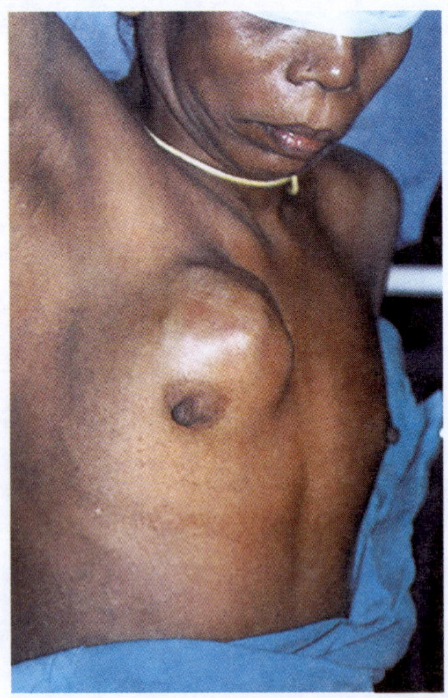

T4a: Chest wall involvement

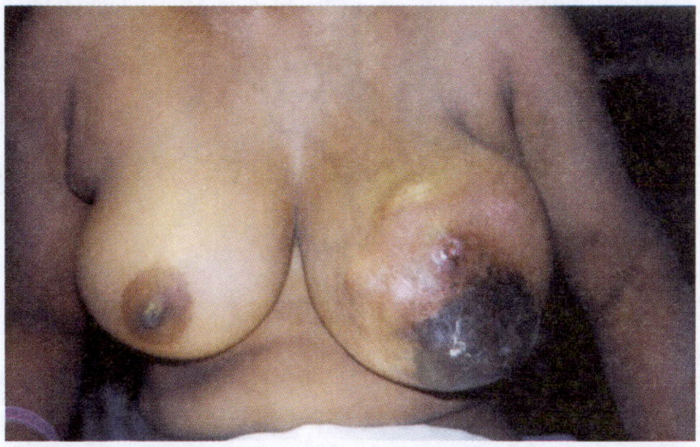

T4b: Skin ulceration by cancer

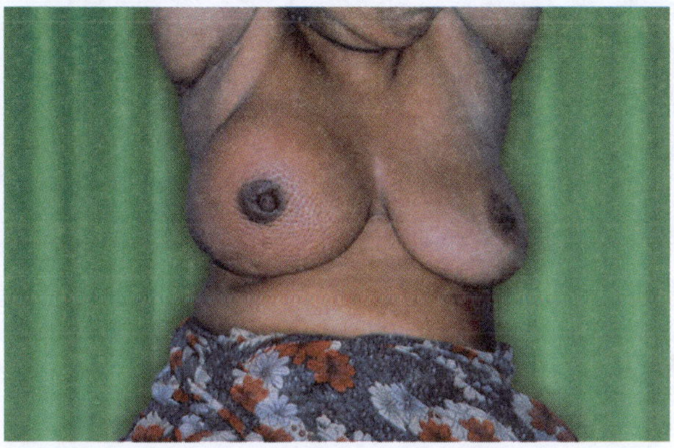

Peau d'orange

AJCC stage categorization:

- **Stage I**: T1N0
- **Stage IIa**: T1N1, T2N0
- **Stage IIb**: T2N1, T3N0
- **Stage IIIa**: All the others including T1N2**
- **Stage IIIb**: T4 and any N
- **Stage IIIc**: N3 and any T
- **Stage IV**: M+

Management of the cancer Breast is based on the AJCC staging:

- **Stage I, IIa, IIb**: Early breast cancer—do modified radical mastectomy (MRM) or breast-conserving surgery (BCS) straight forward
- **Stage IIIa, IIIb, IIIc**: Locally advanced breast cancer—do neoadjuvant chemotherapy followed by MRM + RT
- **Stage IV**: Metastatic cancer—palliative therapy—hormone therapy + chemotherapy

RADIOLOGICAL EXAMINATION

Imaging of Breast

- **Mammography**: Indicated for females >35 years as the breast is less dense for them.
- **Ultrasound**: Indicated for females <35 years due to dense breast.
- **MRI breast**: Indicated for females with silicone implants.

Mammography

- X-ray
- Low voltage and high amplitude
- Bremsstrahlung type of X-ray (not a conventional X-ray)
  - Dose: 0.1 cGy = 4 times chest X-ray
  - No increased risk of cancer
- Screening mammography—advised for >40 years in all females in West (not followed in India)
  - Risk of cancer breast related deaths decreased by 30% by routine screening
- Views to be taken in mammography
  - Craniocaudal view
  - Mediolateral oblique view
  - Done always for both breasts

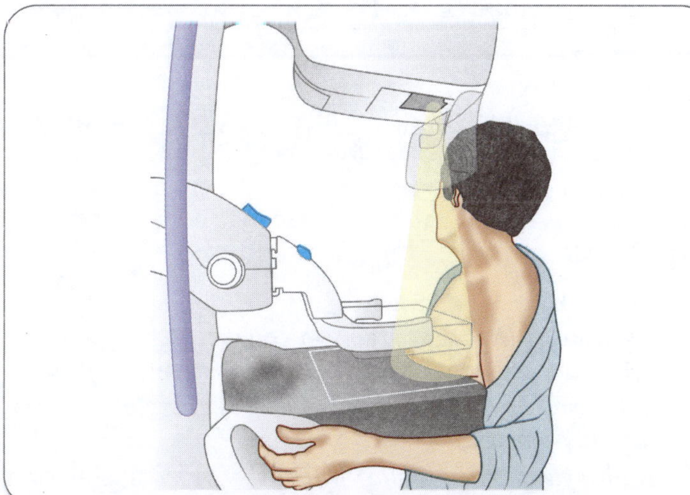

Mammography—craniocaudal view

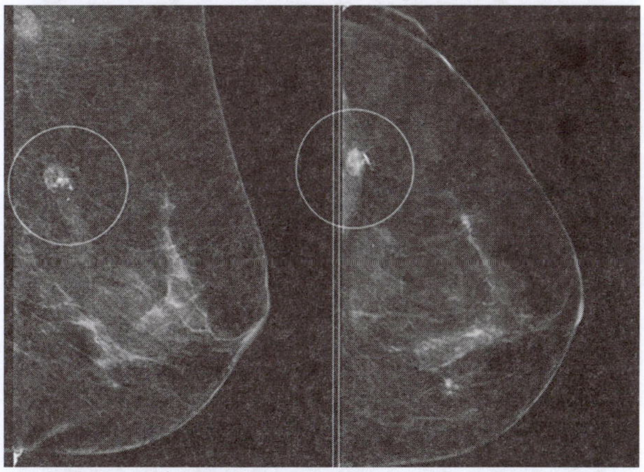

Mammography showing calcification

Breast calcifications:
- **In ductal carcinoma in situ (DCIS):**
  - Microcalcification
  - Scattered calcification
  - Clustered calcification
  - Radiological IOC for DCIS is mammography.
- **Lobular carcinoma in situ (LCIS):** NO radiological finding.
- **Lobular carcinoma (LC) invasive type:** Neighboring calcification
- **Fibroadenoma breast:** Popcorn calcification/ macrocalcification

Extra Mile:

Breast Imaging Reporting and Data System (BI-RADS)** is used to suggest pathological examination based on findings:

Category	Definition	Further plan
0	Incomplete assessment	Need additional imagings
1	Negative	Advised annual screening
2	Benign finding	Recommend annual screening
3	Probably benign	Short interval follow-up
4	Suspicious of malignancy	Biopsy must**
5	Highly suggestive of malignancy	Take appropriate action
6	Known biopsy proved malignancy	

Lesions less than BI-RADS 3 need no pathological investigations**

Mammography:
- Screening investigation of choice for >40 years** for community screening
- IOC for DCIS**

MRI Breast

Indicated in:
- Distinguishing scar from recurrence in women who had previous breast conservative surgery.
- Gold standard for imaging the breasts of women with implants.
- Evaluating the axilla in both primary breast cancer and recurrence.

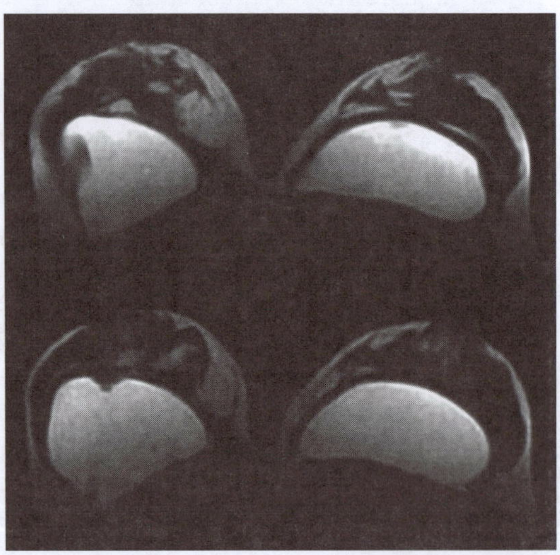

Breasts of women with implants

PATHOLOGICAL EXAMINATION

- **FNAC:** with 22/24 G needle
- **Core-cut biopsy:** 16/18 G needle to diagnose cancer breast—helps to diagnose type of cancer and also hormone receptor status study
- **Excision biopsy**—only with small and inconclusive lesion.

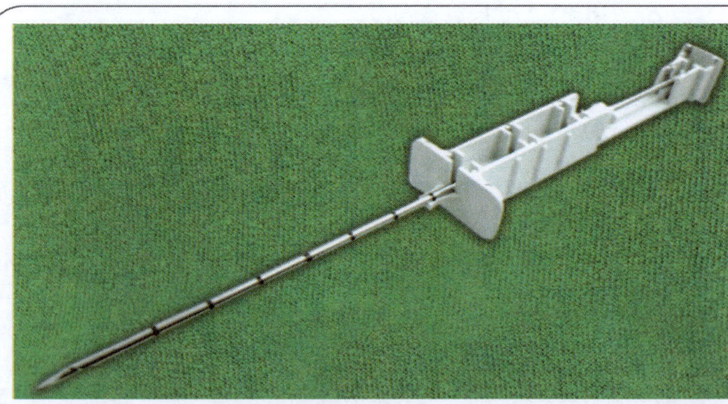

Core-cut (tru-cut) biopsy needle

Ductal Ca—invasive	Lobular Ca—invasive
80%	10%
MC type: • NST (no specific type) or • NOS (not otherwise specified) or • Scirrhous	**Bilateral:** • Multicentric—in all quadrants • Multifocal—multiple foci in same quadrant

Contd...

Ductal Ca—invasive	Lobular Ca—invasive

Types:
• **Medullary Ca**
  ○ Triple negative Ca
  ○ Soft in consistency
  ○ Bad prognosis
• **Colloid Ca**
  ○ Mucinous cancer
  ○ Old age
  ○ Best prognosis
• **Tubular Ca**
  ○ Good prognosis
	• Always advise FNAC of opposite breast
	• Biopsy shows Indian file appearance of cells
	• Mammography shows neighboring calcification
	• **Treatment:** B/L MRM advised

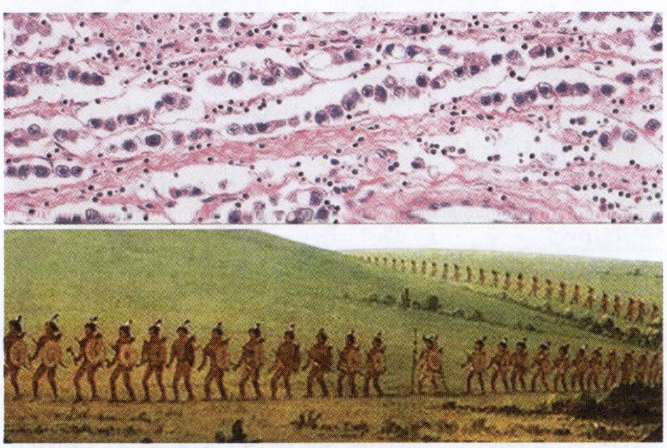

Indian file pattern in lobular cancer

Molecular classification

Luminal A (MC type)	Luminal B (all positive)	HER2 (only HER2 positive)	Basal type (all negative)
ER+	ER+	ER–	ER–
PR+	PR+	PR–	PR–
HER2–	HER2+	HER2+	HER2–
Best prognosis		Poor prognosis	Worst prognosis
a/w BRCA2			Most common cancer in BRCA1**

Classification of breast cancer:

- **Sporadic:** 60–75%
- **Familial:** 20–30%
  - 1st-degree relative has 13% risk
- **Hereditary:** 5%
  - BRCA1—45%
  - BRCA2—35%
  - Li-Fraumeni syndrome—1%
  - Ataxia-Telangiectasia—1%
  - Muir-Torre (Lynch II)—1%
  - Cowden—1%

BRCA1	BRCA2
Chromosome 17q	Chromosome 13q
Poorly differentiated	Well differentiated
Triple negative (basal type)	Triple+/ER+
Bad prognosis	Good prognosis
MC: • Breast Ca (60%) • Ovarian Ca (40%) • Prostate Ca • Colon Ca	MC: • Breast Ca (80%) • Ovarian Ca (20%) • Prostate Ca • Colon Ca • Pancreatic Ca • Gastric Ca • Melanoma • Male breast Ca
Advise them to undergo prophylactic **B/L simple mastectomy** And after completion of family—**B/L salpingo-oophorectomy**	

MANAGEMENT OF CANCER BREAST

Modified Radical Mastectomy

Structures removed are as follows:

- Nipple
- Areola
- Breast tissue (entire)
- Pectoralis fascia
- Axillary dissection procedure (level I, II, III)

Structures preserved are—(ABCDM):

- Axillary vessels
- Bell's nerve
- Cephalic vein
- Nerve to latissimus Dorsi (thoracodorsal nerve)
- Pectoralis major

Axillary dissection boundaries:

- Superiorly—Axillary artery and vein
- Inferiorly—Angular vein
- Medially—Bell's nerve (long thoracic nerve)
- Laterally—Thoracodorsal pedicle (vessels + nerve)

Structures that must be preserved during this dissection:

- Thoracodorsal neurovascular bundle
- Long thoracic nerve of bell

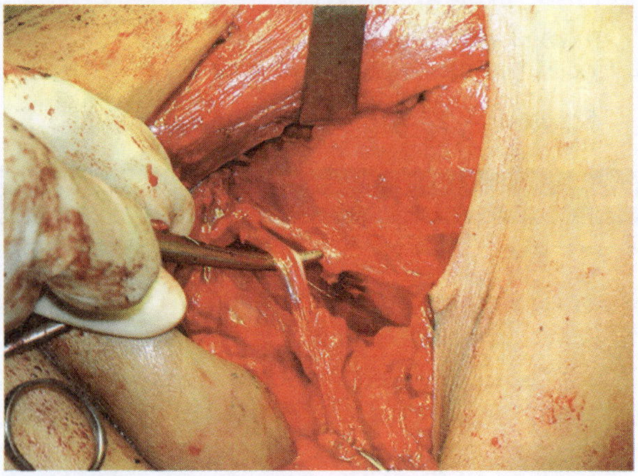

Thoracodorsal pedicle and long thoracic nerve of bell

- Minimum 10 nodes to be removed to call a complete axillary dissection
- Most common nerve injured—**intercostobrachial nerve—only cutaneous supply****
    - Other nerves
        - Bell's nerve—winging of scapula
        - Nerve to latissimus Dorsi—shoulder movements are affected (e.g., medial rotation, climbing trees)
- To deal with pectoralis minor in axillary dissection:
    - **Patey's method**
        - Cut and remove
        - Level I, II, III can be removed
    - **Auchincloss's method**
        - Retract pectoralis minor
        - Level I, II only can be removed
    - **Scanlon's method**
        - Cut and resuture
        - Level I, II, III can be removed
- Place two closed suction drains—one in axilla and another in bed of surgical site
- Closure of skin with subcuticular suture—using monocryl (poliglecaprone)

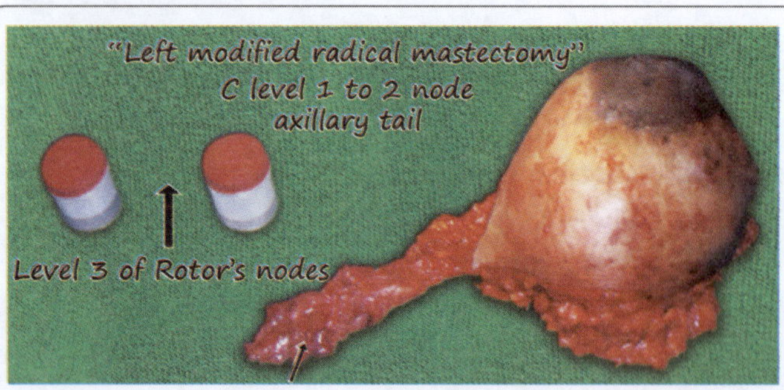

Specimen of modified radical mastectomy

Complications:

- MC complication—seroma**
    - Remove drain on 5th day postoperative
- Nerve related—intercostobrachial nerve injury causing paresthesia.
- Flap necrosis
- Lymphedema of arm
- **Lymphedema of arm + radiotherapy** = lymphangiosarcoma—called Stewart-Treves syndrome.

Sentinel Node Biopsy

- Sentinel node—1st node from Ca breast (axillary node)
- Axillary dissection is the main cause of morbidity.
- To prevent this—sentinel node biopsy is done.
- Therefore, test the 1st node and look for deposit in 1st node.
    - If positive—dissect axilla
    - If negative—do not dissect axilla

Indications:

- Early breast cancer—stage I, IIa, IIb (T1, T2)
- No node palpable (on clinical examination or on USG)

Contraindications:

- T3, T4 lesions (locally advanced breast cancer)
- Palpable node+
- Previous H/o surgery in breast (1st level lymphatic is disturbed—it will have a different pathway)
- Pregnancy
- Contraindications for radiotherapy
    - Collagen vascular disease
    - Previous H/o RT
    - Pregnancy

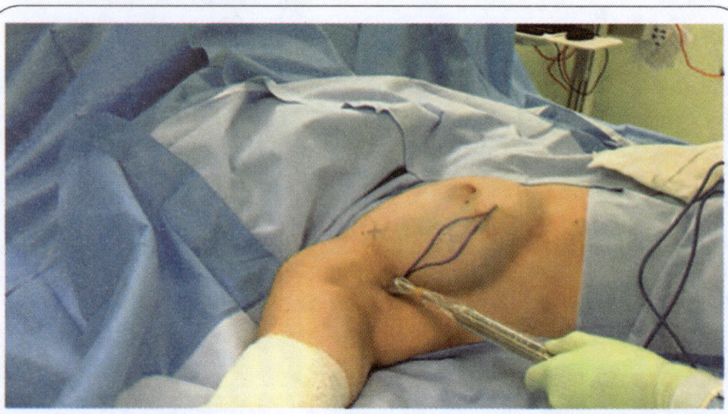

Sentinel node biopsy by radiolabeled colloid

Breast Conservative Surgery

Indications:

- Early breast cancer
- DCIS

Breast-conserving surgery has four components:

1. **Wide local excision (WLE)**
   - Clean negative margin from pathologist on all sides (1-mm negative)
2. **Axillary status should be identified**
   - N0: Sentinel node biopsy
   - N1: Axillary dissection
3. **Radiotherapy** to remaining breast
4. **Keep patient on follow-up**
   - Since only tumor was removed—it may recur.

Contraindications of BCS:

- **If wide local excision not possible like in**
  - Locally advanced breast cancer (skin fixed, chest wall fixed)
  - After 2 times wide local excision—margin is positive—go for MRM
  - Multicentric and multifocal cancer (cannot do WLE)
  - Small breast but tumor is big—cosmetic deformity
- **Where RT is contraindicated**
  - Collagen vascular disease
  - Previous H/o RT
  - Pregnancy—1st and 2nd trimester (in 3rd trimester—we can give RT after delivery)
  - Huge pendulous breast—we'll have to expose abdominal contents while giving radiotherapy to the remaining breast.
- **Patients who tend to loss to follow-up**
  - Low socioeconomic patients
  - Uneducated patients
  - Psychiatry patients

The following are not contraindications:

- Family history
- Central/subareolar tumor
- Node+

Reconstruction of breast: DIEP (deep inferior epigastric perforator) flap

- (Skin + subcutaneous + fat) Free flap—inferior epigastric artery based (from pubic region)—please remember no muscle is used.
- Require microvascular anastomoses

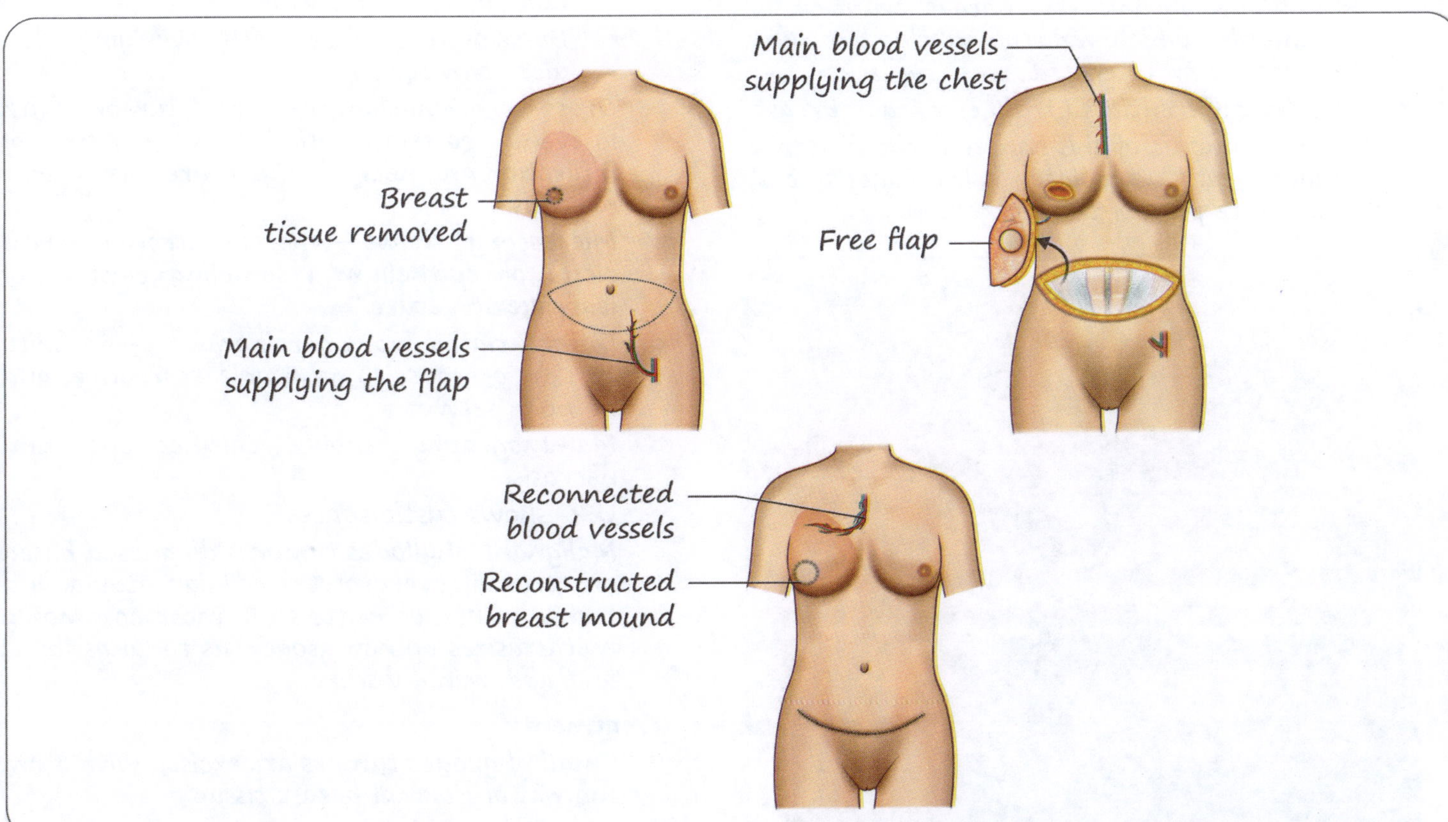

Deep inferior epigastric perforator flap

Must know:

Tamoxifen:
- Partial agonist/antagonist
- Antagonist to estrogen only in breast
- Should be given only in cases of estrogen receptor positive status** but ER negative tumors also respond to some extent**
- Standard treatment for both premenopausal and post-menopausal women**
- Dose: 10 mg BD for **5 years**
- **ASCO guidelines say**—if the patient is premenopausal after completing 5 years of tamoxifen—**offer another 5 years of tamoxifen****

Adverse Effects:
- Bone pain, hot flashes, nausea, vomiting
- Menstrual irregularities, vaginal bleeding, dermatitis**
- **Thromboembolic manifests****
- Hypercalcemia
- **Endometrial carcinoma****
- Increased cataract surgeries, retinal deposits

OTHER LESIONS RELATED TO TUMORS

- **Paget's disease**
  - Present as chronic eczematous eruption of the nipple, which may be subtle, but may progress to an ulcerated, weeping lesion.
  - Must be differentiated from eczema of breast.
  - Pathognomonic of this cancer is the presence of large, pale, vacuolated cells (Paget's cells) in the rete pegs of the epithelium.

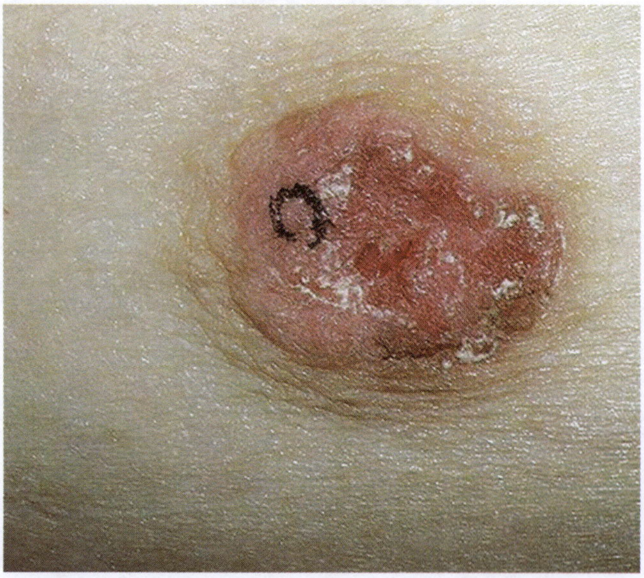

Paget's disease showing nipple erosions

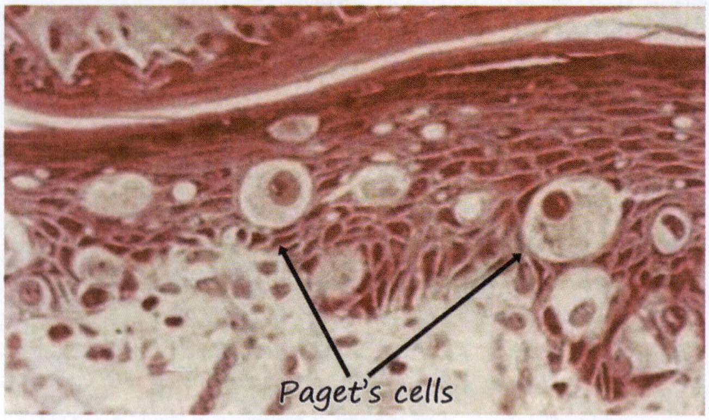

Paget's cells

- **Phyllodes tumor (serocystic disease of Brodie or cystosarcoma phyllodes)**
  - Tumor of mixed connective tissue and epithelium (biphasic proliferation of stroma and mammary epithelium)
  - It may be benign, borderline, malignant.
  - Present at age >40 years.
  - **Clinical examination:**
    - Phyllodes tumor remains mobile on the chest wall.
    - Smooth, rounded and painless multi-nodular lesion is seen.
    - Bosselated surface with overlying skin ulcer can occur.
  - **Gross examination:** Massive tumor with unevenly bosselated surface with areas of infarction and necrosis. Cystic areas represent necrosis.*
  - **Microscopy shows**—whorled stroma forms clefts of epithelium resembling clusters of **leaf-like structure.****
  - Differentiated from carcinoma by—no fixity to skin or muscle, no nipple retraction and no node seen.
  - **Mammography** shows calcifications and necrosis.
  - **USG** shows cystic spaces.**
  - **Malignant phyllodes tumor** is diagnosed based on stromal overgrowth, cellular atypia and high number of mitosis.* It most commonly metastasizes by hematogenous to lungs, bone and abdominal viscera.

Treatment:
- Small phyllodes tumors are excised with 1 cm margin of normal breast tissue.
- Large phyllodes tumors require mastectomy.
- If margins are negative, no radiotherapy is given.*

- For larger tumors, >5 cm, involving chest wall or fascia, margins + irradiation of chest wall is advised.
- No axillary dissection** needed as there is no axillary metastasis.

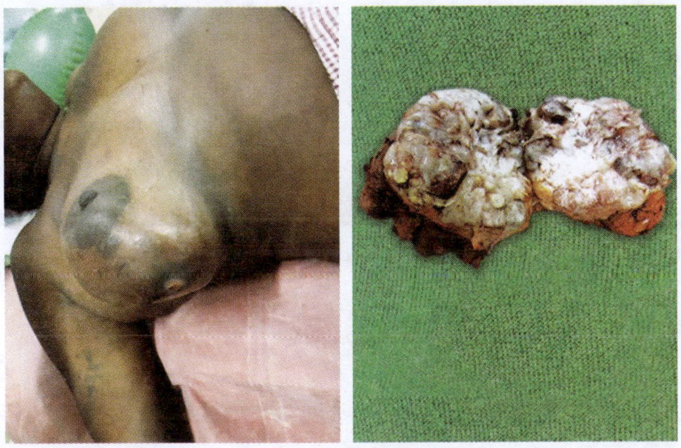

Phyllodes tumor

- **Duct papilloma versus duct ectasia**

Duct papilloma	Duct ectasia (no pain)
Papilloma inside duct	Duct is abnormally dilated
Young female	Middle-aged female
Bloody discharge	Greenish yellow discharge
	Periductal mastitis **(Zuska's disease)**** Pain + Predisposed by smoking females
Ductography—filling defect	Dilated ducts

Contd...

Duct papilloma	Duct ectasia (no pain)
Treatment: Tennis racket-shaped incision (on skin) and microdochectomy	**Hadfield's operation:** • Conical excision of all ducts with apex at nipple • Radical approach • No lactation possible hereafter from this breast • Done only for incurable periductal mastitis

- **Mondor's disease**
  - Superficial vein thrombophlebitis
  - MC vein—**lateral thoracic vein**
    - Thoracodorsal vein
    - Superior epigastric vein
  - **C/F:** Painful, tender, cord like (DDx: lymphatic permeation by tumor)
  - **Management:** Rest shoulder, arm restriction with analgesics.
  - If pain persists—excision.

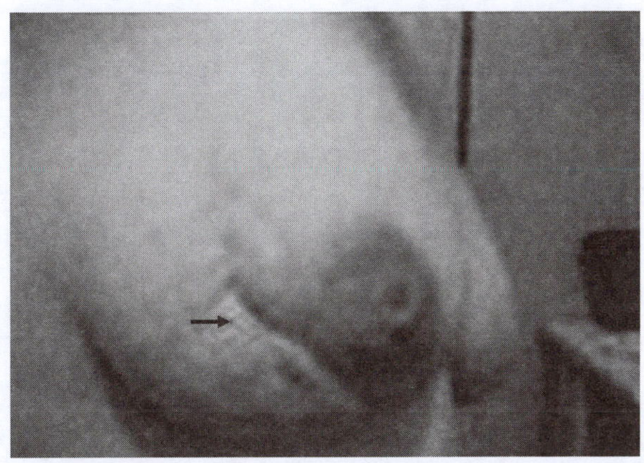

Mondor's disease

6. HERNIAS

INGUINAL HERNIA

Differences between Indirect Hernia and Direct Hernia

Indirect hernia	Direct hernia
Young age Congenital/acquired Due to preformed sac MC in males	Old age Mostly acquired (except Ogilvie) MC in males **Predisposed by** • Collagen vascular disorder • Smoking • Increased intra-abdominal pressure, e.g., Constipation, difficulty in micturition, BPH, chronic cough- COPD
Course: Deep ring to superficial ring Pyriform shaped • Sac is lateral to inferior epigastric artery • Sac is anterolateral to cord structure	Through Hesselbach's triangle Hemispherical shaped Sac is medial to inferior epigastric artery Sac is posteromedial to cord structure
Treatment: • Herniotomy + • Herniorrhaphy/ hernioplasty	• No herniotomy (just push the sac inside) • Only hernioplasty
Complications: High chances of obstruction	Less chance of obstruction (due to wide neck of sac)

Occurrence

In Females

- **Indirect hernia is most** common hernia in females.
- **Direct hernia never occurs**
- Femoral hernia **is more common in females** compared to males.

Males

Indirect **hernia is most common hernia.**

Contents of Sac

Enterocele	Omentocele
Contains bowel	Contains omentum
Reducibility: **Initially:** Difficult (due to narrow neck) **Later:** Easily reducible with gurgling sound	 **Initially:** Easy **Later:** Difficult Due to adhesion of omentum to fundus
Elastic in consistency	Doughy consistency

European Hernia Society Classification

- Primary/Recurrent
- Lateral/Medial/Femoral
- **Defect:** 1 finger = 1.5 cm
  - For example, PL2 hernia = primary lateral 2 finger (3 cm defect)

Surgeries for Hernia

Anatomical repairs (Herniorrhaphy)	Mesh repair (Hernioplasty)	Lap repairs
• Modified Bassini • McVay (Cooper ligament repair) • Moloney Darning • Shouldice	• Lichtenstein • Gilbert's Plug repair • PHS - Prolene Hernia System	• TEP • TAPP

Herniorrhaphy

- No mesh, only suture is used
- Done only in emergency nowadays due to increased chances of mesh infection.

Types:

- Original Bassini—Approximate conjoint tendon with inguinal ligament (intermittent sutures)
- Modified Bassini—Continuous sutures to approximate conjoint tendon with inguinal ligament.
- Shouldice repair—Double breasting of fascia transversalis.

Hernioplasty

Gold standard-Lichtenstein tension free mesh repair
Treatment of choice for direct hernia
(as in direct hernia – posterior wall is already weak-if we put sutures it becomes further weak)

Meshes in Hernia Repair

- ***Mesh types***
  - NET (can be woven or knitted)
    - Adherence is easy (tissue enters mesh-adherence due to friction)
    - Fixation may or may not be done
  - ***Sheet***
    - Adherence is not there
    - Fixation is must to prevent mesh migration
- Materials used for mesh
  - ***Polypropylene mesh***
    - White color
    - Fix with 2.0 prolene/tackers
    - Hydrophobic (Hence, prevents bacterial ingrowth**)
    - Prevents bacterial growth due to hydrophobic nature
  - ***Polyester mesh***
    - Hydrophilic
    - Increases bacterial growth but also increases anti-inflammatory cells reaching there—so it can be used and nothing to worry.
  - ***PTFE (Poly Tetra Fluoro Ethylene)***
    - Flat sheet
    - No tissue ingrowth
    - Used as nonadhesive barrier between layers
- ***Weight of mesh***

Light weight = 40 g/m^2	Heavy weight mesh = 80 g/m^2
• Better tissue integration • Larger pores • Less shrinkage • Better comfort	• Goes for contracture • Other features are opposite to light weight

- ***Biological mesh***
  - It has a scaffold to encourage neovascular ingrowth and collagen deposition.
  - Expensive
  - Derived from
    - Human/animal dermis
    - Bovine pericardium
    - Porcine submucosa
  - Contraindicated in infection (mesh will be dissolved)
  - Prevents attachment of bowel to mesh
  - Used in burst abdomen
- ***Absorbable mesh***
  - Used for temporary closure of abdomen in burst abdomen
  - No role in hernia repair
  - Made up of polyglycolic acid = also called "VICRYL MESH"
- ***Dual mesh/Tissue separation mesh***
  - One side by prolene (toward skin)
  - Other side by vicryl/collagen/PTFE/cellulose (visceral side)
  - Prevents bowel adhesion

Complications of Hernia Surgery

- Surgical site infection
- Nerve injuries

  Most common nerves injured:
  - Laparoscopic hernia repair – lateral cutaneous nerve of thigh > genitofemoral nerve
  - Open repair – ilioinguinal nerve > genital branch of genitofemoral nerve
- Ischemic orchitis due to testicular artery injury (most serious complication)
- Injury to vas deferens
- Recurrence are most common in direct hernia repairs – most commonly near the floor.

NAMED HERNIAS IN INGUINAL REGION

Sliding Inguinal Hernia

- Sac + intraperitoneal structures + some retroperitoneal structures (e.g., cecum, descending colon)
- Most commonly on left side
- Most common content sigmoid colon
- If on right side - content is cecum (MC)

Maydl's/W-Shaped Hernia

- Most distal part is B - present inside the abdomen (more prone for ischemia)
- If we see A and C being viable and push bowel inside
  - Delayed bowel leak from B can occur
  - ***Retrograde strangulation****

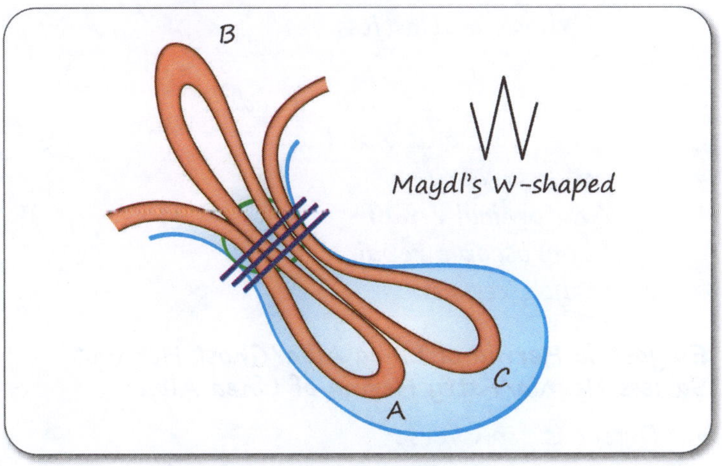

Maydl's hernia

Scrotal Abdomen

- Huge indirect hernia
- May be associated with sliding hernia

Richter's Hernia

- Seen in femoral and obturator hernia
- One circumference of bowel is obstructed
- Fluid is secreted in response, hence, presents as **diarrhea**.

Internal Hernia

- **Stammer's Hernia:** Hernia through defect in transverse mesocolon
- **Peterson hernia:** Hernia behind Roux limb

Extra edge—Named Hernias

- **Ogilvie:** Gap in conjoint tendon. Only congenital direct hernia
- **Laugier's hernia:** Lacunar ligament
- **Beclard hernia:** Type of femoral hernia with defect in saphenous vein area
- **Narath hernia:** Gap due to congenital dislocation of hip.
- **Berger's hernia:** Hernia in pouch of Douglas. Also called sigmoidocele.

OTHER HERNIAS

Umbilical Hernia

In children:

- Congenital (umbilical ring fail to close)
- Defect is not so tight
- No strangulation
- Wait for two years
- Ideal age for surgery: Simple anatomical repair

In adults:

- Abdominal pathology:
  - Obesity
  - Cirrhosis and ascites
  - Pregnancy
- Strangulation is common in adults
- <2 cm – wait and watch
- >2 cm – surgery
  - Anatomical repair
  - Laparoscopic repair
  - Mayo's repair

Epigastric Hernia of Linea Alba/Ghost Hernia/Sacless Hernia/Fatty Hernia of Linea Alba

- Defect is transverse
- Preperitoneal pad of fat comes out first
- Undergoes strangulation—hence, presents with pain
- Pain mimics peptic ulcer disease
- Young males (25–40 years)
- Cough impulse may or may not be present (based on strangulation)
- Ghost/Sacless hernia—only preperitoneal fat pad comes (no peritoneum)
- **Management:**
  - Open entire linea alba while operating—look for minor defects
  - Recurrent due multiple defects missed during previous surgery
  - Adult—close with nonabsorbable sutures
  - Child—absorbable suture

Incisional Hernia

- 10–50% incidence
- Port site hernia (laparoscopy)—1–5%
- Broad necked—less risk of strangulation
- We can operate electively
- Factors causing incisional hernia

Management

- Linea alba closure—polypropylene/polydioxanone **(longest absorbable suture)**
  - Continuous sutures used
  - Intermittent sutures used (give less gap <1 cm between sutures)

  Burst abdomen happen on 6th day post op.

Treatment

- **Mesh repair**
  - Onlay technique (by open method)
  - Laparoscopic—IPOM (intraperitoneal onlay mesh)—dual mesh is used.
  - e-TEP (extended—total extraperitoneal repair)
  - Abdominoplasty (remove excess fat)

Spigelian Hernia

- Occurs in spigelian fascia (connecting xiphisternum to suprapubic)
- Interparietal hernia—between muscles
- Occurs at any age
- Most common site—infra umbilical
- Seen mostly above arcuate line** > below arcuate line.
- **C/F:**
  - Young age—Pain + and lump may or may not be palpable
  - Old age—Pain seen with cough impulse + and defect palpated.

- IOC: CT abdomen/USG
- High incidence of strangulation
- Repair:
    - IPOM
    - Open method—close the defect

> **Note:** Hernia with decreased incidence of strangulation:
> - Umbilical hernia
> - Incisional hernia

Lumbar Hernia

Superior lumbar triangle boundaries (Grynfeltt Hernia – Rare)	Inferior lumbar triangle (Petit's triangle) boundaries (Petit's Hernia – Most common)
• **Superolateral:** 12th rib • **Inferolateral:** Internal oblique muscle • **Medially:** Sacrospinalis tendon of erector spinae	• **Superolateral:** External oblique (defect) • **Inferolateral:** Iliac crest • **Medially:** Latissimus dorsi

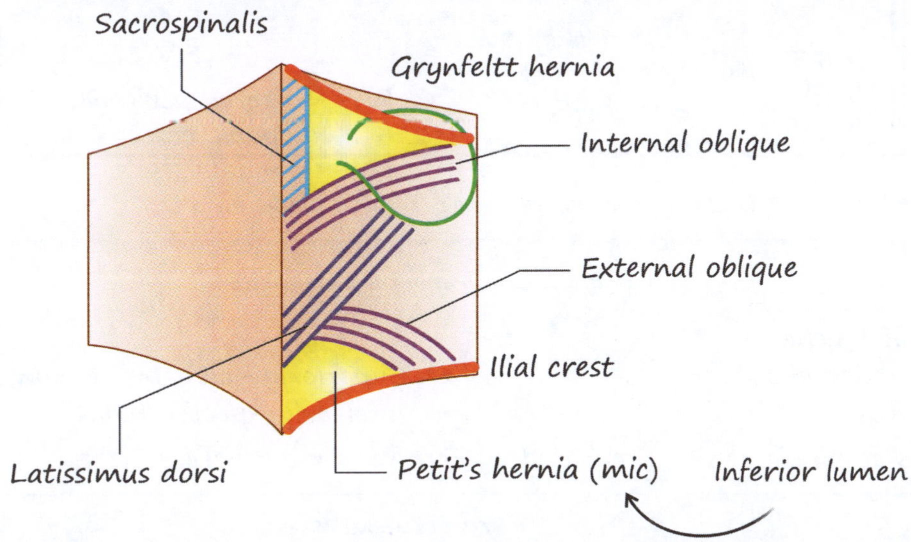

Lumbar Hernias

LAPAROSCOPIC ANATOMY AND SURGERY FOR HERNIA

Triangle of Doom

- Apex—deep inguinal ring
- Medial—vas deferens
- Laterally—gonadal vessels
- Base—reflected peritoneum
- Content—external iliac artery and vein
- When we damage the vessels here, person may die (hence, doom)

Triangle of Pain

- Laterally—iliopubic tract
- Medially—gonadal vessel
- Base—reflected peritoneum
- **Contents:**
    - Lateral cutaneous nerve of thigh
    - Anterior cutaneous nerve of thigh
    - Femoral branch of genitofemoral nerve
    - Femoral nerve

Importance of this Triangle

- If trackers are put below iliopubic tract—it causes severe pain
- Most common nerve injured—lateral cutaneous nerve of thigh—meralgia paresthetica

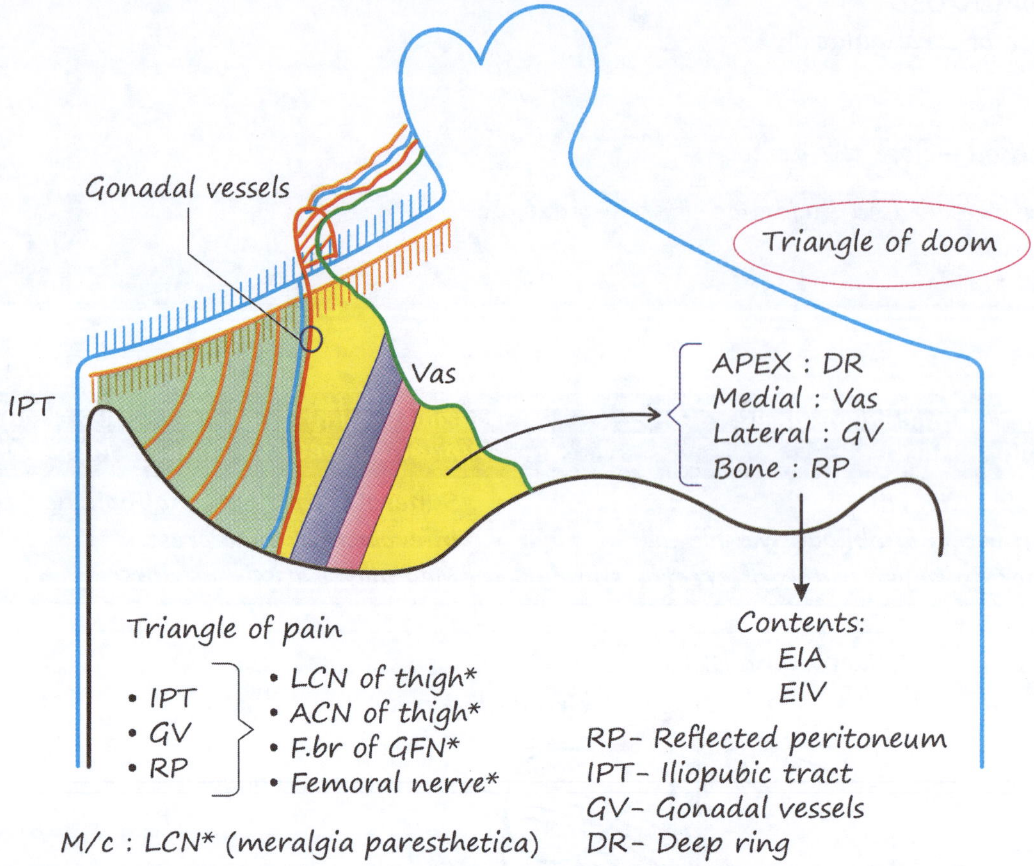

Showing the two important triangles

Myopectineal orifice of Fruchad

- Medially—rectus abdominis
- Laterally—iliopsoas
- Superiorly—conjoint tendon
- Inferiorly—pecten pubis

Application: All types of hernia can be prevented by keeping a mesh here.

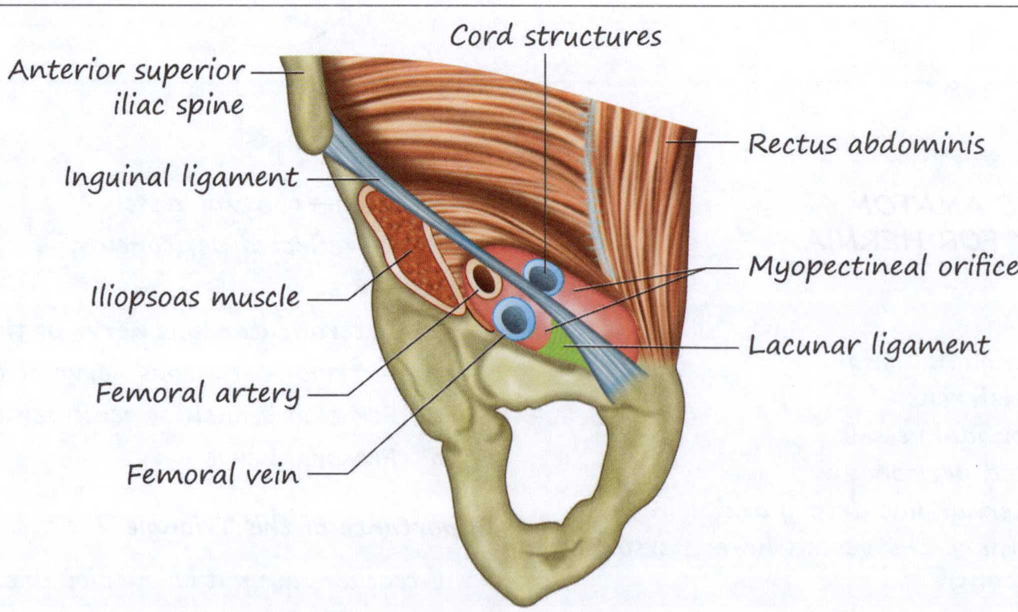

Note: Treatment of choice for mesh infection is laparoscopic repair—laparoscopic removal of mesh

7. GASTROINTESTINAL TRACT

ESOPHAGUS

Narrowest parts in Esophagus on Endoscopy from Incisor Teeth: Natural constrictions:

- 15 cm—Crico pharynx (Narrowest part)
- 25 cm—Arch of aorta
- 27 cm—Left bronchus
- 40 cm—OG junction

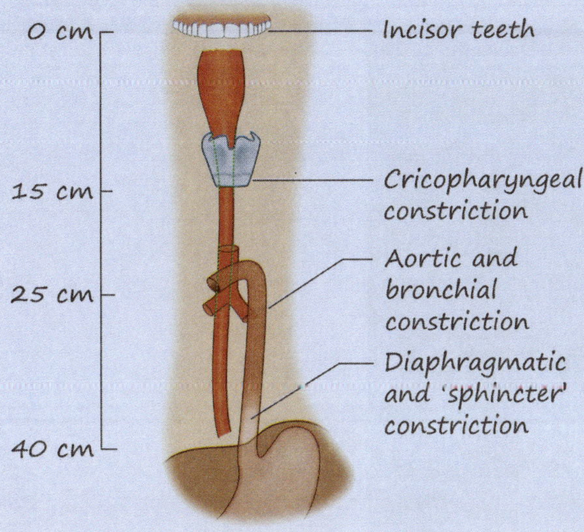

Endoscopy USG

IOC for T and N staging of Esophageal Cancer

Layers in Endoscopic Ultrasound

There are five layers seen in endoscopy.

- **Layer 1:** Mucosa (Hyperechoic)
- **Layer 2:** Muscularis Mucosa (Hypoechoic)
- **Layer 3:** Submucosa (Hyperechoic)
- **Layer 4:** Muscularis Propria (Hypoechoic)
- **Layer 5:** Adventitial layer (Hyperechoic)

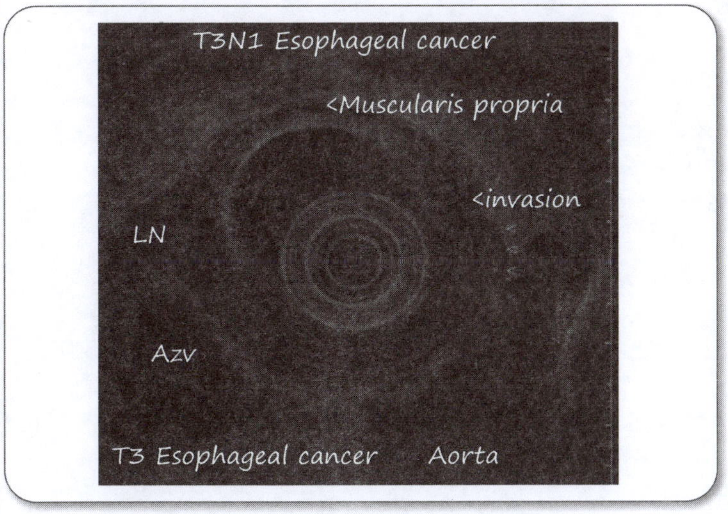

EUS showing esophageal cancer

Must know:

Dysphagia

- 1st Investigation to be done is Barium Swallow**
- Investigation of Choice is Endoscopy**

Clinical features

- Benign Corrosive Strictures—Slow progressive dysphagia (Months to years)
- Malignant Corrosive Strictures—Rapid Progressive dysphagia (weeks to months)
- Slow Progressive dysphagia, Late presentation—Achalasia
- Simultaneous Liquid and Solid Dysphagia—Achalasia
- Intermittent Non-progressive Dysphagia (Episodic)—Schatzki ring
- Dysphagia Lusoria—by Aberrant Right Subclavian Artery

MOTILITY DISORDERS

Gold standard IOC for Motility disorder = High Resolution Manometry** (Uses 36 Sensors)

Classification of Motility Disorders

Chicago Classification

Hypomotility disorders	Hypermotility disorders
Achalasia (Most common overall) **Type 1:** Most common **Type 2:** Best prognosis **Type 3:** Rare type	DES **NCE—Most common hypermotility disorder**

Achalasia and esophagogastric junction disorders	
Type 1 Achalasia (Classic)	• Mean IRP >15 mm Hg • 100% failed peristalsis • Distal contractile integral (DCI) <100 mm Hg.s.Cm
Type 2 Achalasia with Esophageal Compression	• Mean IRP >15 mm Hg • 100% failed peristalsis • Pan esophageal pressurization** • DCI is difficult to measure. • In manometry—ISOBARIC Contraction seen at 30 mm Hg

Contd...

Type 3 (Spastic Achalasia)	• Mean IRP >15 mm Hg • No normal peristalsis • Segmental increased DCI seen • Spastic contractions with distal contractile integral (DCI) >450 mm Hg.s.Cm • Rarely pan esophageal pressurization seen

Contd...

Major disorders of peristalsis	
Distal esophageal spasm	• Mean IRP—Normal • DCI >450 mm Hg.s.Cm • >20 premature contractions
Jackhammer Esophagus (Hypercontractile Esophagus)	• DCI >8000** for at least 2 swallows** • IRP is normal

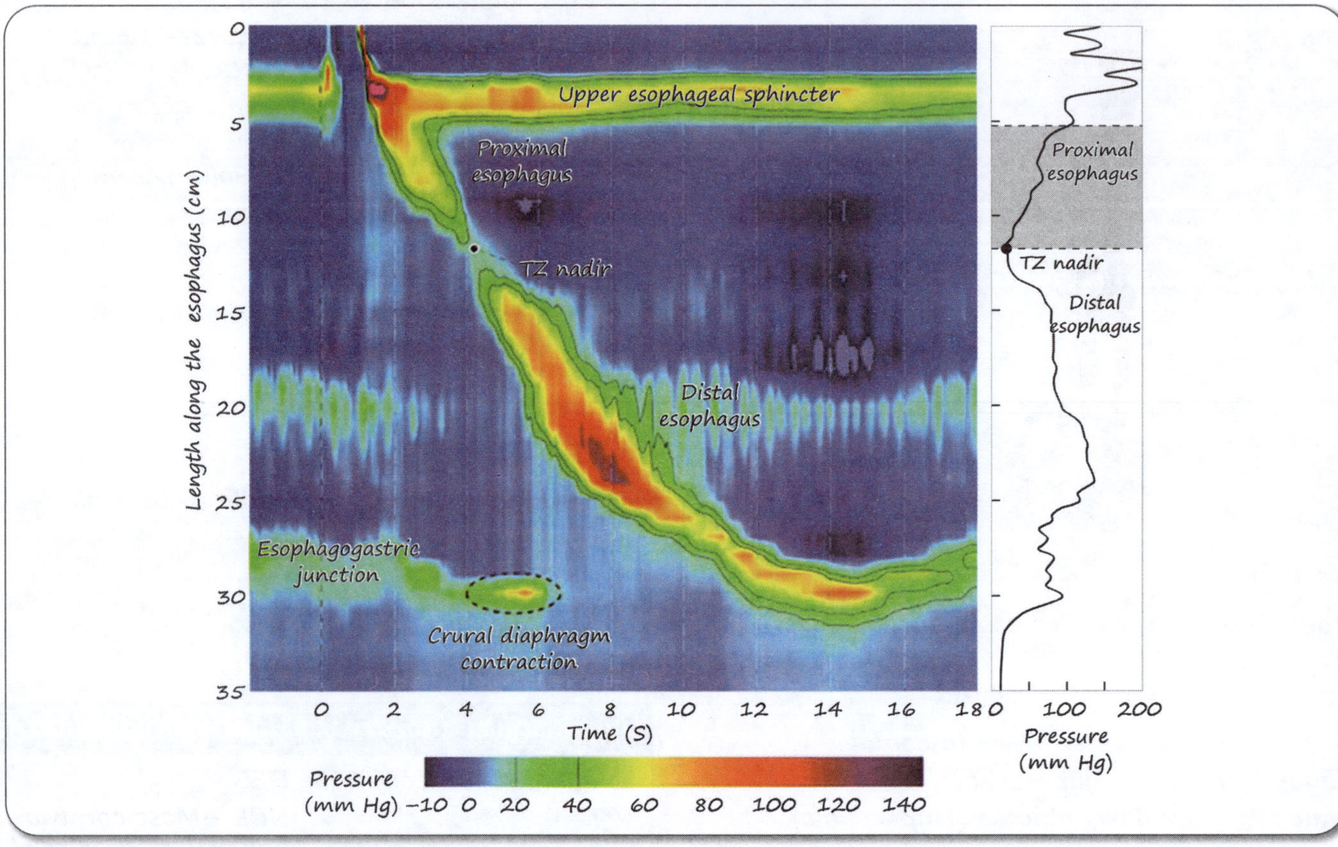

HRM image

ACHALASIA CARDIA

Clinical Features

- MC in young females
- **MC symptom:** Dysphagia (both Solids and Liquids – More for Liquids); Slow Progressive type
- **Triad of achalasia:** Dysphagia + Weight loss + Reflux
- Nocturnal asthma (Also seen in GERD cases)

Investigations

- Barium Swallow—Bird beak appearance, pencil tip, Abrupt Cut off
- Hurst Phenomenon—Flow of contrast beyond bird beak due to contrast load and weight

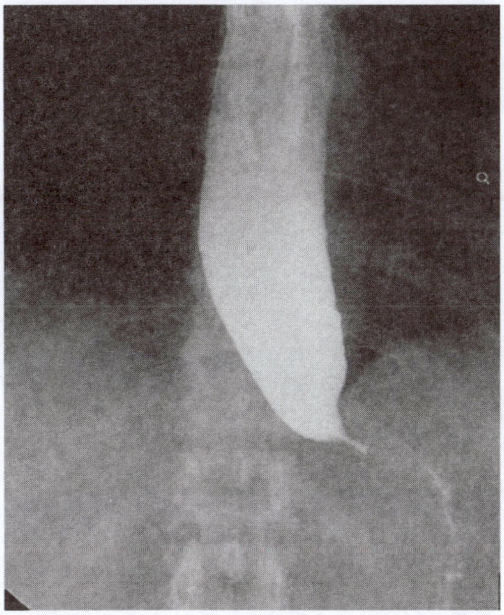

Bird beak

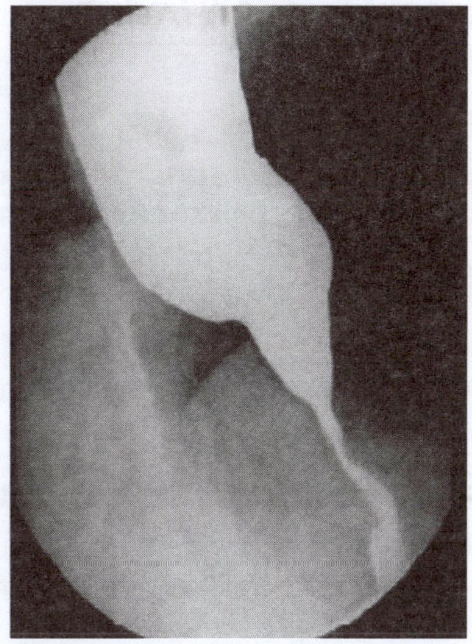

Hurst phenomenon

Complications of Achalasia Cardia

- MC complication—Reflux Esophagitis
- Aspiration
- MC Tumor—SCC (8%)**
- Adenocarcinoma—Below Air fluid level (NEET SS question)
- Sigmoid Mega esophagus

Management

Medical management	Endoscopic	Surgical
• CCB (Nifedipine) • Sildenafil citrate	• Botox injection • Pneumatic balloon dilatation • Recent advance—POEM** (Peroral Endoscopic Myotomy)—**Best method for Type 3 Achalasia**	• Modified Heller's cardio myotomy—Gold Standard Treatment • Complication is GERD—hence, we also do fundoplication. • The best method for fundoplication is DOR'S type (Anterior 180°)

Bailey 28th Edition Update:

ECKARDT Score—Post-treatment score of achalasia to assess the response following endoscopic procedures like Dilatation or POEM.

Diffuse esophageal spasm
• Middle aged female • C/F—Dysphagia + Chest pain • Aggravated by cold fluids and stress • Treatment is Medical—CCB • Surgery can be done—Long esophagomyotomy is advised up to Carina • **Barium Swallow—CORK Screw Esophagus**

Contd...

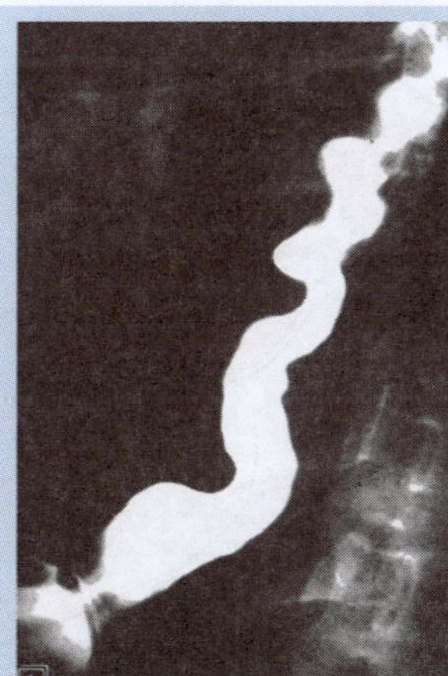

Cork screw esophagus seen in Barium swallow

DIVERTICULUM IN ESOPHAGUS

Kilian's Dehiscence

- Defect in Inferior Constrictor muscle between thyropharyngeal and cricopharyngeal muscle.
- Diverticulum via this defect is Zenker's diverticulum.

Clinical Features

- MC in old men, MC on left side
- MC symptom—Dysphagia
- MC complication—Aspiration
- Other features—Halitosis, Lung abscess, etc.
- IOC—Lateral Oblique view of Barium Swallow.

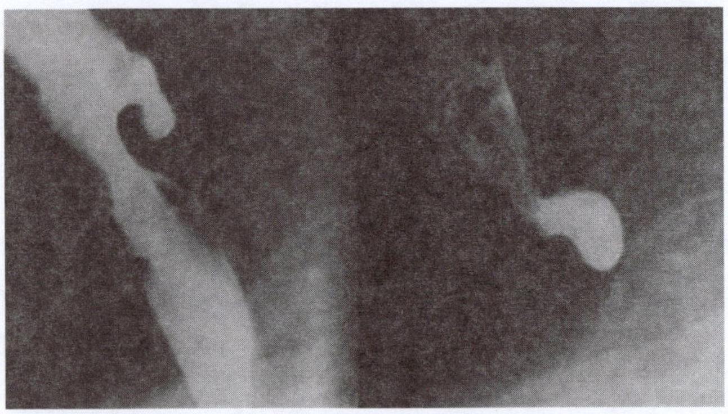

Barium swallow lateral oblique view showing Zenker's diverticulum

- Treatment is Diverticulectomy
- Dohlman's procedure—Stapling method for diverticulum using a special scope.
- Diverticulopexy—For old unfit patients, the diverticulum is made upside down and fixed to Posterior Pharyngeal wall.*

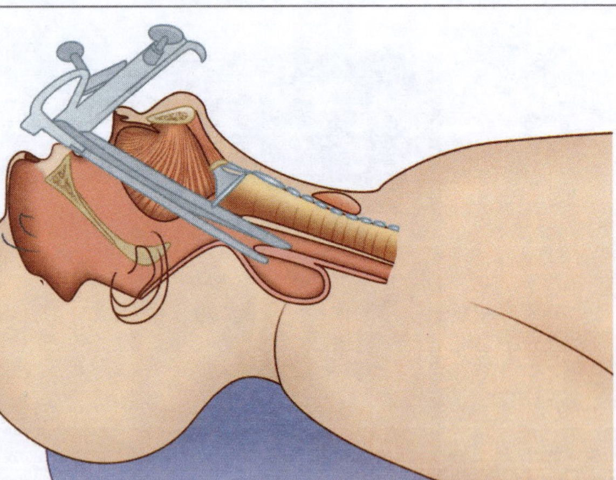

Dohlman's procedure

Traction Diverticulum

- MC in middle of esophagus due to Tuberculous nodes
- True diverticulum
- MC on right side
- MC cause in West—Histoplasmosis
- Treatment is Diverticulopexy
- Nowadays even in middle of esophagus—MC type of diverticulum is pulsion diverticulum.

GASTROESOPHAGEAL REFLUX DISEASE (GERD)

Clinical Features

- MC Symptom—Heart Burn
- MC complication—Reflux esophagitis—MC presentation is Retrosternal Discomfort.
- Nocturnal asthma/Paroxysmal Nocturnal Cough—Laryngopharyngeal Reflux (LPR)

Investigations

- Gold Standard—24 Hours Ambulatory pH monitoring**
- Sensor kept 5 cm above OG junction
- Reflux of Acid at pH <4 is counted every time.
- **Prerequisites to do this test:**
  - Stop PPI for 7 days before test
  - Patient comes in empty stomach and he/she is sent back to do routine activities after keeping the catheter inside.
  - Every time pH <4 strikes, the sensor will get a count.
- With all the values, we calculate a score known as **DeMeester Score; a score of >14.7** is** diagnostic of GERD.

Complications of GERD

- **MC reflux esophagitis**—IOC to find by Endoscopy
- **Laryngopharyngeal reflux causing**—Nocturnal Asthma.
- **Peptic stricture**—MC in lower end of esophagus, thick stricture involving all layers and hence, needs surgical excision and keep Jejunal Conduit interposition.
- **Schatzki ring**—MC in Squamocolumnar Junction. Thin submucosal ring- and hence, can be easily treated by Dilatation+ Fundoplication.
- **Barrett's Esophagus:** Metaplasia of Squamous epithelium to Columnar epithelium. The type of Columnar epithelium is Intestinal Columnar Epithelium with Biopsy showing GOBLET CELLS**.

To confirm dysplasia, we must take Biopsy in all four quadrants at every 1 cm of Barrett's esophagus—Known as SEATLE BIOPSY PROTOCOL.

- **Adenocarcinoma:** 40 times risk in Barrett's Esophagus. Incidence = 0.5 to 1%/year. Hence, keep Barrett's cases under surveillance.

Management

Initial

- Conservative management with lifestyle modification
- 6–8 weeks of PPI given—Responders are given PPI Continuously.

Surgical Treatment

Named surgeries**

- **Nissen Fundoplication**—360° posterior wrap-Can cause GAS BLOAT Syndrome**
- **Toupet**—270° posterior wrap
- **Dor**—180° Anterior wrap
- **Belsey Mark IV repair**—Thoracoscopic approach.

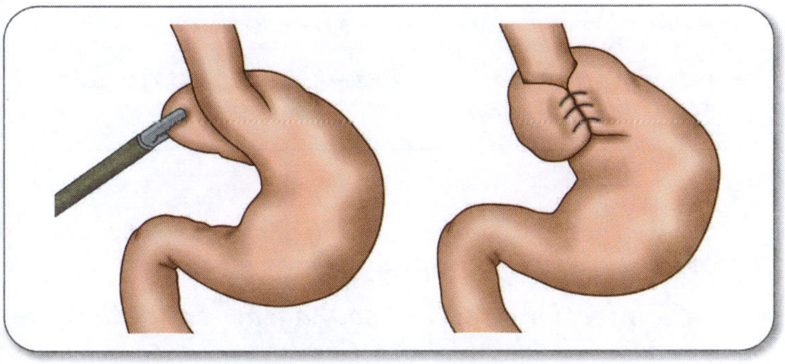

Nissen 360° fundoplication

- **MC complication after Fundoplication—Paralytic ileus > Pneumothorax****

Newer devices used for GERD

- Radio frequency ablation device—**STRETTA procedure****
- **LINX** is a new device made of magnets kept at OG junction to prevent reflux delivered laparoscopically

HIATAL HERNIAS

Four Types

- **Type 1:** Sliding
- **Type 2:** Paraesophageal/Rolling
- **Type 3:** Mixed
- **Type 4:** Massive (Along with Stomach—Small bowel, colon, etc. will go up)

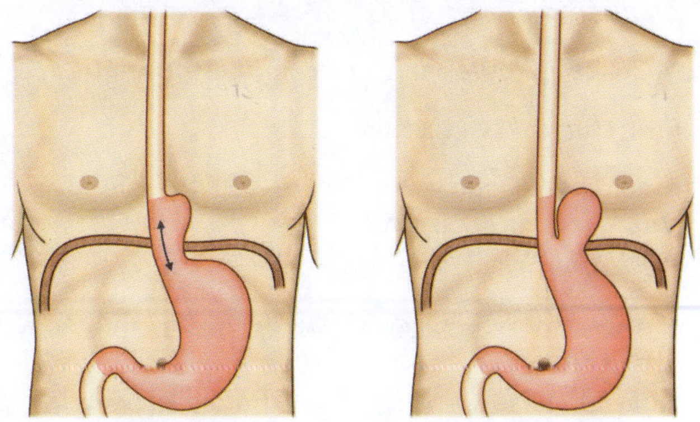

Sliding hiatus hernia — Paraesophageal hiatus hernia

Complications

Sliding hernia	Paraesophageal hernia
• Esophagitis due to reflux [MC]* • Barrett's esophagus • Aspiration and pneumonia	• Hemorrhage MC** complication • Incarceration, strangulation, perforation • Respiratory complications—Dyspnea from mechanical complications
• Conservative medical • Nissen fundoplication if medical treatment fails	• Due to dangerous complications, surgery is must (anterior gastropexy) • Biological mesh is used to close the defect.

ESOPHAGEAL INJURIES

Causes of Esophageal Perforation

- Iatrogenic—MC cause
- Barotrauma (Boerhaave syndrome)
- Corrosive—Alkali ingestion
- Trauma

Most common site by endoscopy in olden days was cervical esophagus, now the common site is thoracic esophagus—Latest update**

Highest mortality of all GIT perforations is with esophageal perforation by BAROTRAUMA.**

Barotrauma (Boerhaave syndrome)	Mallory Weiss tear
• Vomiting after a binge alcohol or spontaneously against a closed GLOTTIS**	Vomiting against a closed LES results in Mallory Weiss tear
• MC site is lower left posterior esophagus	MC site in lesser curve near OG junction at Cardia
• Full thickness rupture	Partial tear
• Mackler's Triad: Vomiting, Chest pain and Left side pleural effusion • Mediastinitis	Characterized by Hematemesis—Self-limiting in 90%
• Management—Urgent surgery by thoracotomy and repair • Golden period = within 24 hours primary repair done	Endoscopic Coagulation is advised
Alkali poisoning	**Acid poisoning**
Consumed in large amounts	Only few sips they swallow due to severe pain in mouth
Liquefactive necrosis	Coagulative necrosis
Destroys all the layers and can cause esophageal perforation	Forms eschar and limited to superficial layers and no perforation
Esophagus is more damaged than stomach	Stomach is more damaged than esophagus
Long-term damage is seen. Develops corrosive stricture for 3–6 months	Long-term damage is rare—Only Gastric antral stricture can develop

Investigations for Esophageal Perforation

- 1st done investigation—X-ray Chest—Shows Mediastinal Air known as **Naclerio's V sign***
- **Early and suspected Esophageal perforation IOC-CT thorax with oral GI contrasts.**

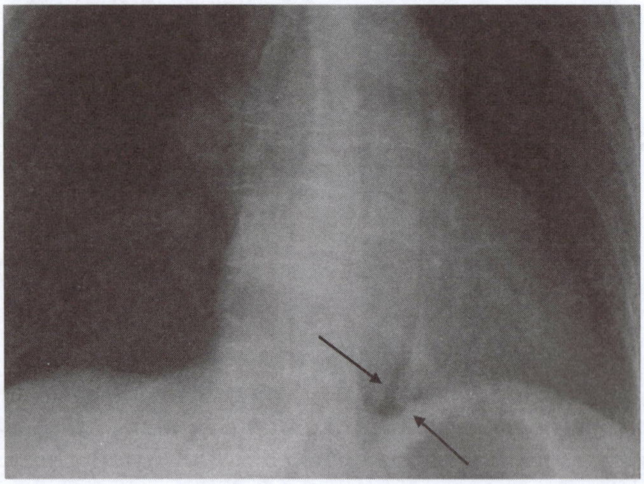

Naclerio's V sign

Infective causes of Dysphagia

- MC infection seen—Esophageal candidiasis**—Characterized by White Curdy patches
- Herpes simplex virus (HSV)—Punched out ulcers
- CMV esophagitis—Serpentine ulcer/Geographical ulcer

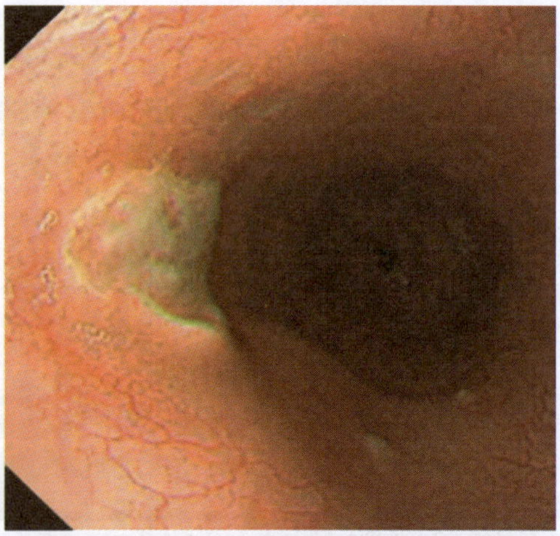

Punched out ulcer in HSV

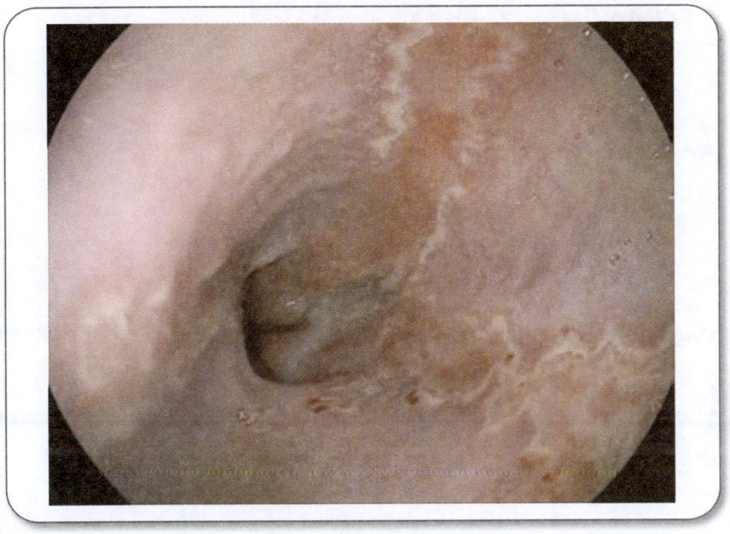

Serpentine ulcer in CMV

Eosinophilic Esophagitis

- Barium swallow shows—FELINE Esophagus**
- Endoscopy shows—Trachea like or Ringed Esophagus
- Treated by steroids

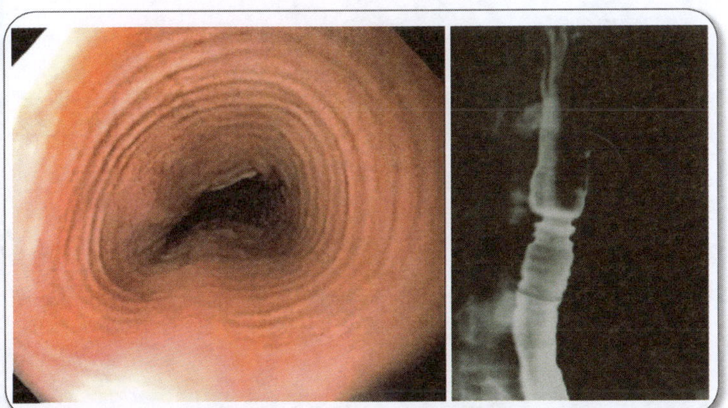

Eosinophilic esophagitis showing trachea like esophagus/feline appearance

TUMORS IN ESOPHAGUS

Malignant Tumor

- MC site—Middle third in World level and in India
- MC type is SCC in world/India
- MC type in Western countries—Adenocarcinoma

Investigations

- IOC to diagnose—Endoscopic Biopsy
- IOC for T, N staging—EUS
- IOC for M staging—PET CT
- Overall staging of cancer esophagus—CECT thorax

Management

- Types of esophagectomy:
  - Transthoracic
  - Transhiatal

Ivor Lewis two stage procedure	McKeown three stage procedure
• Subtotal esophagectomy • Two stage Lymphadenectomy (abdominal and thoracic Nodes) • Two Incisions—Abdominal and thoracic (Two regional nodes removed) • Intrathoracic anastomosis** • Leak percentage is less • Mortality if leaks is high	• Total esophagectomy • Three stage LN dissection (all three) • Three incisions—Abdominal, Thoracic and Cervical (Three regional nodes removed) • Neck Anastomosis • Leak percentage is more • Mortality is less as the contamination into the mediastinum never happens and secretions can be drained out.

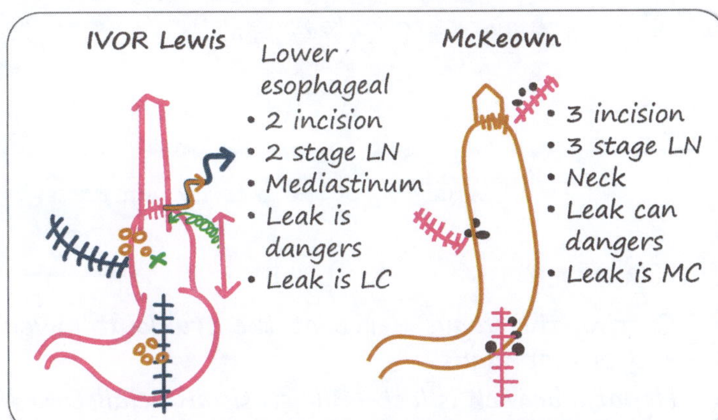

Ivor Lewis and McKeown procedures

Transhiatal Esophagectomy (THE): Orringer Operation

- Two incisions—Neck and abdomen
- Neck anastomosis
- Mortality is less as thorax is not opened
- Nodal clearance is less.
- Post Op radiotherapy is given after THE.

Conduits for Surgery

- Best conduit for esophageal replacement-Stomach as it is highly vascular and has less chances of necrosis.
- Best conduit in cases of corrosive injury to stomach and esophagus and for LONG SEGMENT replacement—Colon
- Best conduit for short segment replacement of esophagus—Jejunum, especially in peptic stricture cases.
- Gastric conduit is based on right gastroepiploic artery and right gastric artery.

STOMACH

Vagus Nerve Branches

Anterior Gastric Nerve (Left)

- Hepatic branch
- Gastric branches
- Crow's foot (Nerve of Latarjet)*

Posterior Gastric Nerve (Right)**

- Criminal nerve of Grassi
- Crow's foot
- Coeliac branch

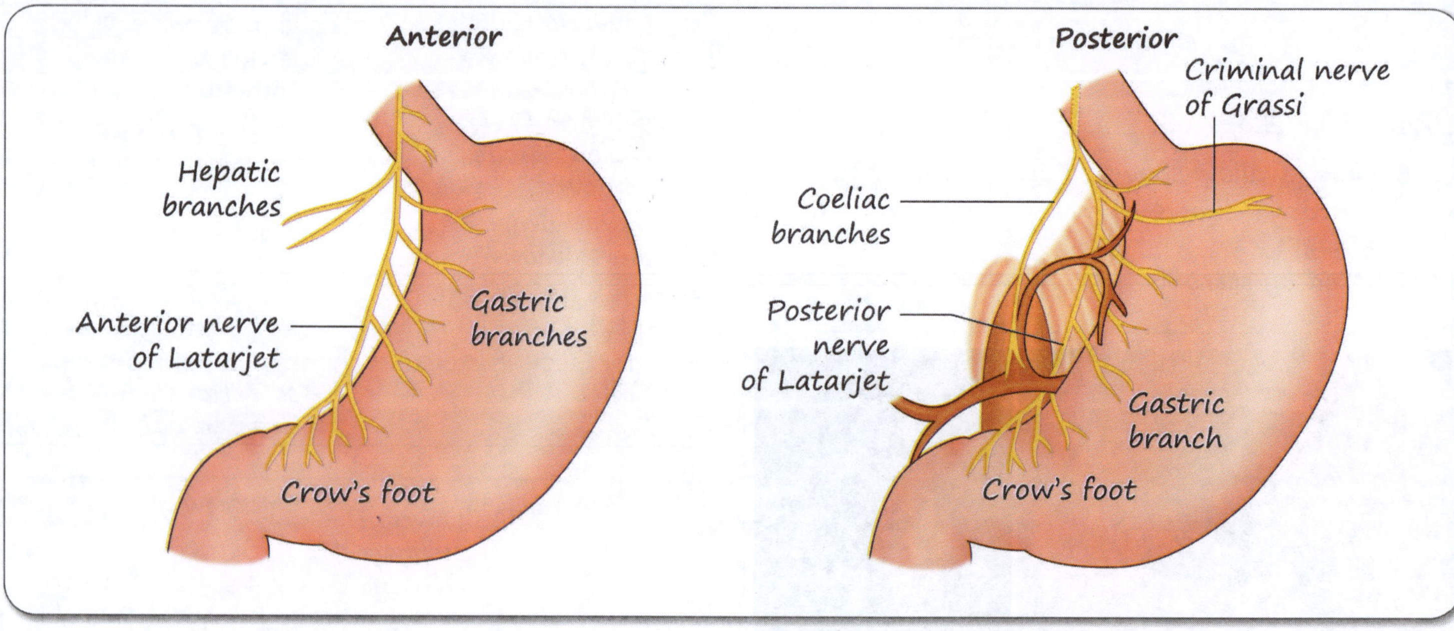

Anatomy of the anterior and posterior vagus nerves in relation to the stomach

Truncal Vagotomy

- Cutting the vagus nerve at the trunk at lower end of esophagus.
- Hepatic branch is lost—Bile stasis and Gallstones.
- Since pyloric Branches—Crow's Foot function is lost and hence, there will be pylorospasm (Function of Nerve of Latarjet is to do Pylorus relaxation)
- Coeliac branch is lost—Postvagotomy diarrhea
- Gastric branches lost—Loss of gastric tone

Complications of Truncal Vagotomy

- Bile stasis + Gallstones
- Pylorospasm
- Post-vagotomy diarrhea

Since there is pylorospasm, we must do drainage procedures:

- Posterior Gastrojejunostomy
- Heineke-Mikulicz Pyloroplasty

These drainage procedures have their own list of complications.

High Selective Vagotomy (Parietal Cell Vagotomy)

- Only the gastric branches are selectively cut.
- No need of drainage procedure in this operation.
- But the problem is we may miss a few branches during surgery and hence, risk of recurrence is more (5%–10%)

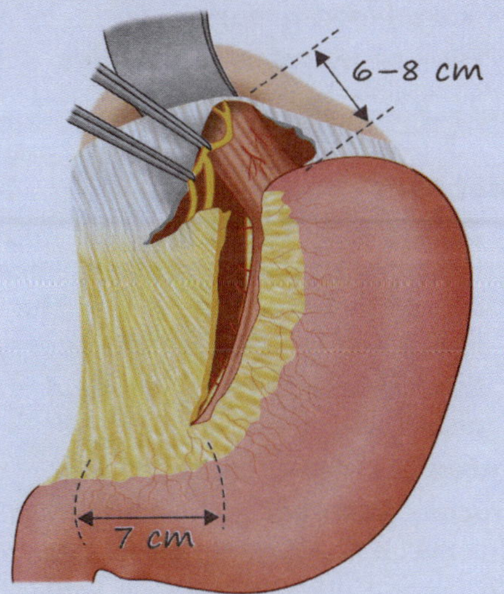

HSV—The gastric branches are cut 7 cm proximal to pyloric orifice

Complications of TV with GJ

- Complications of losing the Vagus nerve—discussed in previous page
- **Problems due to GJ:**
  - Malabsorption syndromes
  - Afferent and efferent Loop syndromes
  - Dumping syndrome

Malabsorption

- Iron Deficiency Anemia (MC deficiency in Gastric surgeries)
- Calcium Deficiency—Osteoporosis
- Vitamin B12 deficiency

Dumping Syndrome/Postcibal Syndrome

Early dumping syndrome	Late dumping syndrome
• Happens in half an hour after meal • Massive fluid shift toward hypertonic food particles	• Happens in 2–3 hours after meal • This happens due to reactive hypoglycemia**
C/F—Dehydration, Thirsty and Giddiness	C/F—Palpitation, Tremors and sweating
Diagnosis by PCV—there will be hemoconcentration	Diagnosis by PPBS value—Hypoglycemia

Dietary advice to prevent Dumping Syndrome

- Low carbohydrate diet
- High fat diet and protein diet
- Frequent small meals.
- Never drink too much water during eating.

Treatment of Dumping Syndrome

- Conservative treatment
- DOC—Octreotide**
- Revisional surgeries—Reverse Roux limb interposition.

Helicobacter Pylori

Two toxins produced: Cag A toxin and Vac A toxin**

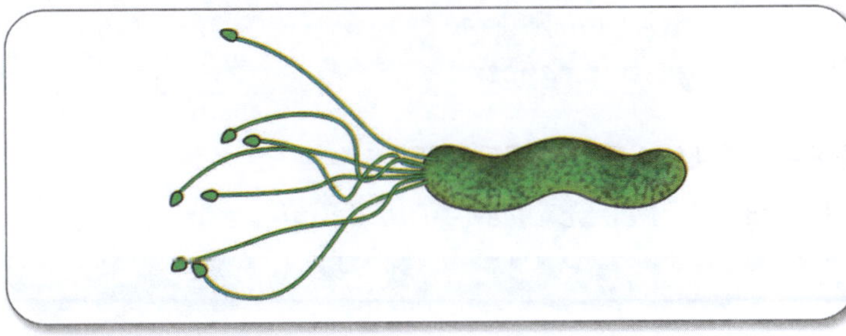

Investigations

- IOC (If endoscopy done)—Invasive test—Rapid Urease Test**
- IOC—noninvasive test—ELISA for Serology
- IOC to look for eradication—C13/C14 Urea Breath Test
- New investigation for Eradication—Stool for *H. Pylori* Antigen
- GOLD STANDARD to diagnose *H. pylori*—Staining and Culture
- Stains used for *H. pylori*—**Silver Starry Stain, Giemsa Stain, Warthin Starry stain****

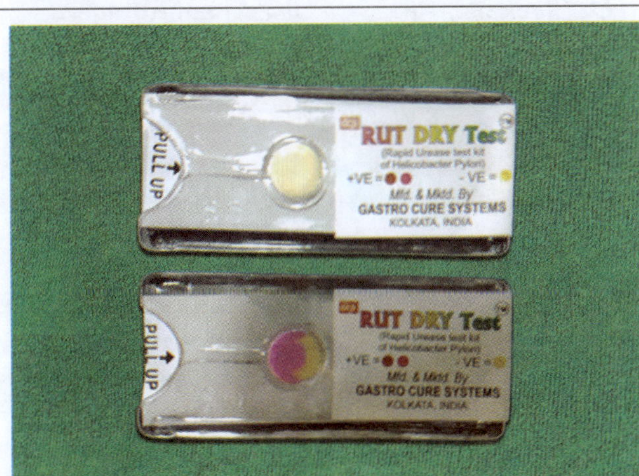

RUT positive

Treatment

- Triple drug regimen: 14 days
- LAC-Lansoprazole+Amoxycillin+Clarithromycin (US FDA Approved regimen)

Diseases Caused by *H. Pylori*

- Peptic ulcer diseases—Duodenal Ulcer (90%) >Gastric Ulcer (80%)
- Type B gastritis
- Nonulcer dyspepsia
- MALTomas (100% association)
- Distal Gastric cancer
- Menetrier's disease
- Intestinal Gastric cancer (Diffuse gastric cancer may or may not be associated)

Not associated with

Proximal gastric cancer

PEPTIC ULCER DISEASE

MC type of Peptic ulcer—Duodenal ulcer

Duodenal ulcer	Gastric ulcer
MC site is 1st part of Duodenum • Anterior Located—Perforate • Posterior located—Bleed • Bleeding is MC from Gastroduodenal Artery	**MC in lesser curve near incisura angularis**
Etiopathology Increased acid production	**Etiopathology** Due to loss of mucosal barrier
Management • Antiulcer drugs like H2 Blockers, PPI will be beneficial for duodenal ulcers. • Give them 6–8 weeks of PPI	**Management** Heals very well with Ulcer healing agents or coating agents like Sucralfate* and reduce the risk factors
Surgical treatment: Indications: • Intractable ulcer (when not healing within 8 weeks) • Bleeding—MC indication of surgery** • Perforation • Gastric outlet obstruction	**Surgical Treatment: Indications:** • Intractable ulcer • Bleeding • Perforation • Obstruction

Complications of Duodenal Ulcer

- **Bleeding Duodenal ulcer:** Endoscopic Management—Adrenaline injection/Coagulation.
  - **Indications of Surgery in Bleeding Duodenal Ulcer**
    - Failed Endoscopy >2 times
    - Rare blood group
    - Hemodynamically unstable
    - >6 units of Blood transfused
    - >3 units transfused per day
  - **Treatment**
    - Duodenotomy and Three-point U suture ligation of GDA and its branch. After duodenotomy, we close the duodenum like a Heineke-Mikulicz Pyloroplasty.
    - In stable patients, truncal vagotomy is also done.
- **Perforated Duodenal Ulcer**
  - **Clinical Features:** Guarding, rigidity and obliteration of liver dullness*, Hippocratic facies—Sick looking face in septic shock.
  - **Investigations**
    - **X-ray Chest/Abdomen including diaphragm in ERECT view:** Air under diaphragm—1 mL air can be detected
    - 70% of the cases will have air under diaphragm (30% will have no air)
    - **Gold standard investigation:** CECT abdomen (100% sensitive)
    - **X-ray left lateral view:** 5–10 mL air detected

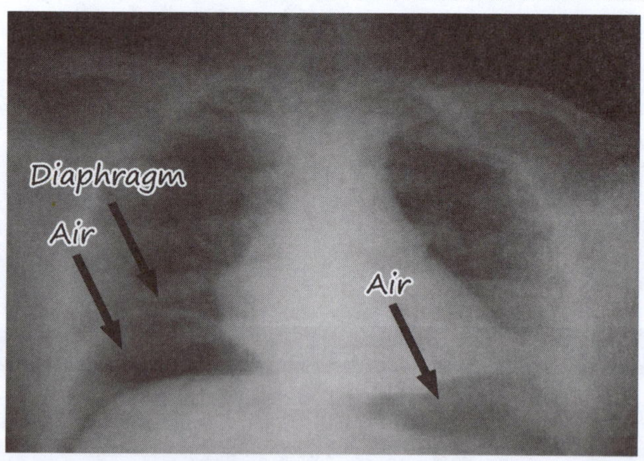

Air under diaphragm

  - **Treatment**
    - Emergency laparotomy, lavage, identify the perforation.
    - **Size <1 cm (Small):** Direct closure can be done with polyglycolic acid suture.
    - **Size >1 cm:** Omental patch is used. (Modified Graham's Patch is a Live patch).

- ***Gastric Outlet Obstruction***
  - *Correct the electrolyte imbalance- Hypokalemic, Hyponatremic, Hypochloremic, Hypocalcemic Metabolic alkalosis + Paradoxical renal aciduria.*
  - ***Fluid of Choice:*** *Normal saline + Potassium Supplements.*
  - ***Surgery:*** *TV + GJ*

Extra Points

Named Gastric Ulcers

- ***Cushing Ulcers: Stress ulcers in Head injury, MC in Proximal stomach near Cardia, more chances to perforate***
- ***Curling Ulcers: Stress ulcers in BURNS, MC in stomach now than duodenum***
- ***Cameron Ulcers: Vertical Riding Ulcers in Sliding/ Rolling Hiatus hernia, MC in fundus****

GASTRIC CARCINOMA

- *MC site in India/World—Incisura (Antrum)*
- *MC site in western countries- Proximal Stomach (Bailey gives Western statistics only)*
- *MC type is Adenocarcinoma.*

Premalignant Risk Factors

6–S	4–A
S – Smoking	A – Adenomatous polyps
S – Spirit	A – Atrophic gastritis
S – Spicy foods	A – Anemia (Pernicious anemia)
S – Salted foods	A – Blood group A
S – Smoked foods	
S – Stored foods	

GENETIC SYNDROMES

- *Li-Fraumeni syndrome*
- *Lynch syndrome*
- *FAP*
- *E-Cadherin mutations*

Clinical Features

STOMACH - features	5 MCQs
S – Silent T – Tumor O – GOO M – Melena C – Cachexia H – Hematemesis	**Krukenberg Tumor:** • Bilateral ovarian deposit • Superficial deposit • Seen in premenopausal women only • On C/S—inside ovary is normal • Transcoelomic spread** **Sister Mary Joseph Nodule:** • Transcoelomic spread • Umbilical deposit **Blumer's Shelf:** • Per rectal deposit in POD** • Transcoelomic spread **Virchow's Node—Left supraclavicular node (Troisier sign)** **Irish node—Left axillary node** **The two nodes are due to lymphatic spread**

Must know:

Minimum number of nodes removed in each GI tumor

- ***Stomach:*** *16 nodes*
- ***Breast:*** *10 nodes*
- ***Esophagus:*** *15 nodes*
- ***Small Bowel:*** *8 nodes*
- ***Colon:*** *12 nodes*

Early gastric cancer

- Tumor involving only mucosa and submucosa
- With or without lymph nodes
- Diagnosed by CON FOCAL Endoscopy and Narrow Band Imaging scopy
- Japanese classification is used
- **Treatment:** EMR (Endoscopic mucosal resection) and ESD (Endoscopic submucosal dissection)

Classification

Borrmann classification: Based on Gross examination

I. Polypoid
II. Ulcero proliferative (Fungating)
III. Ulcerative
IV. Diffuse Linitis Plastica

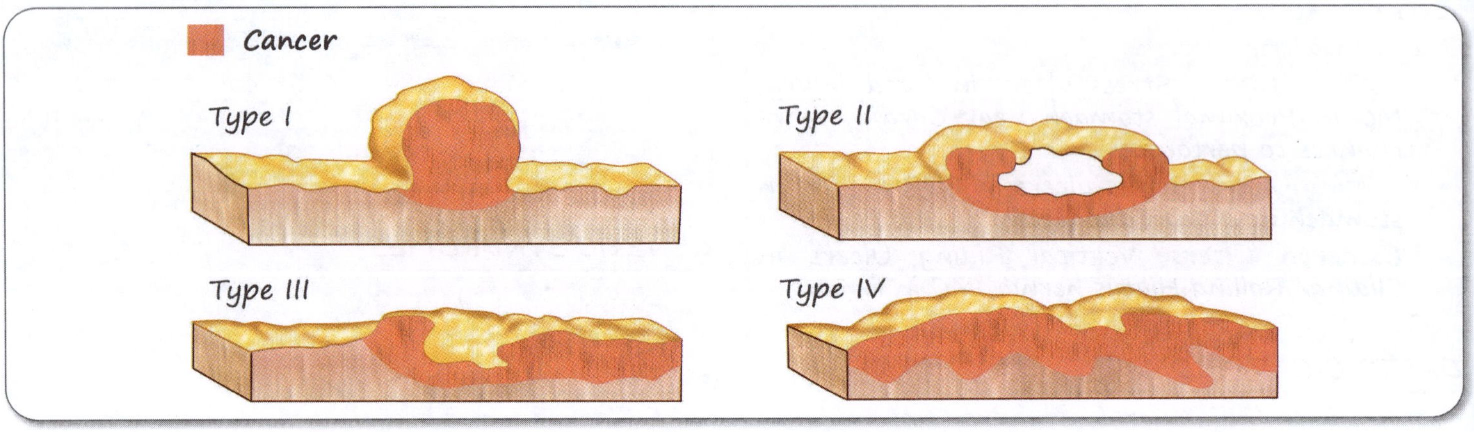

Borrmann classification of advanced gastric cancer

Lauren's Classification: Based on Microscopic appearances

Histology	Intestinal	Diffuse
Epidemiology	MC in sporadic	MC in familial
Sex incidence	Males more common	Females more common
Age incidence	Elderly	Young
Risk factors	Environmental *H. Pylori* positive	Genetic Family H/O Blood group A Pernicious anemia E-Cadherin Mutation—Prophylactic gastrectomy advised in these patients
Metastasis	**Hematogenous Mets Common****	**Lymphatic Mets MC** **Transcoelomic Spread is more common**** **Peritoneal mets are MC**
Prognosis	Good	Bad*
Pathology	Gland formation + **MC in distal Stomach**	**Poorly differentiated** **Signet Ring cells.** **MC in Proximal Stomach**
Genetics*	**APC gene mutation**** P53 and P16 inactivation Microsatellite instability	Decreased E-Cadherin** **P53 and P16 inactivation**

Surgical resection

- Proximal margin—5 cm clearance proximal (NCCN guidelines says—4 cm margin proximal).
- Distal up to duodenal 1st part.
- We either do subtotal gastrectomy or total gastrectomy.

Billroth-2 Reconstruction:

- Gastrojejunal anastomosis after subtotal gastrectomy.
- No more gastroduodenal anastomosis (Billroth 1 done now).
- Increased Bile reflux is seen in this reconstruction.
- Duodenal stump Blow out:
  - Happens on 4th/5th POD
  - Bile and pancreatic juice leaks
  - No need for urgent surgery
  - USG guided drainage is enough

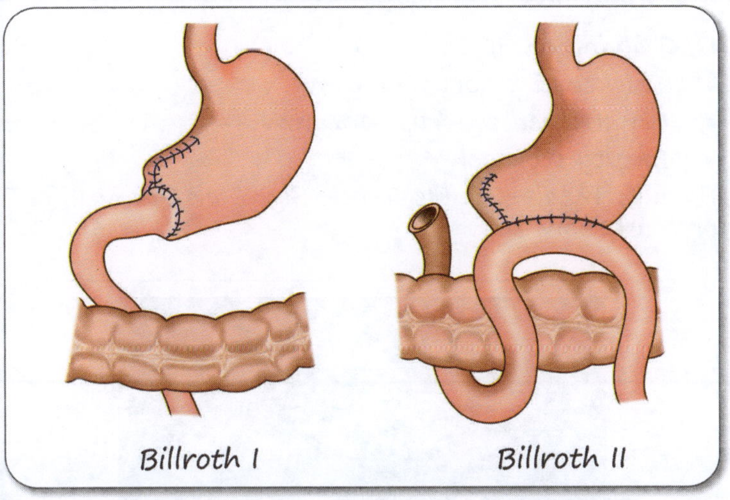

Roux-en-Y reconstruction:

- Done after total gastrectomy
- Two anastomoses: Esophago-jejunal and jejuno-jejunal anastomoses done
- Herniation behind Roux Limb is known as PETERSON Hernia**

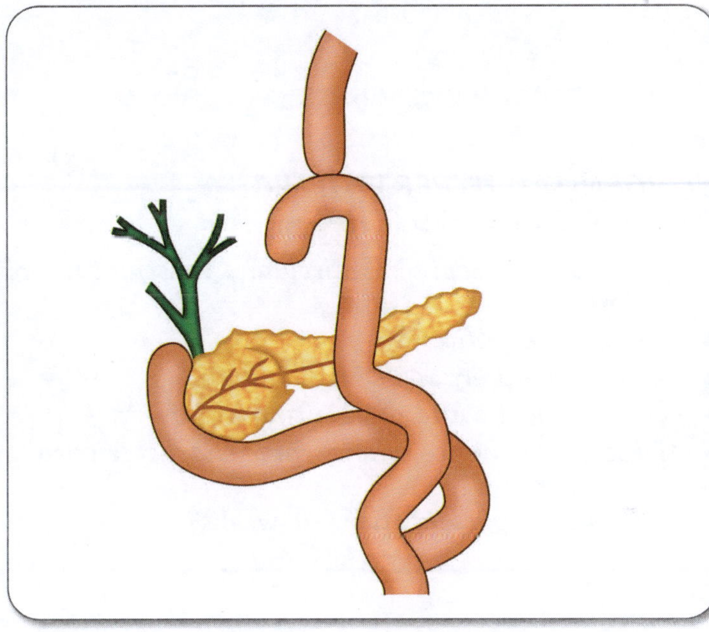

Roux-En-Y anastomosis

Non-Hodgkin Lymphoma	Gastrointestinal Tumors (GIST)
MC in stomach MC site—Antrum In Burkitt alone, it is MC in fundus	MC in Stomach MC in Proximal stomach in gastric curve side near fundus
Types: • MC is Diffuse large cell • MALT (2nd MC) • Mantle • Burkitt	**Types:** Wild type—CD117 negative, CD 34 negative Normal GIST—Both are positive
Origin—Lymphatic tissues on gut wall	Origin—Cells of Cajal or Pacemaker cells
Diagnosis: for both • **Endoscopy is difficult to diagnose due to normal mucosa** • **Hence, IOC—EUS guided Biopsy or CT guided Biopsy**	
	Tumor markers: • CD 117—Tyrosine kinase receptor mutation positive in 90% • CD 37—40% positive • PDGFRA—Platelet derived Growth factor receptor antibody • **Latest - DOG—Discovered on GIST**

Contd...

Management:

- **MALTOMA early—*H. pylori* eradication alone is enough**
- **Advanced cases—R – CHOP regimen**
    - R – Rituximab
    - C – Cyclophosphamide
    - H – Hydroxy adriamycin
    - O – Oncovin
    - P – Prednisolone

Treatment:

- Surgical resection with clear margin.
- No lymph node dissection needed.

After surgery:

For high-risk tumors—will give Imatinib mesylate or Sunitinib

CONGENITAL HYPERTROPHIC PYLORIC STENOSIS (CHPS)

- Gross hypertrophy of **Circular** ****musculature** of pylorus.
- Acquired Condition.
- Incidence—1 in 3000 live births
- M/c surgical cause of vomiting in infants
- First born male infants are characteristically affected more**.
- **M/c age of presentation—4 weeks**.**

Clinical Feature

- **Nonbilious vomiting** increasingly projectile may also be nonprojectile*
- Inspection—shows VGP (Must be done during feeding time**)
- Palpation—Right hypochondrial olive like mass+ (Done during nonfeeding time)
- **Palpation of an olive-like structure in right upper quadrant is pathognomonic.****
- **Hypochloremia, hypokalemia and metabolic alkalosis happen due to severe vomiting.**

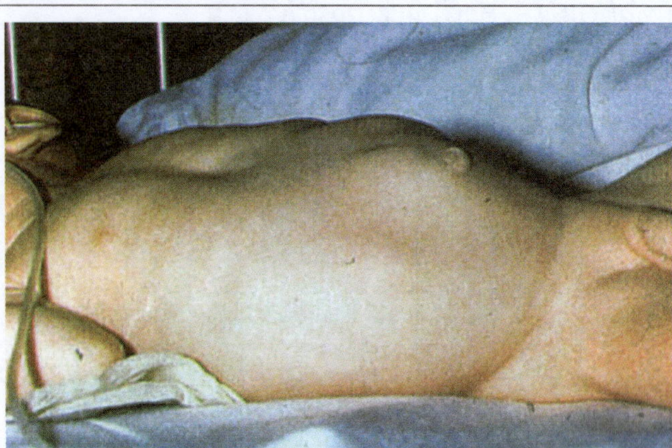

CHPS with nonbilious aspirate and note the VGP**

Investigations

USG abdomen: IOC

- Thickened pylorus >4 mm
- Lengthened pylorus >16 mm
- Empty stomach

Barium meal—Double Track Sign** or String Sign** or Mushroom sign

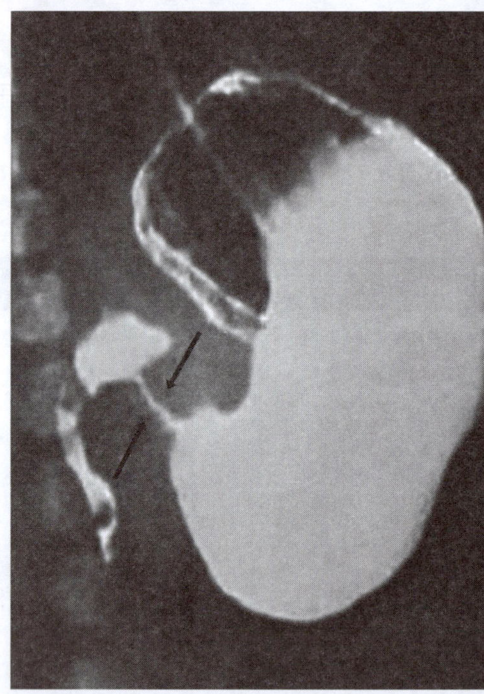

String/Mushroom sign in CHPS

Extra mile

- Lump is not always palpable. But if it is palpable, no other investigation is needed*
- Babies look healthy and not malnourished—as they consume enormous milk during disappearance of mass time.

Treatment

- Ramstedt's pyloromyotomy*—pyloric mass is split horizontally without penetrating the mucosa
- If the mucosa is inadvertently opened during surgery—close mucosa alone and keep baby nil per oral for 48 hours. (In normal cases, we start oral in 6 hours)
- Opened mucosa is repaired by 3'0 Vicryl sutures.

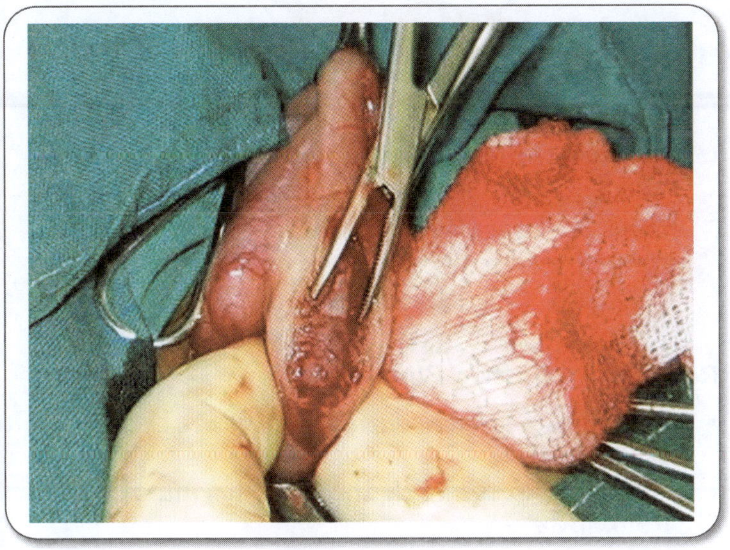

Ramstedt's pyloromyotomy

WILKIE'S DISEASE OR SUPERIOR MESENTERIC ARTERY (SMA) SYNDROME

- SMA compresses the third part of duodenum and this results in GOO*
- **Predisposing factors:**
  - MC in tall and thin young females on severe diet and weight loss.
  - Cast syndrome-due to spine immobilization body cast.
  - Chronic immobilization.
  - Tight dresses.
- Aortomesenteric angle (Angle between SMA and Aorta = Normal: 35°–65°).
- If the angle becomes <22°, it results in Wilkie's disease.
- **Management:**
  - Conservative therapy
  - Weight gain
  - Ifnotresponding,wedo—Duodenojejunostomy
  - **Strong Procedure**—Cutting Ligament of Trietz and releasing the 3rd part duodenum away from compression.

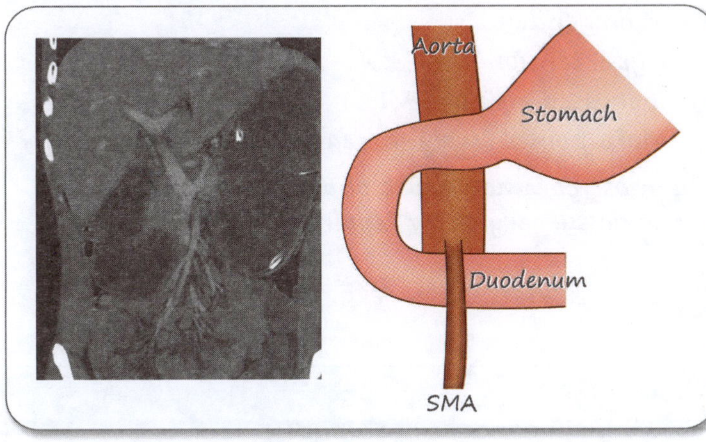

Wilkie's disease

Must know:

- **Double bubble appearance:** Duodenal atresia
- **Triple bubble appearance:** Jejunal atresia
- **Trichobezoar:** Hair in stomach
- **Phytobezoar:** Vegetable particles in stomach
- **Menetrier's disease:** Hypertrophied gastric mucosa looking like brain, TGF Alpha increased.
- **Watermelon stomach:** Gastric Antral vascular ectasia (GAVE)

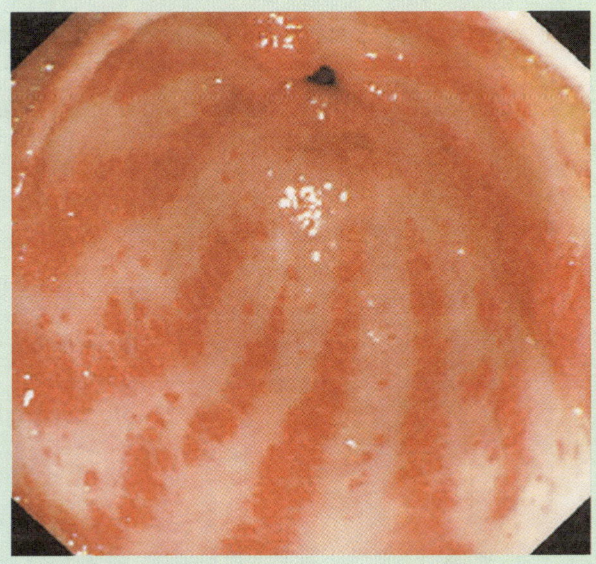

Watermelon stomach

BARIATRIC SURGERY

OS – MRS Scores: (Obesity Surgery—Mortality Risk Score)

Add one point for each of the following factors:

- Age >45
- BMI >50

- Male gender
- Hypertension
- Increased risk of DVT or Pulmonary embolism.
  More points imply increased risk of mortality.

The most common cause of death nowadays after bariatric surgery is DVT/pulmonary embolism.

Types of Bariatric Surgery

Restrictive
- Vertical banded gastroplasty
- Adjustable silicone gastric banding
- Sleeve gastrectomy

Mostly restrictive (and partly malabsorptive)
- Short-limb (50–100 cm) Roux-en-Y gastric bypass
- Long-limb (150 cm) Roux-en-Y gastric bypass

Mostly malabsorptive

Biliopancreatic diversion (BPD) with or without duodenal switch

Sleeve Gastrectomy

- Most commonly performed bariatric operation in world.
- The lesser curve based gastric tube is constructed over a size 32–36 Fr Bougie.

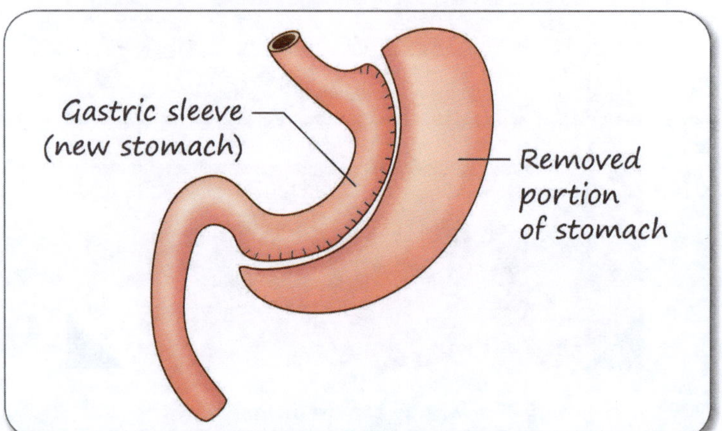

Sleeve gastrectomy

Gastric Banding

Band is wrapped at the upper part of fundus with adjustable subcutaneous port.

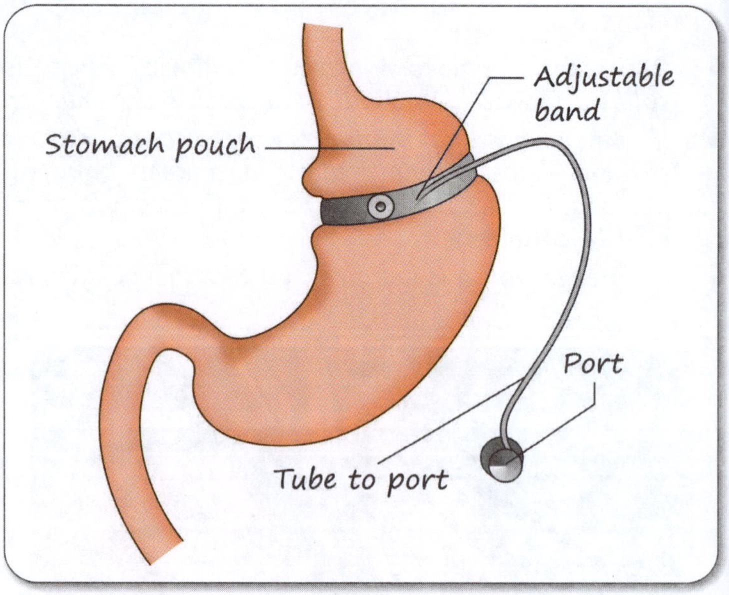

Gastric banding

Roux-En-Y Gastric Bypass

- Roux limb length varies between 100 cm and 150 cm.
- Peterson hernia is the internal hernia behind the Roux limb**.

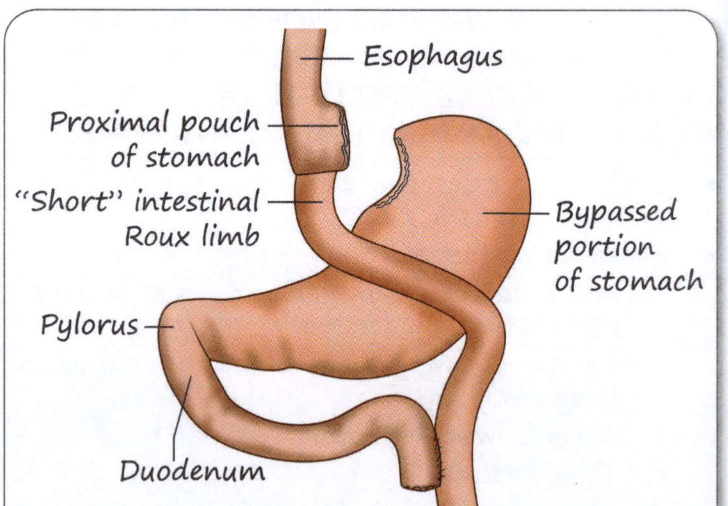

Roux-En-Y gastric bypass

Biliopancreatic Diversion (BPD) without Duodenal Switch

- Distal gastrectomy is performed and 200 cm of jejunum with ileum is anastomosed to stomach remains (150 mL).

- Duodenum and its contents (BILE AND PANCREATIC JUICE) are allowed to join in a common 50 cm of terminal ileum.
- Hence, partly restrictive (stomach removed) and highly malabsorptive (diversion of digestive enzymes).

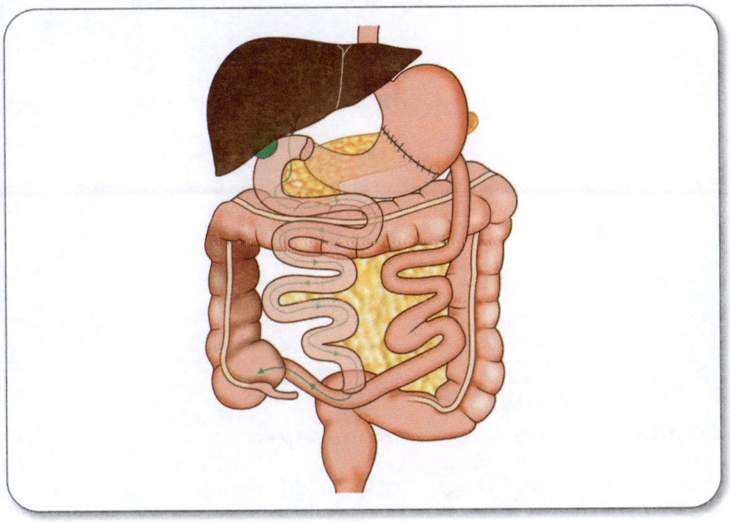

BPD without duodenal switch

BPD with Duodenal Switch

- Sleeve gastrectomy is performed.
- 1st part of duodenum is anastomosed to ileum.
- 2nd part of duodenum and remaining jejunum are allowed to anastomose at terminal 100 cm of ileum.

Advantages of Duodenal Switch

- No marginal ulcers (Duodenum produces feedback inhibition to acid)
- Less incidence of dumping syndrome (Pylorus and Duodenum are preserved, which helps in delaying food entry)
- Staged procedure can be done. We can stop with Sleeve at stage 1, if patient is unstable during surgery.

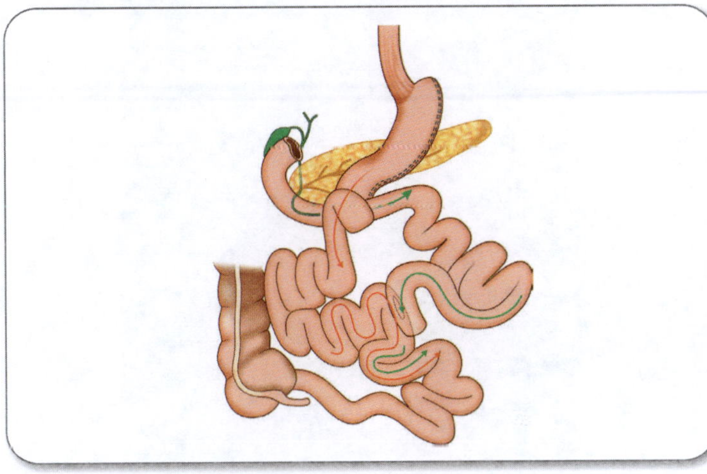

BPD with duodenal switch

MC cause of death in Bariatric surgery:
- **Immediate post op:** Anastomotic leak and peritonitis
- **Within 30 days:** DVT/Pulmonary embolism
- **Overall:** DVT/PE

INTESTINAL DISEASES

Basic Investigations in Intestine

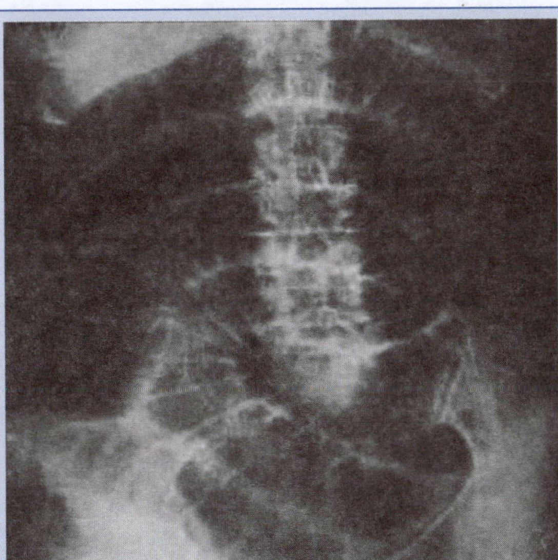

Plain X-ray abdomen erect showing dilated bowel loop

- The dilated bowel shown here is jejunum.
- Based on the appearance of valves of Kerckring/ Valvulae Conniventes.

Contd...

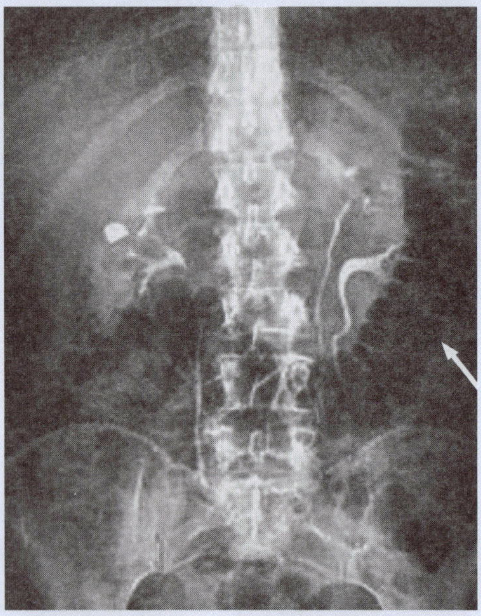	• This is colon. • Identified by the presence of Haustrations.
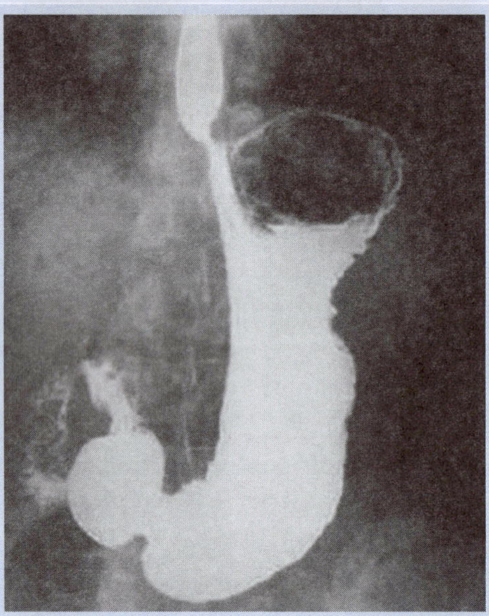 Barium meal	• X-ray taken after half an hour • Shows stomach and duodenum
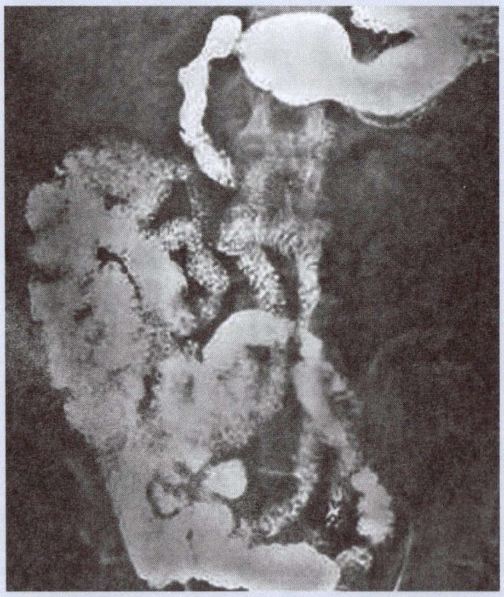 Barium meal follow through	• To study small bowel • X-ray taken at 2, 4, 6 and hours **Extra point:** • Jejunum has bird feather appearance. • Ileum is featureless.

Contd...

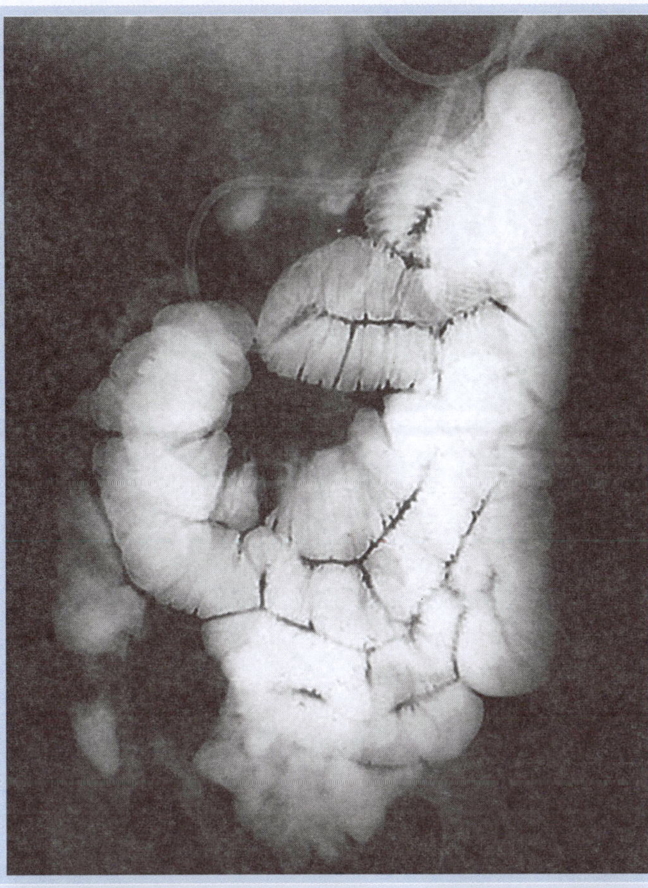

- *Nasojejunal tube put inside and Gastrografin contrast is pushed inside.*
- *ENTEROCLYSIS or Small bowel Enema*
- *Can be done by X-ray, CT or even MRI enteroclysis*

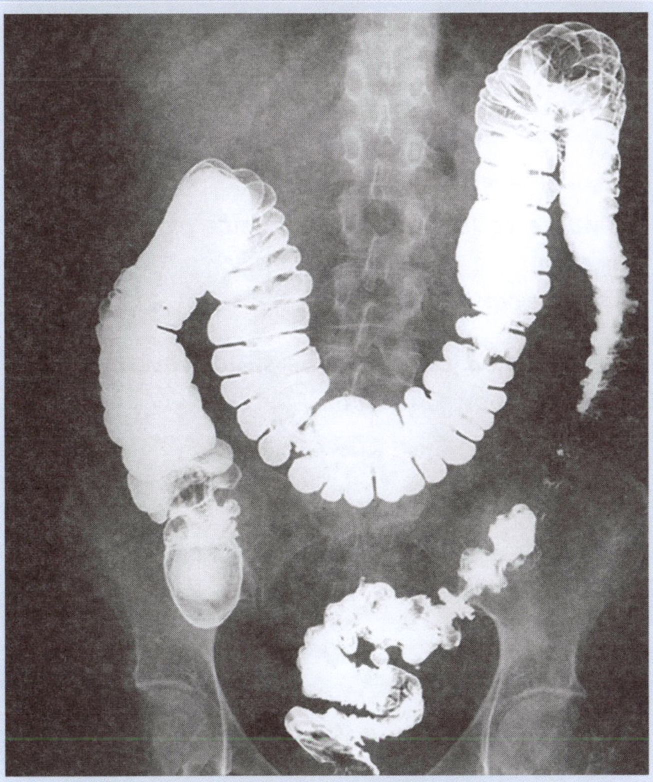

Barium enema

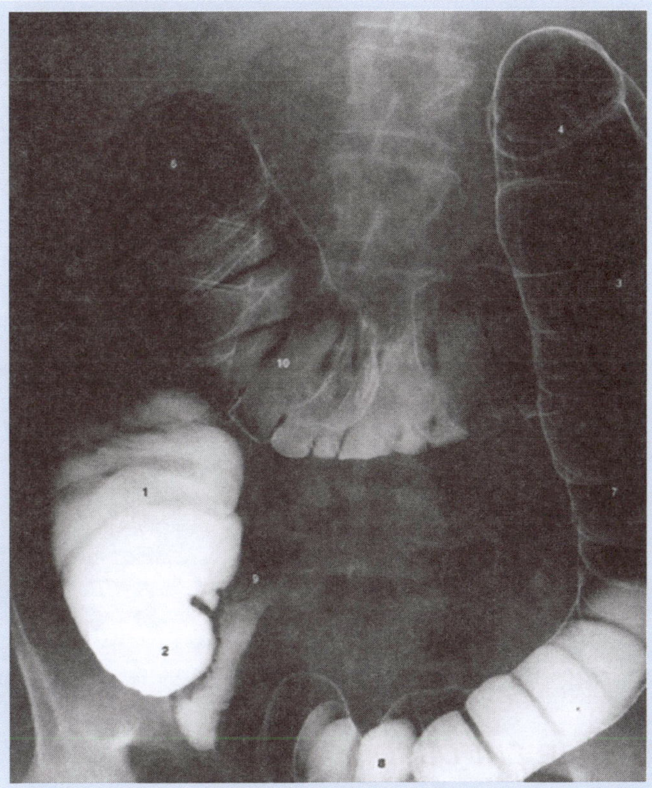

Double contrast Barium enema—Air or CO_2 is used

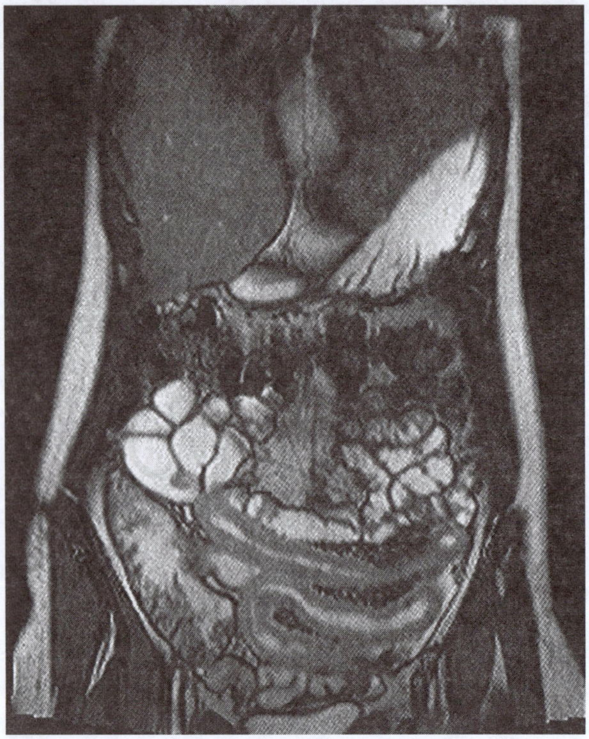

MR Enteroclysis with Ileal Crohn's disease showing thickening of small bowel

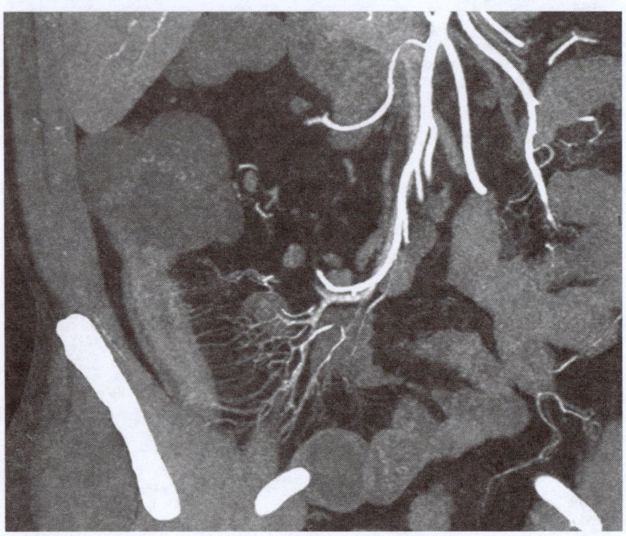

CECT abdomen showing Comb sign—prominent vascularity toward ileum in Crohn's disease

CAPSULE ENDOSCOPY

- **Size = 2.6 cm × 1.1 cm**
- Battery life = 8 hours
- Receiver collects all the images taken—2 images/second (Total 50000 images)
- Swallow the capsule, mild diet can be taken, no sedation needed.

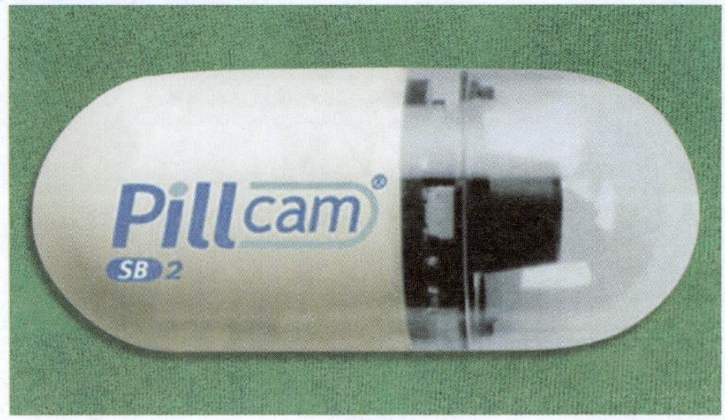

Capsule endoscopy

Indications of Capsule Endoscopy

- SB bleeding obscure GI Bleeding
- SB tumors, polyps
- SB angiodysplasia
- Crohn's disease (this is the IOC)**

Contraindications

- SB obstruction
- SB stricture

Complication

- Capsule retention (13%)—MC in CD patients.

Limitations of Capsule Endoscopy

- Unable to locate the exact site of lesion
- Incomplete study may happen
- Biopsy cannot be taken

Other method to study the small bowel:
Double Balloon Endoscopy 240–360 cm

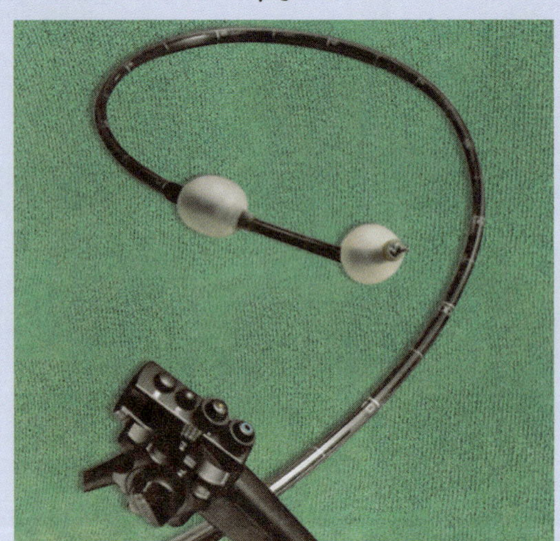

Double balloon endoscopy

MECKEL'S DIVERTICULUM

- Persistence of proximal part of vitellointestinal duct (VID) is Meckel's (Distal part of VID is **Raspberry tumor/Umbilical adenoma**).
- **Follows Rule of 2: for adults**
  - 2% individual
  - 2 inch in length
  - 2 feet proximal to IC junction
- **Ectopic mucosa seen in Meckel's:**
  - Gastric Mucosa (MC)
  - Pancreatic
  - Colonic
  - Brunner's Glands
- Ectopic gastric mucosa disappears as the age advances.
- **Children:**
  - Bleeding is the MC symptom.
  - Ectopic gastric mucosa is seen in adjacent ileum and hence, bleeds due to peptic ulcer.
  - IOC in children: Tc-99m Pertechnetate Scan*
  - While performing resection of Meckel's Diverticulum, we must do Resection and Anastomosis as adjacent ileum contains ectopic mucosa.
- **Adults:**
  - Obstruction is MC symptom.
  - Ectopic mucosa is not there and hence, bleeding is less common.
  - IOC: Enteroclysis
  - Treatment: Wedge resection can be done.

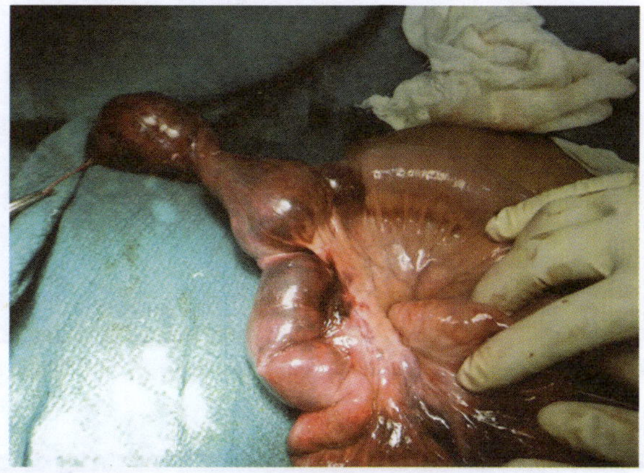

Gangrenous Meckel's diverticulum due to rotation (Volvulus)

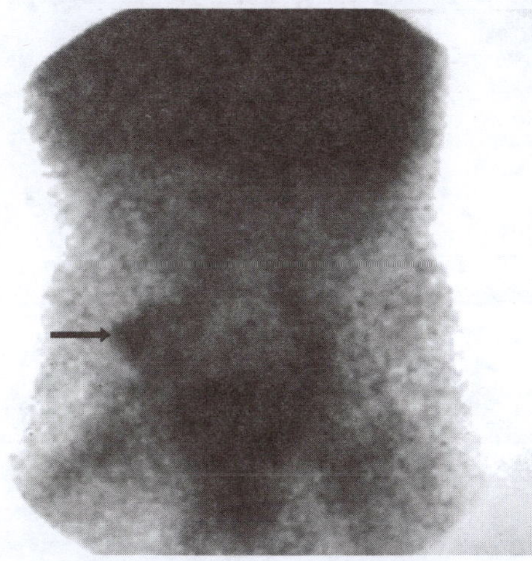

Tc-99m scan showing ectopic gastric mucosa in Meckel's diverticulum

Complications of Meckel's diverticulum: Incidence—6.4%

- Bleeding
- Obstruction
- Hernia—Littre hernia
- MC Tumor—Carcinoid tumor
- Diverticulitis

Direct line from Bailey:

Short, Wide mouthed and no nodularity—Leave it; Narrow mouth and nodularity advised resection

INTESTINAL TYPE OF TB

Intestinal type of TB most commonly involves terminal ileum and ileocecal junction*

Points	Hyperplastic—Primary TB	Ulcerative—Secondary TB
Etiology	• M. bovis primary ingestion from raw milk • When patient's immunity is good.	• Secondary to swallowing infected sputum • Patient having very low immunity*
MC site	Ileocecal valve	Longer parts of terminal ileum

Contd...

Presentation	As obstruction	As transverse ulcers** and on healing causes stricture. (Typhoid presents with longitudinal ulcers)
C/F	• Acute abdominal pain with intermittent diarrhea • Mass in right iliac fossa	Diarrhea and weight loss
Barium meal follow through	• Pulled up cecum • Ileocecal angle becomes obtuse • Stierlin sign • Umbrella sign • Fleischner sign • Goose neck deformity	Absence of filling of lower ileum

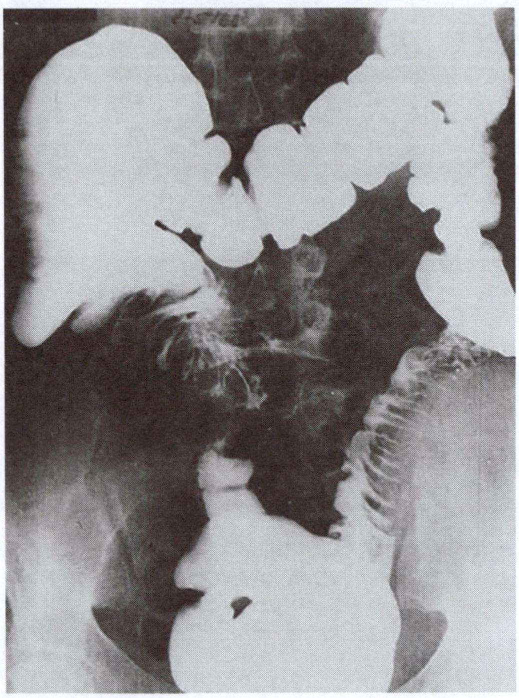

Pulled up cecum in ileocecal TB

Management:

- Both cases present with small bowel obstruction.
- IOC is Ileocolonoscopy and Biopsy from Ileum.
- We start Category I—ATT and under cover of ATT, we do limited resection of ileocecal TB.

SHORT BOWEL SYNDROME

- Length of small bowel is 600 cm. After resection and it becomes <200 cm, it results in short bowel syndrome.
- **Adult causes:** Acute SMA ischemia, Trauma, CD

Clinical Features

- **Watery diarrhea:** Unabsorbed bile salts into colon
- Malabsorption of fat-soluble vitamins
- Failure of Enterohepatic circulation: Bile salt is reduced
- **Steatorrhea:** Reduction in bile salt pool
- Fat-soluble vitamin deficiency (A, D, E, K)
- ***Oxalate kidney stones:*** Unabsorbed fatty acids bind with calcium
- **Cholesterol gallstones:** Decreased bile salt in bile

Other problems

- Megaloblastic anemia
- **Increased gastrin secretion**:** Increased Gastrin is seen as there is no feedback inhibition for acid from small intestine. This results in Peptic ulcer disease due to increased acid.

Medical management	Surgical management
• Fluid electrolyte correction • TPN initially • Enteral nutrition once ileus gets settled • High dose PPI/H_2 Blockers to reduce gastric acid secretion • Loperamide • Octreotide reduces intestinal secretions • Recent drug-TEDUGLUTIDE—increases bowel growth—GLP 2 analogue**	• Intestinal lengthening operation of Bianchi** • Serial transverse Enteroplasty (STEP procedure) • Segmental Intestine reversal • Interposition of colon • Final resort in cases of patients with liver failure, catheter-related sepsis and thrombosis of major veins is intestinal transplantation.

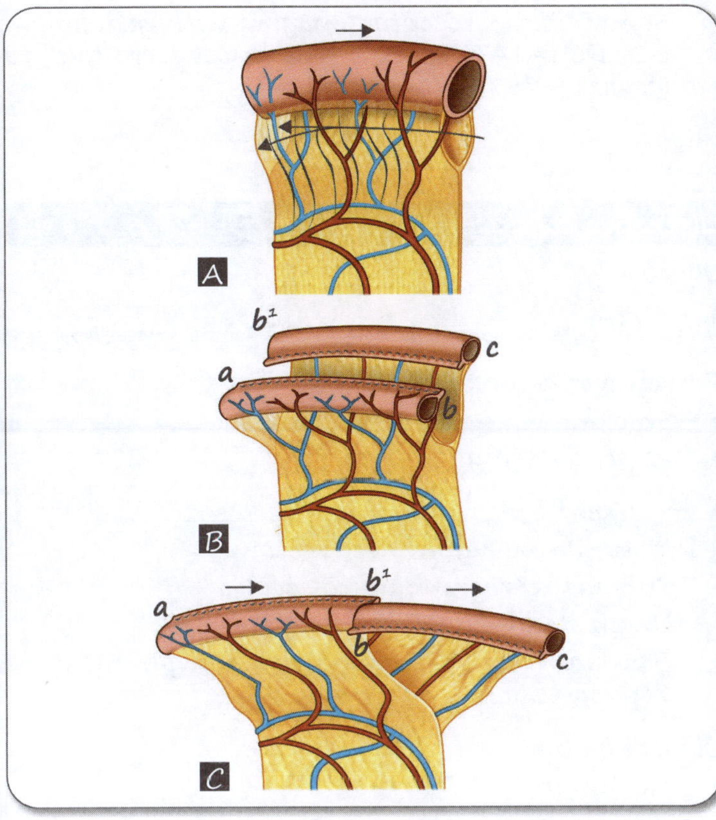

Bianchi procedure

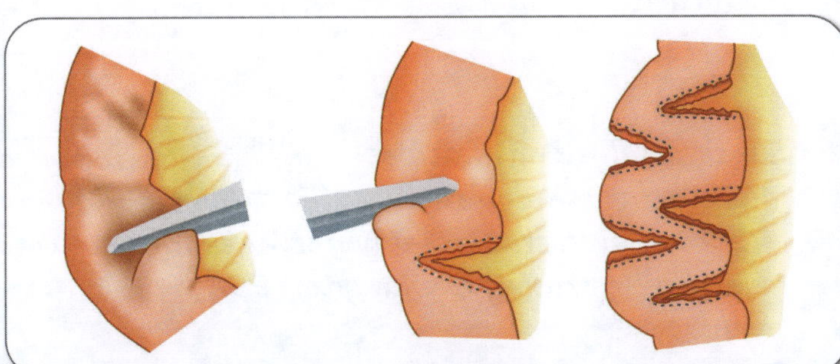

STEP procedure

ENTEROCUTANEOUS FISTULA

- **MC Cause:** Iatrogenic
- **Types:** High output (>500 mL/day); Low output (<200 mL/day)
- MC complication of high output fistula—Skin excoriation**, fluid electrolyte imbalance, sepsis.
- **Highest electrolyte imbalance:** Duodenal fistula

Principles in Management of Enterocutaneous Fistula: (SNAP)

- S – Sepsis Elimination
- N – Nutrition—a period of TPN
- A – Anatomical assessment
- P – Planned Surgery after 6 weeks

Factors Preventing Healing of Fistula: (Mnemonic—High FRIENDS)

- F – Foreign body in tract
- R – Radiation enteritis
- I – Inflammatory bowel disease
- E – Epithelialization of tract
- N – Neoplasm
- D – Distal obstruction
- S – Short tract (<2.5 cm tract)
- H – High output fistulas also

CARCINOID TUMORS

- Neuroendocrine tumors of GIT are known as carcinoid tumors.

Location	Site	Predominant hormone
Foregut	Bronchus and thymus	5-Hydroxy Tryptophan and ACTH (Low serotonin)*
Midgut	Stomach, proximal duodenum, ileum, jejunum, right colon	Serotonin, Histamine, Bradykinin
Hindgut	Left colon and rectum	**Somatostatin or Peptide YY****

- **MC site:** Bronchus > Appendix > Ileum (Terminal)
- **MC in GIT:** Appendix
- MC system affected is GIT system > Bronchus

Carcinoid Syndrome

- **Vasomotor symptoms (80%)—cutaneous flushing** is the MC symptom**.
- GIT—explosive diarrhea. Due to serotonin.
- Cardiovascular—Right heart problems are more common. **The three most common cardiac lesions are pulmonary stenosis (90%), tricuspid insufficiency (47%) and tricuspid stenosis (42%)** MC valve affected is Tricuspid Valve.**
- Asthmatic attacks—Bronchospasm
- Malabsorption and pellagra (dementia, diarrhea, dermatitis) due to excessive diversion of tryptophan.

Investigations

- 24 hour urinary 5-hydroxyindoleacetic acid (5-HIAA)** is highly specific.
- Neuroendocrine tumor marker—chromogranin A and synaptophysin.

- Localization of tumor—Somatostatin receptor scintigraphy with indium-111 labeled pentreotide was used previously.
- Somatostatin receptor imaging with gadolinium 68 DOTATATE CT is the most sensitive to localize—95% cases.

INFLAMMATORY BOWEL DISEASE

Crohn's disease	Ulcerative colitis
Incurable	**Curable**
Bimodal	Bimodal (one at young and another at old age)
Predisposing factor is smoking	**Preventive factors:** • Smoking • Appendectomy
Involvement • Mouth to anus • Unaffected—rectum** • Most commonly involved—terminal ileum**-known as Terminal ileitis or regional enteritis.	**Involvement** • Most commonly involves rectum. • Spreads retrograde up to cecum. • Unaffected—Anus** • **Backwash Ileitis—Terminal ileum involvement in 20% cases.**
Clinical features • MC symptom—Pain abdomen • Others—Bleeding and Diarrhea • Earliest feature—Aphthous ulcer** • Strictures+ • Fistulas+ • Intestinal obstruction+	**Clinical features** • MC symptom—Diarrhea • Bleeding is MC here • Rare feature—Toxic Megacolon • Perforation
Extraintestinal manifestations • MC—Erythema nodosum** • Ankylosing spondylitis • Peripheral arthritis • Kidney stones • Cholesterol gallstones	**Extraintestinal manifestations** • MC—Hepatic manifestation (Fatty liver) • MC skin manifestation—Pyoderma gangrenosum • Primary Sclerosing Cholangitis (PSC)** • Uveitis • Scleritis **All the extraintestinal manifestations disappear on treatment—except PSC > Ankylosing Spondylitis**
Pathological features • Serpentine Ulcer**/Bear claw ulcer • Aphthous ulcer • Transmural involvement • Skip lesions • Fistula • Noncaseating granuloma • Mesenteric fat wrap • Cobble stone appearance • Death—MC due to malignancy	**Pathological features** • Collar button ulcer • Partial thickness only involved • Continuous lesion • No fistula, Stricture, Granuloma or fat wrap • Pseudopolyps appearance of uninvolved areas (they are not premalignant) • Crypt abscess, cryptitis • Toxic megacolon—Full thickness involvement

Contd...

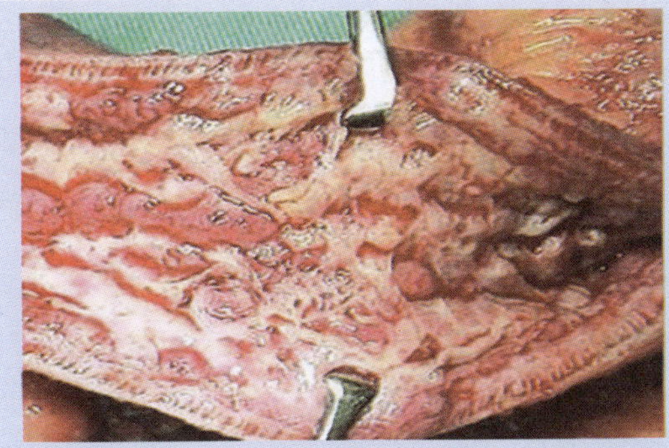 Serpentine ulcer 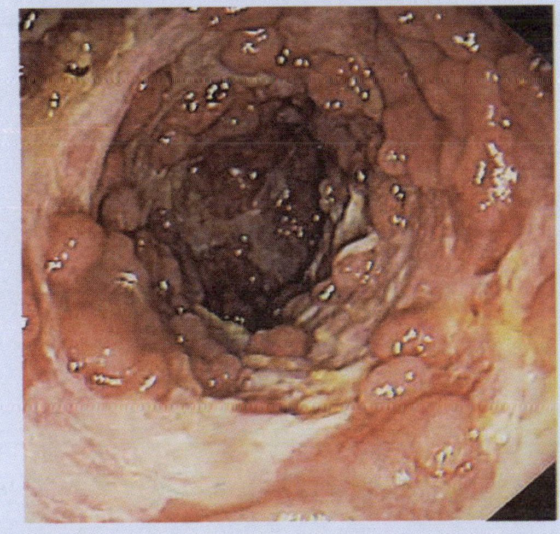 Cobble stone appearance	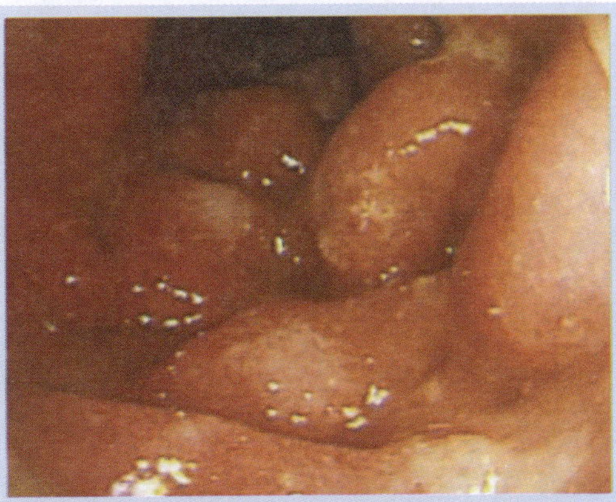 Pseudopolyps
Investigations: • **IOC/Gold standard**—Capsule endoscopy will show ≥ three ulcers in absence of NSAID **Biopsy:** Ileocolonoscopy (Terminal 50–80 cm can be entered) Stool for Lactoferrin and Calprotectin tests • **ASCA (Anti-Saccharomyces cerevisiae antibody)+ in 90%**	**Investigations:** • IOC—Colonoscopic Biopsy • **Antibody test: P-ANCA is positive (Antineutrophil Cytoplasmic antibodies)**
Barium Investigations: • String sign • Stierlin sign • Garden hose pipe appearance	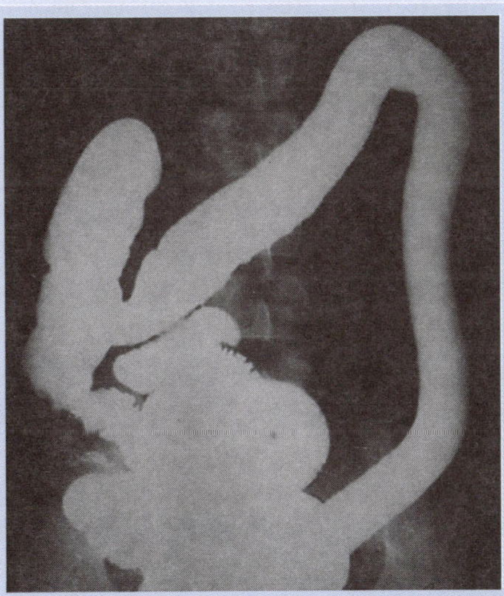 Barium enema showing loss of haustration and known as Pipe stem/lead pipe appearance

Contd...

CECT Abdomen: **Comb sign**—Increased vascularity to bowel shown as comb sign* 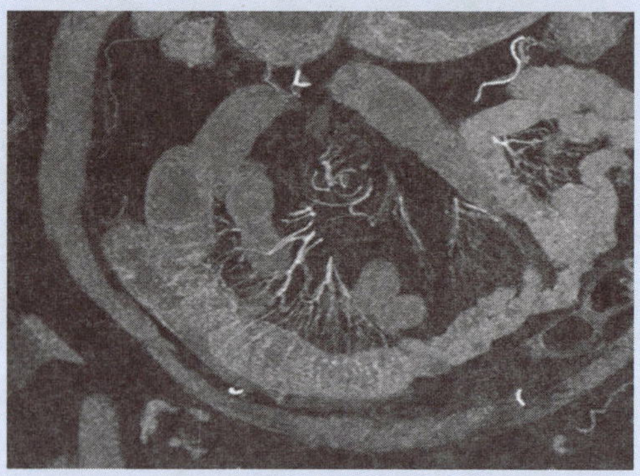 Comb sign	
Complications • Fistula • Perforation • Abscess • Stricture • Intestinal obstruction (MC due to stricture) • Cancer (MC in Terminal Ileum*) **MC indication for surgery is Stricture causing obstruction**	**Complications** • Intractability • Toxic megacolon • Perforation • Bleeding PR • Cancer **MC cause of death in Both CD and UC – Cancer**
Management of stricture • Single stricture—Resection • Multiple short strictures—Stricturoplasty by Heineke—Mikulicz type • Multiple long strictures (>10 cm)—Stricturoplasty by finney's type	**Gold standard surgery** Total proctocolectomy + Ileal Pouch Anal Anastomosis is advised after 8 years in pancolitis or 12 years in Left Colitis. If they are not willing, they are advised to be in screening surveillance.

ACUTE APPENDICITIS

- MC emergency done in worldwide—Acute appendicitis.
- MURPHY'S TRIAD—Migratory pain, vomiting, fever.

Common Signs in Appendicitis

- **McBurney's Point tenderness**: tenderness at the point (Medial 2/3rd and lateral 1/3rd of spino umbilical line—McBurney's point)
- **Blumberg sign:** Rebound tenderness
- **Rovsing's sign:** Palpation of left iliac fossa produces pain in right iliac fossa by shift of bowels.
- **Sherren's triangle hyperaesthesia:** (triangle formed by ASIS, umbilicus and pubic symphysis) due to irritation of lower abdominal nerves.
- **Copes psoas sign:** Retrocecal appendicitis* on extension of hip produces pain due to irritation over psoas major [muscle that flexes the hip]
- **Copes obturator sign:** Pelvic appendicitis*, flexion and medial rotation produce pain.

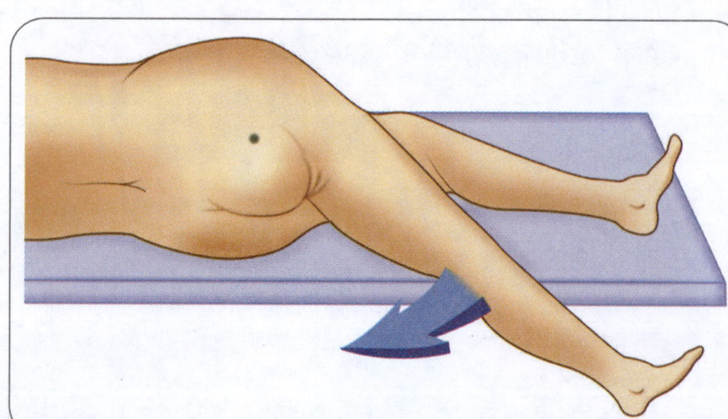

Copes psoas test for retrocecal appendicitis

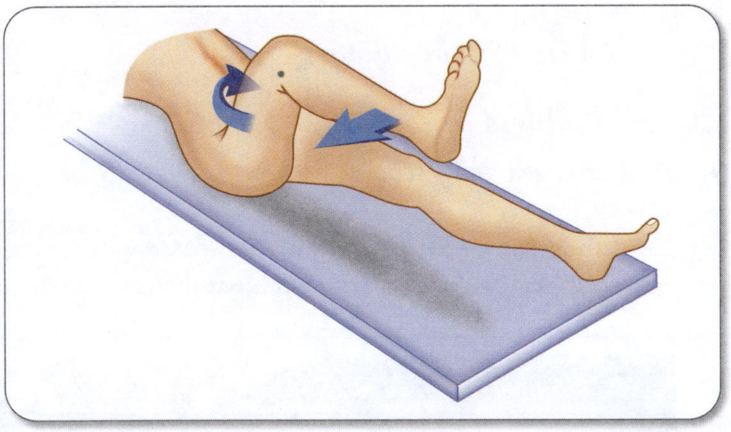

Copes obturator test for pelvic position appendicitis

ALVARADO SCORING in Acute Appendicitis (Mnemonic—MANTRELS)

- M – migratory pain
- A – anorexia
- N – nausea and vomiting
- T – tenderness* (2 points)
- R – rebound tenderness
- E – elevated temperature
- L – Leukocytosis* (2 points)
- S – shift to left, segmented neutrophils
- All are given 1 point except tenderness and leukocytosis that are given 2 points**
- SCORE OF ≥7 IS STRONGLY SUGGESTIVE OF APPENDICITIS

Investigations

1st done—USG abdomen: Findings in Acute appendicitis—80% sensitive

- Blind ending
- Nonperistaltic
- Noncompressible
- >7 mm Thickness

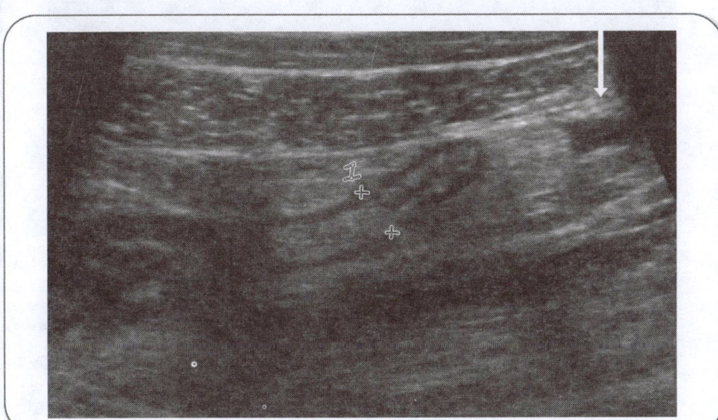

Acute appendicitis

IOC for Acute Appendicitis: CECT Abdomen

- Extremes of age
- Doubtful cases
- 2nd trimester of pregnancy (If MRI is not available as MRI is the IOC**)

Etiology for Acute Appendicitis

- MC – fecolith**
- Ascaris
- Tumors

MC organism isolated—**Bacteroides fragilis****

MC aerobe—*E. coli*

Complications of Acute Appendicitis

- Rupture/perforation
- Abscess
- Appendicular mass

Appendicular Rupture

- MC in extremes of age, fecolith, diabetic and immunocompromised patients.
- MC in antimesenteric border at the tip.
- MC in pelvic position of appendix**
- **Rupture in <24 hours:** Diffuse peritonitis
- **Rupture in >24 hours:** Due to omental covering of the perforated area—there is only localized peritonitis. Hence, delayed rupture is better.
- Early antibiotics do not prevent rupture.
- **C/E:** Guarding and rigidity+
- Emergency appendectomy done.

Appendicular Abscess

- Retroperitoneal or pelvic abscess happens.
- **C/E:** fever + Chills and rigors.
- **Treatment:** USG guided drainage of abscess.
- **Retrocecal abscess:** Retroperitoneal drainage.
- **Pelvic abscess:** Via PR/PV
- Index appendectomy during same admission advised.

Appendicular Mass

- The regimen followed is OCHSNER SHERREN REGIMEN**
- After a gap of 6 weeks, we must give interval appendectomy**

Ochsner Sherren Regimen

- Conservative treatment of mass
- The mass is formed by surrounding omentum, small intestine and dense inflammation; if we dissect at this time, EC fistula can happen.
- In case you open the abdomen and find a mass– don't dissect and follow this regimen.
- Nil oral until paralytic ileus recovers
- IV Fluid, antibiotics and Input/output monitoring, electrolyte correction.
- Charts for Pulse temperature and mass size.
- Once symptoms resolve, discharge and ask them to come after 6 weeks for surgery Interval appendectomy.

Surgical Treatment

Conventional Open Method

- Grid iron Incision at McBurney's point known as GRID IRON Incision—Injury to iliohypogastric nerve can happen and patient may develop DIRECT HERNIA.
- Females—LANZ horizontal cosmetic incision.
- Usually, we reach the appendix by muscle splitting.
- Muscle cutting incision—Rutherford-Morrison Incision*.

Laparoscopic Method

- Three ports are used
- 1st Done by KURT SEMM**

INTUSSUSCEPTION

- MC in age group 6 months—6 years
- MC cause due to Rhinovirus infection causing Hypertrophic Peyer's patches and that pulls the bowel and causes intussusception.
- **Anatomy:**
  - Apex: Lead point
  - Inner tube: **Intussusceptum**
  - Outer tube: **Intussuscipien**

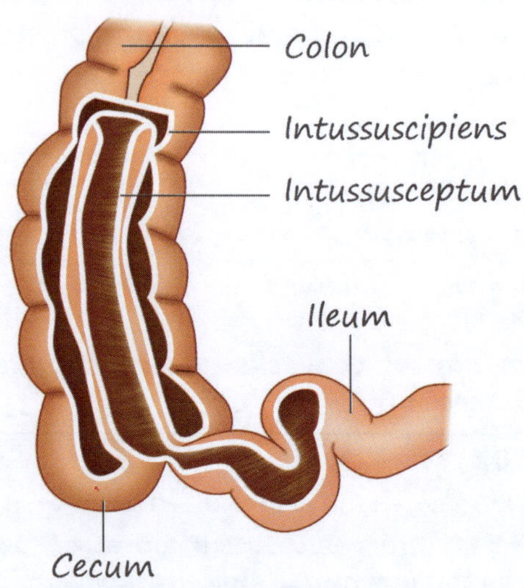

Anatomy of intussusception

- MC type is Ileo colic
- MC type in old age – Colo colic
- Apex: Lead points:
  - MC lead point: Hypertrophied Peyer's patches
  - Benign tumors
  - Meckel's
  - Cancer (MC in old age)

Clinical Features in 6-Month-Old Baby

- Red currant jelly stool
- Vomiting
- Le dance sign—Empty right iliac fossa
- Sausage shaped mass toward umbilicus

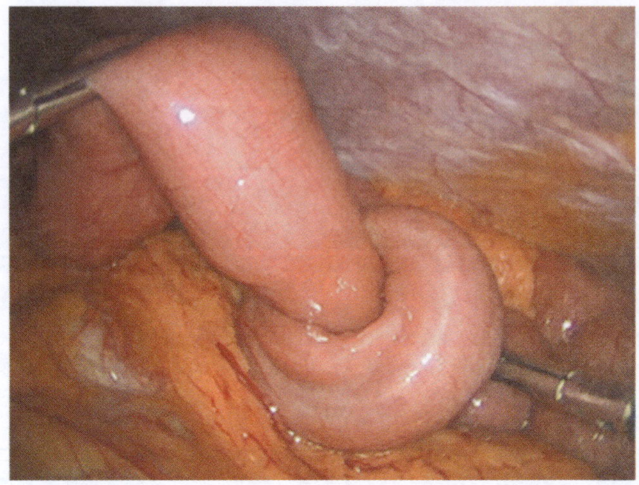

Intussusception

USG Features/CT Features

- Target sign
- Pseudo kidney sign
- Bull's eye sign

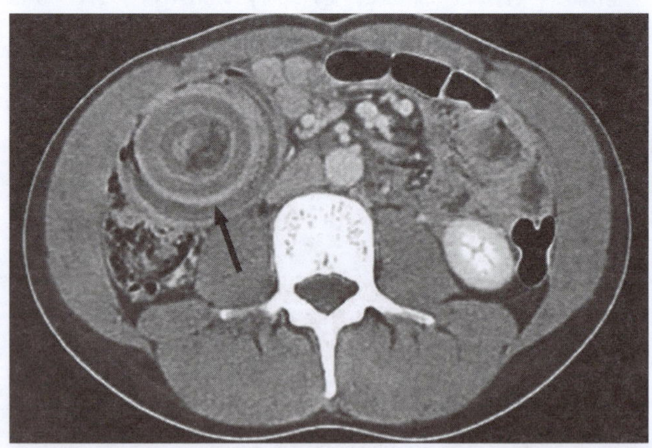

Target sign

Barium Enema

- Claw Sign/Pincer sign
- Coiled Spring sign

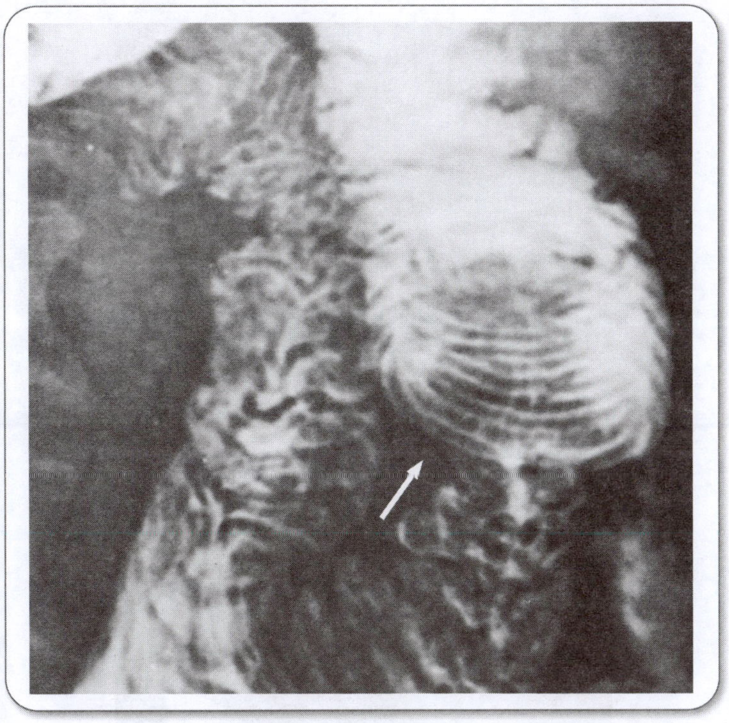

Coiled spring sign

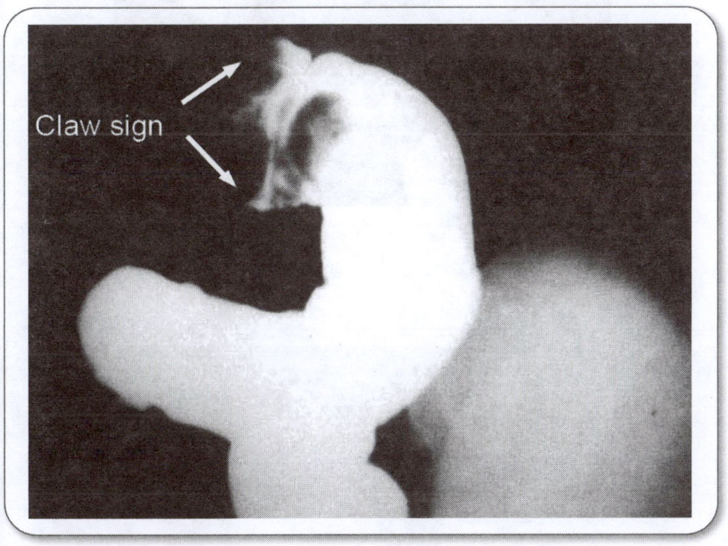

Claw sign

Management

- **Infants:** USG guided saline or air enema is done.
- **Others:** Surgical reduction is done—Don't pull the inner tube from back, always push it from above downward by milking.

ADULT CAUSES OF SMALL BOWEL OBSTRUCTION

Erect X-ray Findings

- Normal air fluid level: 3–5
- >5 air fluid level is pathological.
- Air fluid level with vertical diameter: >2.5 cm it is pathological**.
- Step Ladder pattern is seen**.
- String of pearls appearance is also seen if more fluids are present and less gas is seen.
- X-ray shows—No gas on Colon and rectum

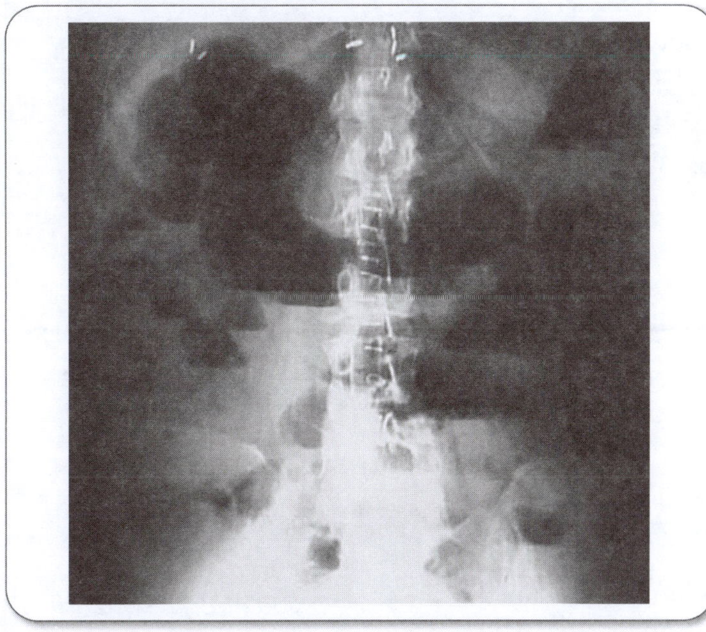

Step ladder pattern

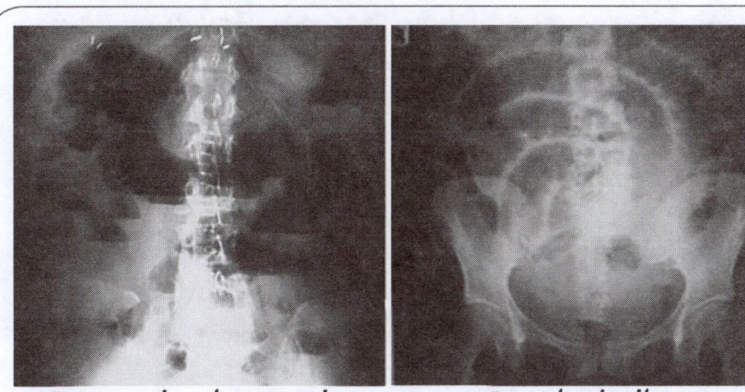

Dynamic obstruction | Paralytic ileus

Note the presence of gas in left colon and in rectum in paralytic ileus

Dynamic obstruction	Nondynamic obstruction (paralytic ileus)
MC cause—Adhesions*	MC cause—Postoperative patient** **Electrolyte imbalance:** • MC hypokalemia** • Na, Mg, Cl disturbances Hypothyroidism Neurological causes
Four cardinal features are seen	Pain is absent**
Bowel sounds +++ (borborygmi)	Absent bowel sounds
X-ray shows: • Multiple air fluid levels • No gas in rectum	**X-ray shows:** Gas + in rectum and colon
Management ***Adhesive obstruction:*** • NPO, IV Fluid • For 24–48 hours • >48 hours: Lap adhesiolysis** ***Other causes:*** Surgery Immediately done** (Sun should never set or rise)	**Management** • NPO • IV Fluid • Electrolyte correction • Wait for 48–72 hours • If not resolved: CATCHPOLE REGIMEN** Injection Neostigmine**

Order of recovery of bowel as per Bailey in Ileus:
- Small bowel—24 hours
- Colon
- Stomach (Last to recover)

Barium enema appearances:
- Thumb print appearance**—Ischemic Colitis
- Lead pipe—Ulcerative colitis
- Hose pipe—Crohn's disease
- Question mark—Hirschsprung disease
- Apple core—Cancer
- Claw sign/Pincer sign—Intussusception
- Ace of Spade appearance/Bird beak appearance—Sigmoid volvulus
- Coiled spring appearance—Intussusception
- Pulled up cecum—Ileocecal TB

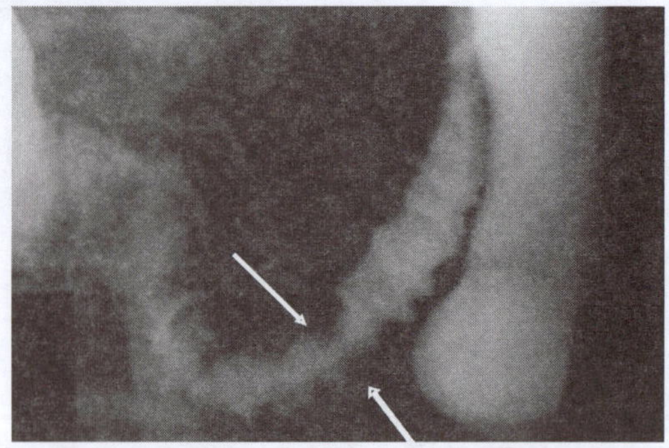

Thumb print sign (Ischemic colitis)

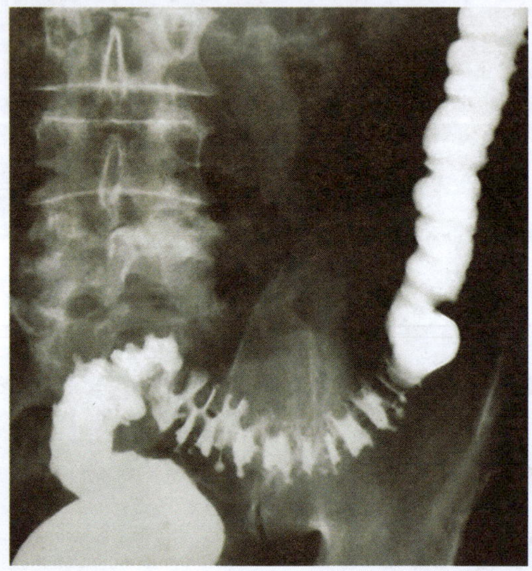

Sawtooth appearance (Diverticulosis sigmoid colon)

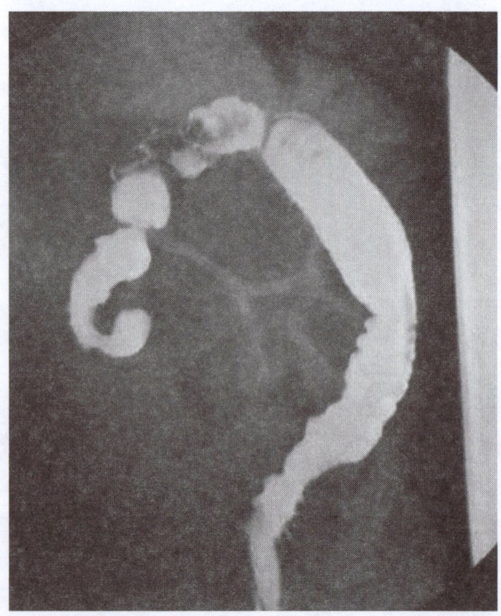

Question mark colon (Total aganglionosis colon)

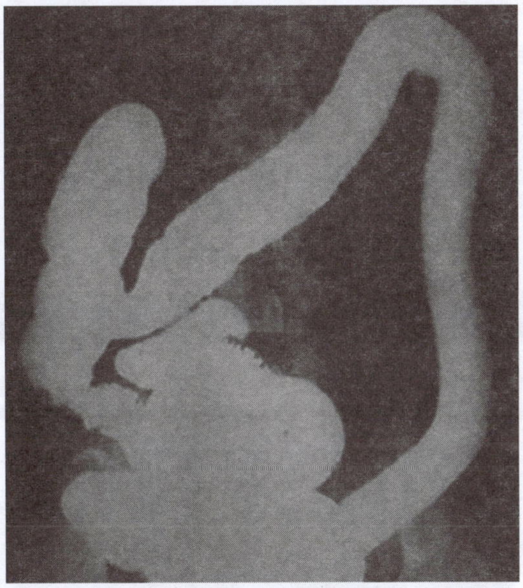

Lead pipe colon in ulcerative colitis

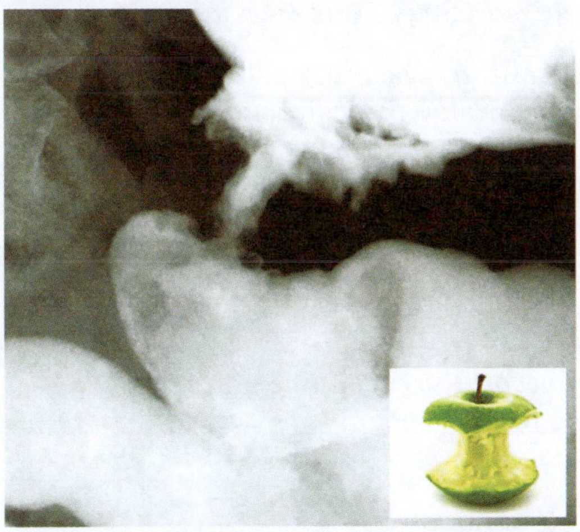

Apple core appearance in cancer colon

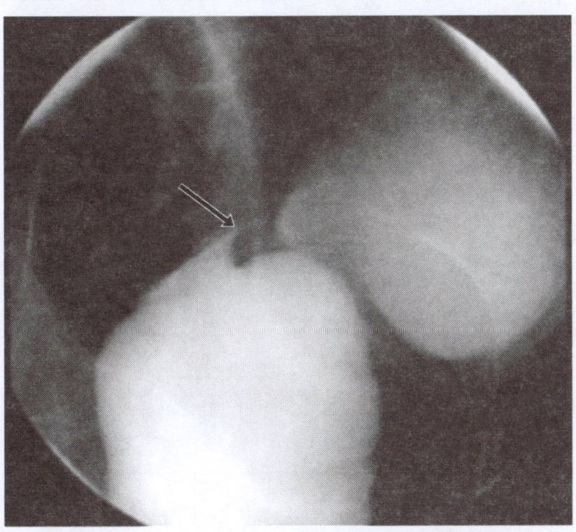

Bird beak or ace of spade appearance in sigmoid volvulus

SIGMOID COLON DIVERTICULUM

- MC site of acquired diverticulum is sigmoid due to highest luminal pressure inside the diverticulum.
- Multiple diverticulum is known as Diverticulosis*.
- IOC for diverticulosis—Barium enema—Shows SAWTOOTH APPEARANCE**
- MC complication—Diverticulitis—Inflammation and perforation seen. Barium enema is contraindicated. IOC for this complication—CECT abdomen.
- Hinchey Classification is used for Diverticulitis.

CONGENITAL MEGACOLON (HIRSCHSPRUNG DISEASE)

- Failure of migration of neural crest.
- RET oncogene mutation is seen.
- Absence of ganglion cells in Auerbach and Meissner's plexuses in constricted part of the colon.
- Dilated part of the colon is absolutely normal.

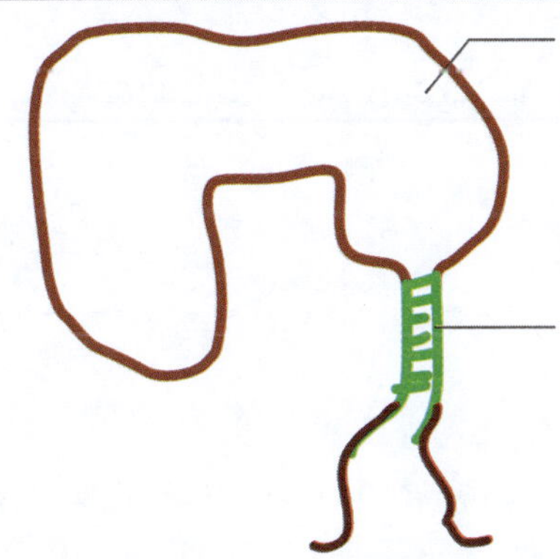

Hirschsprung disease

Locations

- MC site: Rectum
- May involve entire left colon
- May involve entire colon (total aganglionosis)
- May extend up to small intestine also

Presentation

- Newborn: Delayed passage of meconium
- Infants: Constipation without fecal soiling**
- Adults: Habitual constipation (H/O self-enema)

Investigations

- IOC: Full thickness Biopsy of rectum above dentate line
- In newborn by Suction Biopsy
- **Findings in Biopsy:** Absence of ganglion cells in both myenteric and submucous plexus* with

accompanying hypertrophy of nerve trunks and increased acetyl cholinesterase staining is seen**

- Anal Manometry—Recto Anal Inhibitory Reflex (RAIR) is absent** (NEET SS question)
- Barium Enema—Shows Question mark colon in Total aganglionosis**

Management

- Resection of aganglionic segment and pull-through operation.
- Duhamel, swenson and soave operations are types of pull-through operations.

Tubular adenomatous polyps syndromes

Familial adenomatous polyps	HNPCC
5q mutation in APC gene Autosomal dominant syndrome	Microsatellite Instability Mutation of MMR gene MLH-1(MC), MSH-2, MSH-6
More than 100 polyps seen in colon	Polyps <100 number
Incidence—1%	Incidence—3–5%
History of FAP: • Polyps develop around 10 years of age • Before high school (<20 years)—Develops cancer • By 40 years of age, they all die	**History of HNPCC:** • Polyps develop around 20 years of age • Cancer develops around 40–50 years of age • 2nd MC cancer—Endometrial cancer.
Most common mode of screening is by checking for APC Truncation mutation**	To do screening, we must select the high-risk cases by using the following criteria: • Amsterdam criteria • Modified amsterdam criteria • Bethesda criteria ○ Also includes polyps in criteria
Surveillance • Colonoscopy screening—from 10 years of age • Before 20 years, we must do Prophylactic Total Proctocolectomy**	**Surveillance** • Colonoscopy surveillance—From 20 years of age • No prophylactic surgery—Total colectomy done between 40–50 years once the cancer develops.
Associated syndromes: ***Gardner syndrome: AD*** • FAP+ • CHRPE (MC extraintestinal manifestation)—Congenital Hypertrophy of Retinal Pigment Epithelium • Desmoid tumors • Exostosis of bone • Epidermoid cyst (Multiple sebaceous cysts) ***Turcot Syndrome: AR*** • FAP + Brain tumor (Medulloblastoma)	**Associated syndromes:** ***Lynch—1:*** • Only CRC ***Lynch—2:*** • CRC associated with other cancers • MC brain tumor is Glioblastoma **Muir-Torre syndrome:** HNPCC with multiple sebaceous cysts
Management Prophylactic TPC + IPAA	**Management** Once they develop cancer at around 40–50 years of age, we do total colectomy and ileorectal anastomosis

CARCINOMA COLON

MC site is Rectum > Sigmoid colon

Right colon [Cauliflower/ fungating type]	Left colon [Stenosing type or stricture type]
• Chronic blood loss • Anemia • Melena • Mass in RIF	• Alteration in bowel habits • Hematochezia • Obstruction

Fearon Vogelstein sequence of adenoma carcinoma

- Initiation—APC gene (5q gene)—1st hit
- Promotion—HNPCC gene (MSI)
- In between—K ras (12p); DCC (18q);
- Last hit—P53 gene (17 p)—MOST COMMON MUTATION IN CRC**

Predisposing Factors for Carcinoma Colon

Dietary Factors

- High Animal fat diet
- Low fiber diet
- Low Carbohydrate diet
- Lack of antioxidants

Inflammatory Bowel Disease

- Ulcerative colitis
- Crohn's disease

Iatrogenic

- Radiotherapy to colon
- Ureterosigmoidostomy after bladder resection

Investigations for Colorectal Cancer (CRC)

- Diagnosis—Colonoscopic Biopsy
- T, N and M staging—CECT abdomen (MC site of Distant mets—Liver)
- Tumor marker—CEA** (Normal value <5 ng/mL)
- Apple core in Barium enema

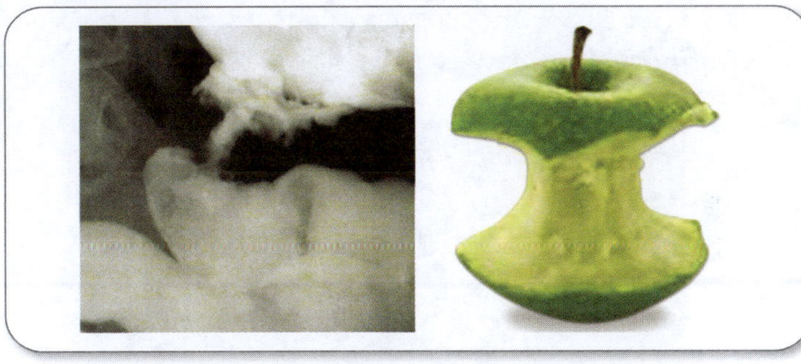

Apple core

Surgical Treatment of Colon Cancers

Right hemicolectomy	Extended right hemicolectomy	Left hemicolectomy
Last 30 cm ileum Cecum Appendix Ascending colon Up to right $2/3^{rd}$ colon Ligation of ICA, RCA and right branch of MCA done All four level lymph nodes removed	Extended resection up to splenic flexure is done Main trunk of MCA ligated	Removal of Left $1/3^{rd}$ transverse Descending Sigmoid Upper part of rectum Ligation of LCA and Sigmoid arteries
Indications: • Cecal cancer • Ascending colon cancer	**Indications:** • Transverse colon growth • Hepatic flexure growth • Splenic flexure growth	**Indications:** • Splenic flexure • Descending colon • Sigmoid colon

FOLFOX therapy is given nowadays for six cycles as adjuvant therapy.

- Folinic acid (Leucovorin)
- 5-FU (Continuous infusion advised) or Oral form Capecitabine can be used, **Oxaliplatin**.

Follow-up of Colorectal Cancer

- **CEA:** 3 monthly for 2 years, 6 monthly for 2–5 years
- **Colonoscopy:** Yearly once for 5 years. (No need after 5 years)
- **CECT abdomen:** 1–3 years annually (No need after 3 years)

Sigmoid Volvulus

- MC type
- MC in old men
- Predisposed by high fiber diet**
- MC in Anticlockwise > Clockwise
- **X-ray shows:** Coffee bean shaped
- **Barium enema:** Ace of spade or Bird beak appearance
- **1st line:** Sigmoidoscopic reduction
- **Definitive treatment:** Sigmoid colectomy

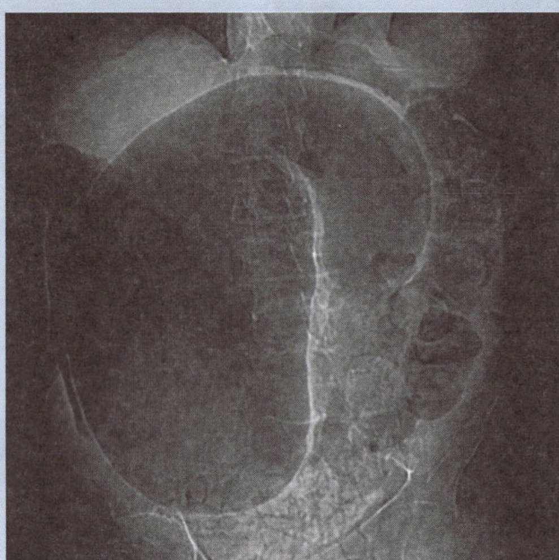

STOMAS

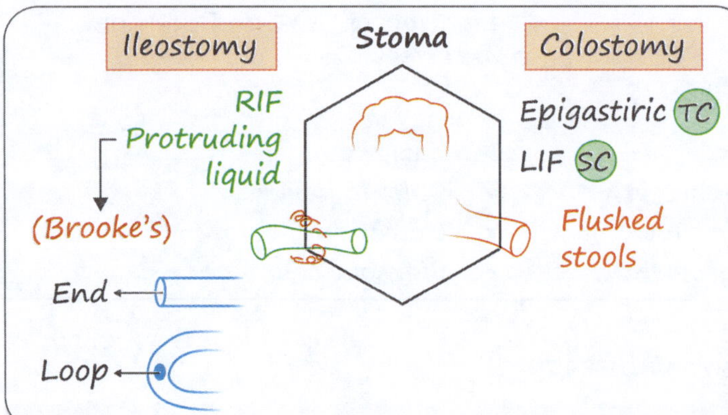

Stomas

- Content from ileostomy is liquid and more damaging to skin.
- Content from colostomy is solid stool and no skin damage occurs.
- Types of stoma: End or loop type

Complications of Stoma

Ileostomy

- **MC complication:** Skin excoriation
- **MC early complication:** Ileostomy necrosis
- Fluid electrolyte imbalance
- Parastomal hernia
- Stoma prolapse

Colostomy

- Stoma prolapse
- Parastomal hernia

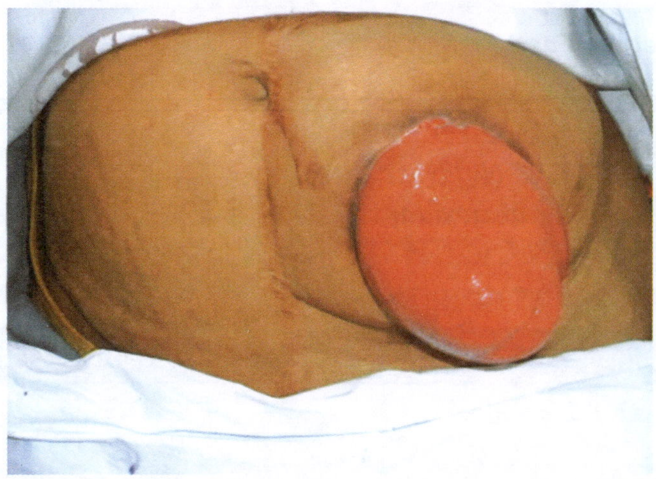

Stoma prolapse

- **MC complication of Colostomy:** Parastomal hernia**
- **MC indication of redo surgery in Colostomy:** Parastomal hernia.

MESENTERIC CYSTS

- MC in small intestine mesentery 60%
- **Four types are there:**
  - i. Chylolymphatic (MC)
  - ii. Enterogenous
  - iii. Urogenital remnant
  - iv. Dermoid

Chylolymphatic cyst	Enterogenous cyst
Usually congenital as a result of sequestration of lymphatics	Derived from diverticulum of mesenteric border that has become sequestrated
Cyst wall is thin, lacks muscular wall, not lined by mucosa	Thick wall lined by mucosa
Usually solitary, often unilocular with clear lymph or chyle	Content is mucinous
Most frequently seen in mesentery of ileum	
Independent blood supply	Common blood supply as adjacent bowel
Enucleation is enough**	Resection anastomosis needed**
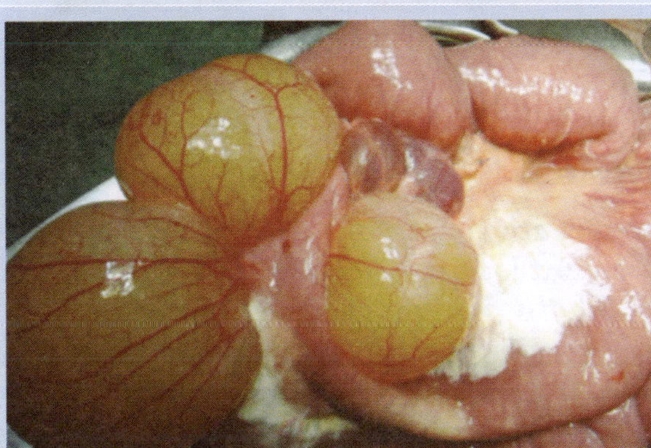	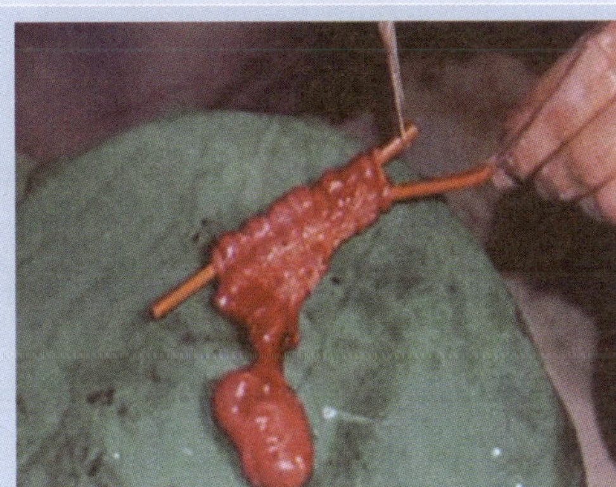

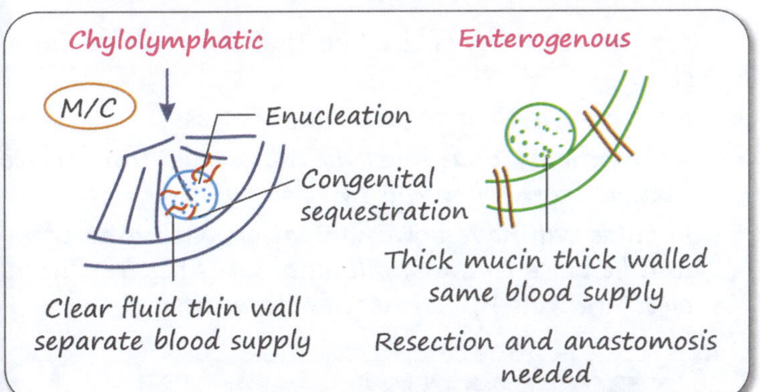

Chylolymphatic and Enterogenous cysts

Tillaux Triad

- Central area of dullness with zone of resonance all around.
- Swelling moves perpendicular to mesentery freely.
- Soft fluctuant swelling in the umbilical region.

Complications of Mesenteric Cyst

- **Acute abdominal pain due to:**
  - Torsion of mesentery
  - Rupture of cyst
  - Hemorrhage into cyst
  - Infection of cyst

RECTAL AND ANAL DISEASES

Hemorrhoids

- Prolapsing anal cushion is known as hemorrhoids
- Painless bleeding PR seen in Grades 1 and 2
- Painful bleeding PR seen in Grades 3 and 4
- Please note; 5 day self subsiding hemorrhoid is thrombosed external hemorrhoids.

Grade 1—No prolapsing mass.
Grade 2—Prolapse via anus but gets reduced spontaneously
Grade 3—Prolapse via anus and gets reduced manually by himself
Grade 4—Prolapsed and not reducible

- Grades 1 and 2 Hemorrhoids are treated during office visit (OP procedure).
- Grade 1—using GABRIEL Syringe, we can inject 5% phenol in almond oil as sclerosant.
- Grade 2—We can do Banding.
- Grades 3 and 4 are operated under spinal anesthesia.

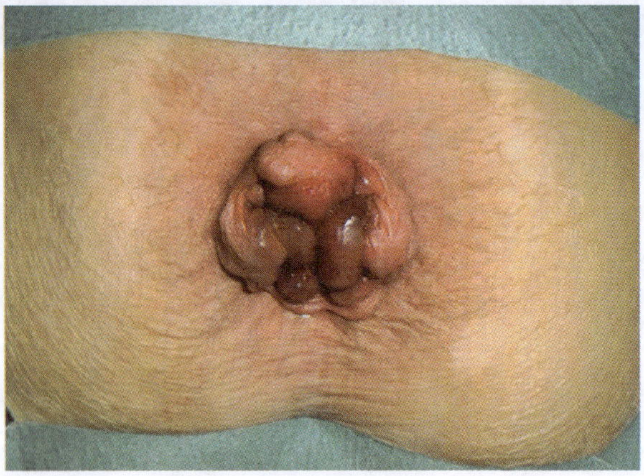

Hemorrhoids

Surgical Techniques

- Milligan-Morgan operation—Open hemorrhoidectomy—removal of hemorrhoids at 3, 7 and 11 O'clock position. After the surgery, "anus looks like a clover the problem is over"—it means there will not be stricture in future.
- Ferguson operation—Closed hemorrhoidectomy*

Newer Operations

- LONGO procedure (Using circular stapler)
- HALO—Hemorrhoidal artery ligation operation
- THD—Transanal hemorrhoidal dearterialization

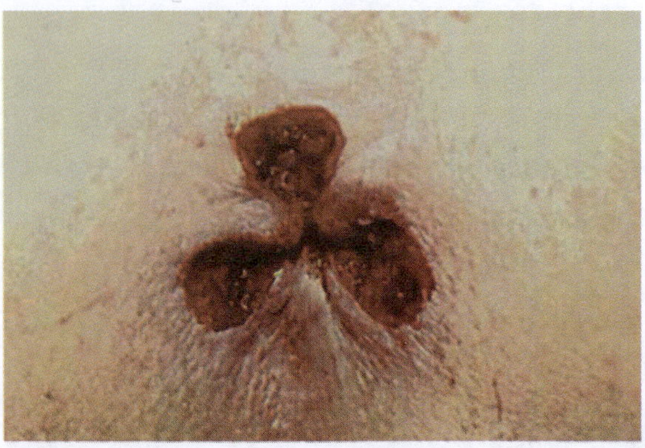

Milligan-Morgan operation—Clover shape Anus

Fissure in Ano

- Fissure in ano is a tear in anal mucosa which is pain sensitive.
- MC in 6 O'clock
- In pregnancy—12 O'clock
- In Crohn's—Lateral positions
- C/F—Severe painful defecation with spasm and Bleeding P/R
- Sentinel tag—Protective tag present in chronic fissure.

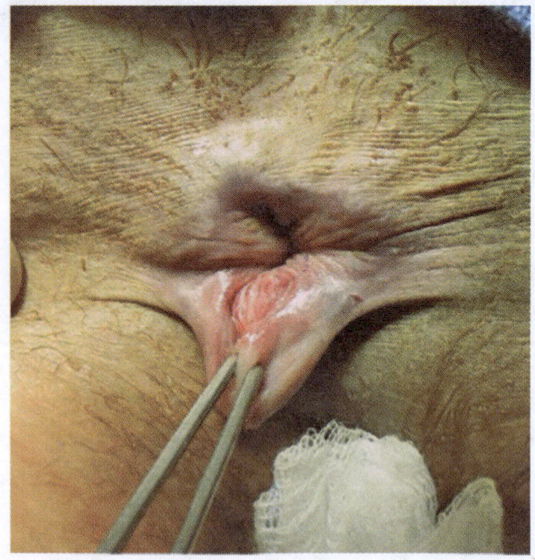

Posterior fissure in ano

Management

- **Conservative:** Laxatives, Glyceryl trinitrate ointment local application, Diltiazem Application, SITZ bath
- Surgical treatment of Choice—Lateral Sphincterotomy**—Internal sphincter cut at lateral position (3/9 O'clock position)—NOTARO'S Operation.

Fistula in Ano

- Communication of anal epithelium with perianal skin.
- MC cause is Cryptoglandular Abscess*
- As medicos, you must be able to differentiate fistulas from pilonidal sinus.
- Fistulas will have communication with anal canal and lie close to anus; pilonidal sinus lies in Gluteal cleft and has no connection to anus.

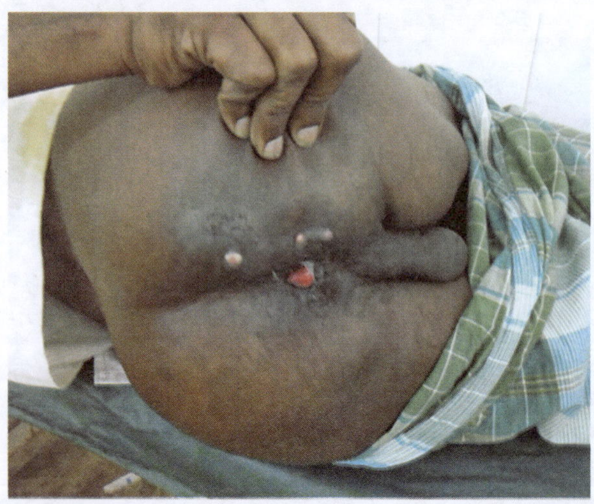

Multiple fistulas in ano at 7 O'clock, 10 O'clock and 11 O'clock positions

- **Park's Classification of Fistula in Ano**
  - **Type 1:** Inter sphincteric Fistula (MC type)
  - **Type 2:** Trans sphincteric Fistula
  - **Type 3:** Supra sphincteric fistula
  - **Type 4:** Extra Levator Fistula
  - **Type 1 and 2:** Low Fistula
  - **Type 3 and 4:** High Fistula

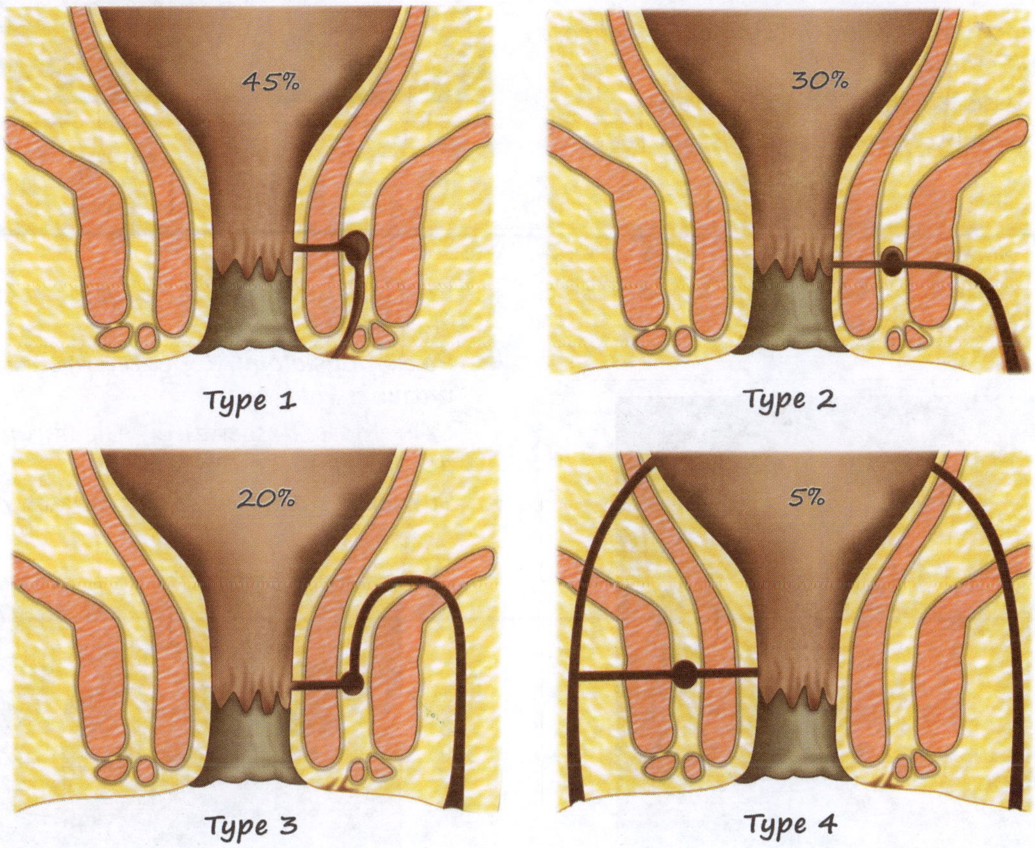

Park's classification of fistula in ano

Goodsall's Rule

- Anterior fistulas drain straight.
- Posterior fistulas drain by forming a horseshoe tract.
- If tract is >3.5 cm anteriorly—it is an exception—It forms a long tract and drains posteriorly.

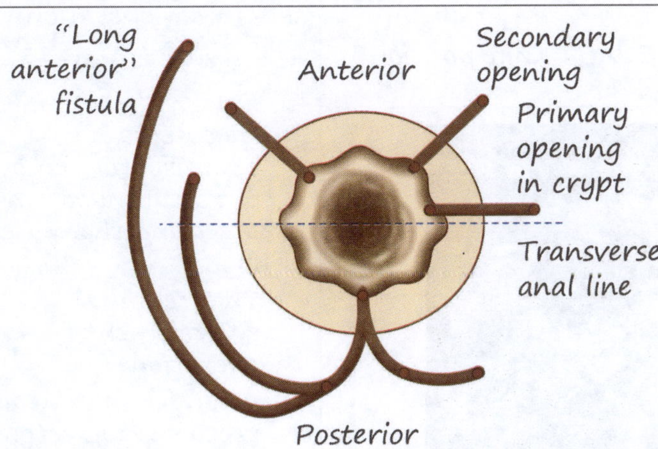

Goodsall's rule

Management of Fistula

- **Types 1 and 2:** Fistulectomy or fistulotomy
- **Types 3 and 4:** Seton application done

Newer Treatments

- **Biological treatment:** Small intestine Submucosa of Porcine (SIS Plug)
- **VAFT:** Video assisted fistula tract excision
- **LIFT:** Ligation of Intersphincteric fistula tract

Pilonidal Sinus

- Hair in the gluteal region enters gluteal cleft in jeep drivers and hence, known as JEEPER'S Bottom or Pilonidal sinus.

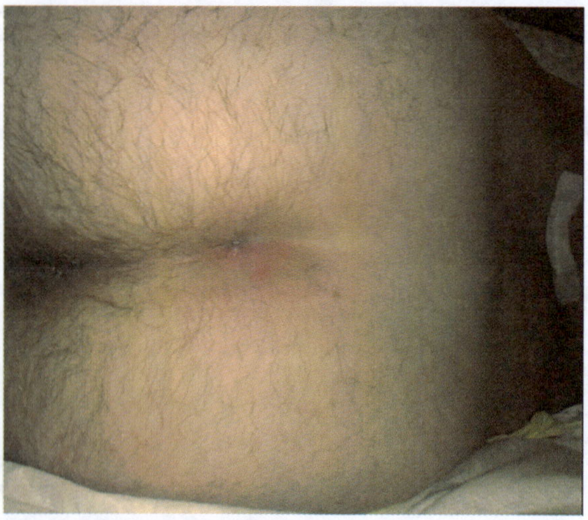

Pilonidal sinus

- The tract will have hair.
- They get infected and cause pain and discharge*.
- Lay open the tract and core the tract completely.
- **Treatment for recurrence:** Bascom's technique or Karydakis flap or Rhomboidal flap (Limberg flap) operations are done.
- Operation is done in PRONE JACK Knife position**

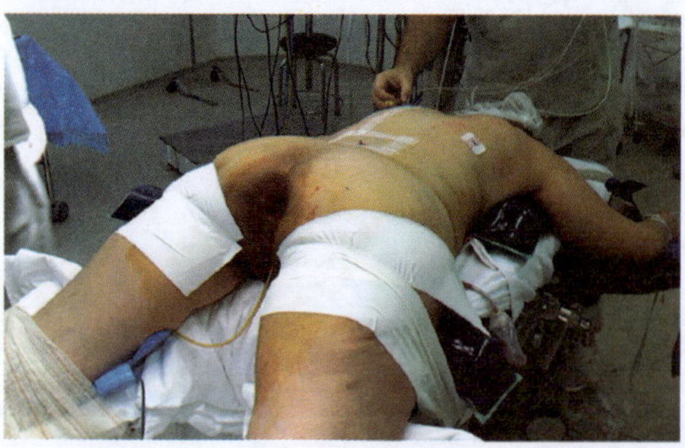

Prone Jack knife position to operate Pilonidal sinus

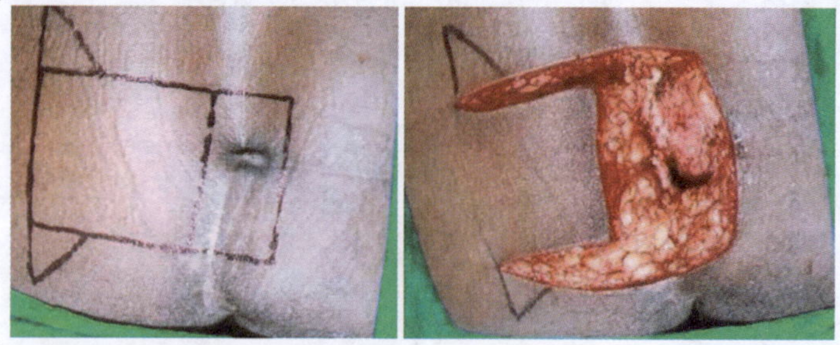

Limberg flap

Rectal Prolapse

- Partial and complete type of rectum descending via the anus.
- **Pathophysiology:** Repeated pregnancy, psychiatric patients, old age.
- **C/F:** Mass descending, Bleeding, discharge and decubitus ulcers.
- Surgery is advised for complete rectal prolapses.

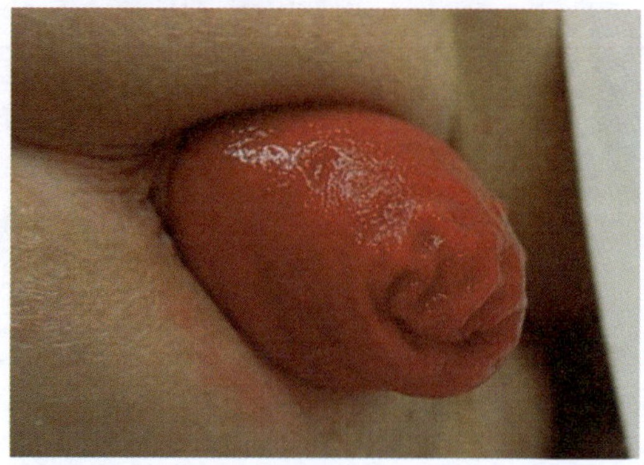

Rectal prolapse

Perineal approach	Abdominal approach
Useful for very old people who cannot withstand abdominal operation	Procedure of choice in young age
Recurrence is more (>20%)	Least recurrence
• Delorme's mucosectomy operation of removal of rectal mucosa and placating the muscle layer* • Thiersch anal encirclement operation • Altemier's perineal recto sigmoidectomy procedure with Colo anal anastomosis*—Resection procedure**	• Ripstein's anterior rectopexy • Well's posterior rectopexy • Resection rectopexy (Frykman and Goldberg) for redundant sigmoid colon • Anterior resection

LIVER

Anatomy of Liver

Portal Triad Structures

- Posterior—Portal vein
- Anterior to right—CBD
- Anterior to left—Hepatic artery
- Epiploic foramen of Winslow is seen posterior to these three structures
- Pringle maneuver is done *via* this foramen, where we compress the inflow vessels (Hepatic artery and Portal vein by a soft clamp)

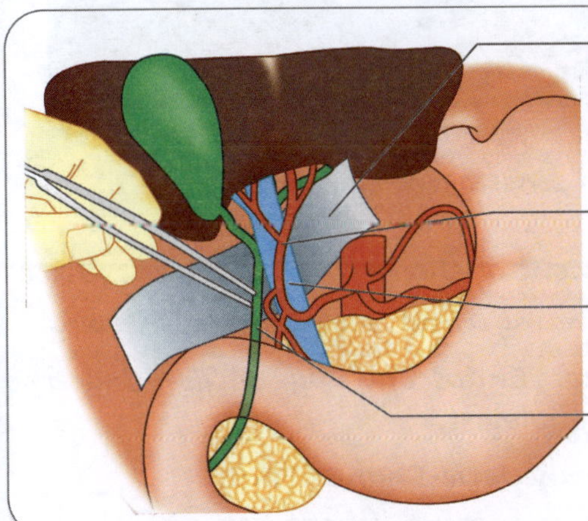

Portal triad and epiploic foramen

Couinaud Surgical Segments of Liver

- Total segments in liver—8 segments
- The Middle Hepatic vein corresponds to an imaginary line CANTLIE'S Line—runs from gall bladder fossa to right of IVC. (Cantlie's line—Cholecystocaval line)

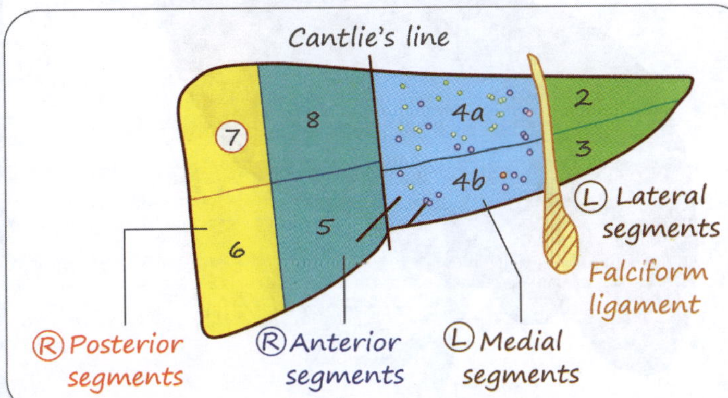

Liver segments

Brisbane 2000 is the latest naming for hepatectomy:

- Left hemihepatectomy = 2, 3, 4a, 4b
- Right hemihepatectomy = 5–8
- Left lateral hepatectomy = 2, 3 removal (lateral to Falciparum ligament)
- Right posterior hepatectomy = segments 6 and 7 removed
- Radical cholecystectomy = 4b + 5
- Pediatric liver transplant donated segments 2 and 3 are used
- Adult liver transplant donated segments—5, 6, 7, 8

Scoring Systems in Liver

Modified Child Pugh Score (Mnemonic - BAAPE)

Clinical**	1	2	3
Encephalopathy	None	1 or 2	3 or 4
Ascites	None	Mild	Moderate
Bilirubin (mg/dL)	1–2 mg/dL	2.1–3 mg/dL	≥3.1 mg/dL
Albumin (g/dL)	≥3.5 g/dL	2.8–3.4 g/dL	≤2.7 g/dL
Prothrombin time (increase in seconds)	1–4	4.1–6	≥6

- **Grade A: 5–6**
- **Grade B: 7–9**
- **Grade C: 10–15 points**

MELD: Modified End Liver Disease Scoring: Based on "CBI"

- Creatinine
- Bilirubin
- INR
  - Recently waiting list for transplant is made on the basis of MELD score*
  - **Initially MELD score was used to predict mortality after TIPSS**
  - Values vary from 6–40*. Liver transplant is allowed only for MELD >15**

Cirrhosis with Portal Hypertension

Causes of Portal Hypertension

Presinusoidal	Sinusoidal (MC)	Postsinusoidal
• Intrahepatic - Schistosomiasis (MC), NCPF • Extrahepatic - EHPVO	Cirrhosis causing fibrosis (MC)	Extrahepatic - Budd Chiari Syndrome - HV or IVC occlusion

Pathophysiology

- Due to high portal pressure—The collaterals will open.
- Normal portal pressure—5–8 mm Hg
- Collaterals between systemic and portal venous system:
    - Left gastric vein with hemiazygos vein—Esophageal varices
    - Inferior mesenteric vein (Superior rectal vein) with middle and inferior rectal vein—Hemorrhoids develop.
    - Left Umbilical (Paraumbilical vein) opens up—Caput medusae.
- Ascites due to increased SMV pressure
- Splenomegaly

Complications

- MC cause of death—liver failure (only option is liver transplant)
- 2nd MC cause of death—Bleeding**
    - Esophageal variceal bleed (MC)
    - Portal Hypertensive gastropathy
- Varices formed at portal pressure >10 mm Hg
- Varices bleeding occurs at PP >12 mm Hg

Management

1st Step: Massive hematemesis:

- DOC for variceal bleeding—Injection Octreotide** infusion
- Other drugs—Vasopressin or Terlipressin along with GTN to avoid Coronary ischemia*

2nd Step: Ryles tube shows continuous bleed:

- Modified Sengstaken—Blakemore Tube:
    - 1st inflate gastric balloon using 300 mL of air; followed by esophageal balloon up to 60 mm Hg by air
    - Lumens are used to inflate and aspirate the contents
    - Tamponade effect is produced on varices
    - Maximum time to retain the balloon—12 hours
    - Extended pressure results in esophageal necrosis and perforation.

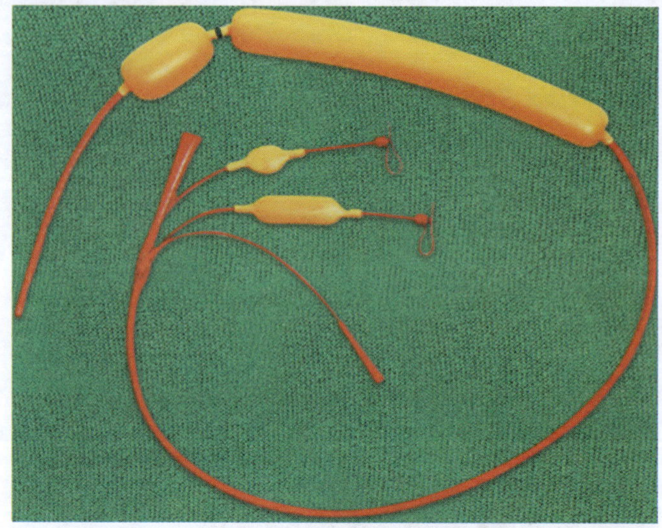

Modified sengstaken–blakemore tube

3rd Step: Treatment of choice for Esophageal varices is Endoscopic Banding >Endoscopic Sclerotherapy.

4th Step: Failed Endoscopy by MGE—Call the Interventional radiologist.

Transjugular Intrahepatic Shunt (TIPS)

- Intrahepatically, a stent is kept between HV and PV by transjugular route**
- The stent will now reduce the Portal pressure immediately and Varices bleed stops.
- Stent is made up of Polytetrafluoroethylene (PTFE)

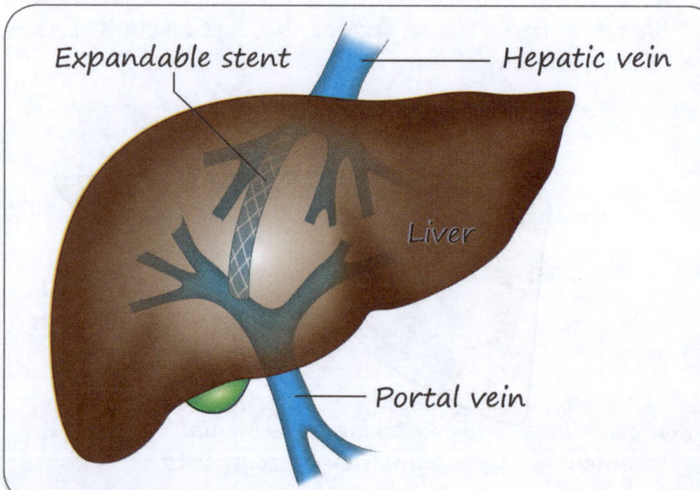

TIPS

Complications of TIPS:

- Early Complication** —Capsule rupture with intraperitoneal hemorrhage.
- Within 1 month—Encephalopathy can happen**
- Shunt thrombosis also develops in one month
- Shunt stenosis occurs in one year (Most common)

5th Step: If TIPS not possible or feasible:

Surgical Shunt Operations

Nonselective shunts	Selective shunts
Entire Portal Blood is diverted into systemic circulation and hence, encephalopathy develops*	Only splenic blood diverted; Portal blood is flowing into liver and metabolized and hence, no encephalopathy; but there is ASCITES formed
Types: • End to side portacaval • Side to side portacaval • 16 mm Interposition portacaval • TIPS also nonselective • LINTON = Conventional = Proximal splenorenal shunt: Splenectomy is done and proximal splenic vein anastomosed to left renal vein	**Types:** Warren's = Distal splenorenal shunt: The distal splenic vein is anastomosed to left renal vein. Increased pressure in SMV causes Ascites**

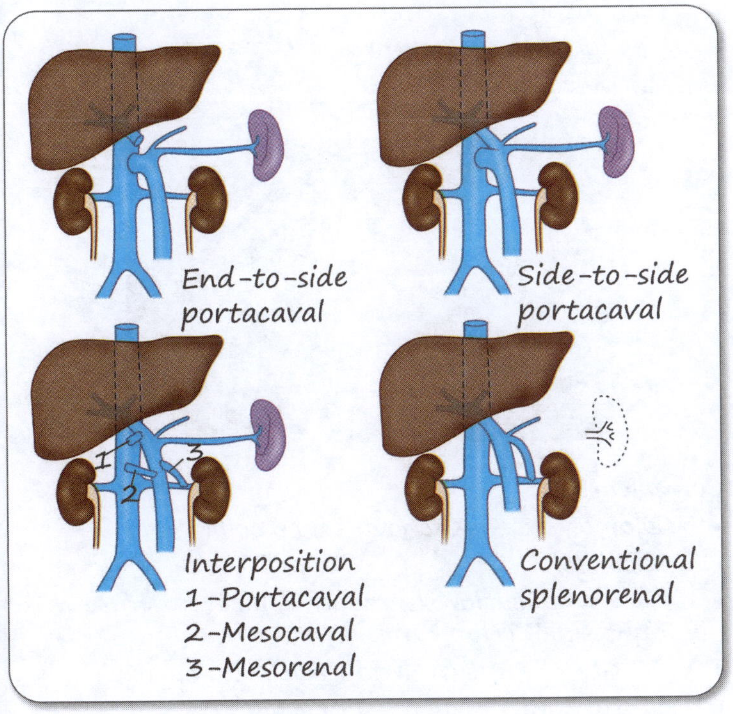

Nonselective shunts

Budd Chiari Syndrome

- Two causes—HV thrombosis and IVC occlusion by Congenital membranous webs
- BCS—MC cause in western is HV thrombosis**—The thrombosis most commonly is due to Polycythemia Rubra vera**
- BCS—MC cause in Asians/Indians is IVC webs
- IOC to diagnose—Hepatic Venography is gold standard—SPIDER WEB appearance**
- CECT abdomen—shows Enlarged Caudate Lobe—HOT SPOT of caudate lobe seen.

Management

- Liver is normal—Shunt operations are planned as shown below:
    - Liver failure cases—Liver transplant is TOC

Shunt operations:

- HV thrombosis—Side to side Portacaval shunt (SSPCS) done
- IVC webs—Double shunt operation done (SSPCS + cavoatrial shunt) or SSPCS with IVC stenting

Surgical Infections in Liver

Pyogenic abscess	Amoebic liver abscess
Sick patient with fever, chills and rigors with Hepatomegaly. Severe Right Hypochondrial tenderness++	Hepatomegaly + Pain (MC symptom – Pain)
M:F = 1.5:1	M>>>>>>>F
Predisposing Factors: • MC in immunocompromised cases • Diabetes mellitus	**Predisposing Factor:** **Alcohol******
Lab Values: Increased AST, ALT, Alk.PO_4, Bilirubin	**Lab Values:** • All values normal • **Only PT may be elevated***
Serology: Negative for Amoeba Blood Culture is positive	**Serology:** Amoebic antigen+ Blood Culture is negative*
CECT Abdomen: • Clustered Abscess seen with Peripheral Rim Enhancement** • They may be 50: 50 single or multiple 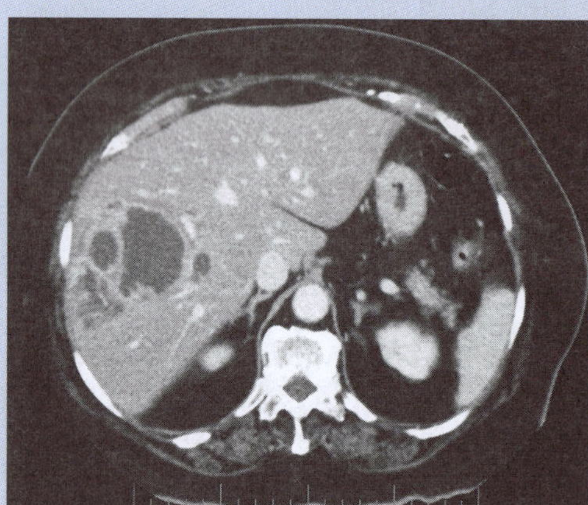	**CECT Abdomen:** • Well defined abscess with no peripheral enhancement but there may be peripheral wall edema++ • Trophozoites are present in the wall. • Mostly they are **solitary**** • MC in segment 7** 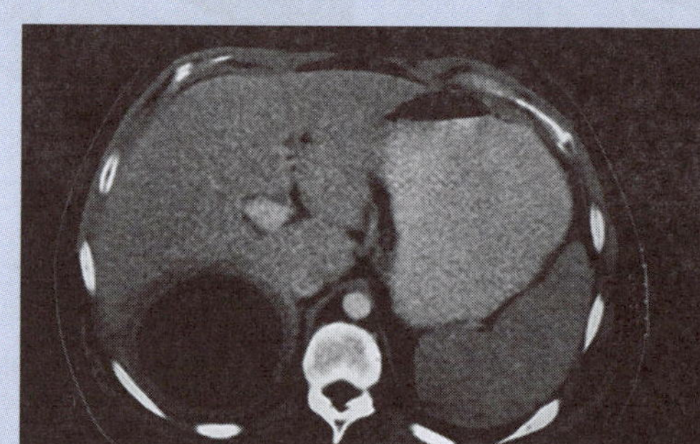
Complications: • Sepsis • Endogenous Endophthalmitis • Osteomyelitis • Infective Endocarditis**	**Complications:** • Color of pus – Anchovy sauce color • Odorless • MC complication is reactive pleural effusion in Right side** (Not rupture) • MC site of rupture into Peritoneal cavity** • Rupture into pleura – Put an ICD** • Rupture into bronchus (Broncho pleural fistula)

Contd...

Treatment:	**Treatment:**

• Immediate Treatment of choice is aspiration of abscess
• Based on Pus C/S and Blood C/S- Higher antibiotics are given.
	TOC – Injection Metronidazole 750 mg TDS for 2 weeks and convert to oral
	• Luminal Amoebicides—Diloxanide furoate, Emetine, etc. × 10 days
	• **Aspiration - Indications:**
	  o Doubtful diagnosis
	  o >5 cm sized abscess
	  o Located on Left lobe
	  o Superficial located abscess
	  o Not responding for >3 days

Hydatid Cyst Liver

- Caused by Echinococcus granulosus, Echinococcus Multilocularis
- E. Multilocularis is very rare and dangerous (Malignant Hydatid Cyst). Always needs liver resection.
- E. Granulosus—Dog Tapeworm.
- Definitive host—Dogs
- Intermediate hosts—Sheep and goats
- Accidental host—Human (End host—Will not spread from one man to other)

Pathophysiology

- The MC site of hydatid cyst—Segment 6 and 7**
- The cyst wall is formed by three layers
  1. **Outer Ectocyst/Pericyst/Adventitial layer:** Derived from host tissue
  2. **Middle laminated membrane:** Thin membrane allows some essential substances
  3. **Inner Germinal layer:** Living layer producing daughter cysts**
- **MC site**—Liver
- **Other sites**—Lungs, brain, kidney
- Ectocyst is derived from host tissues and is **absent in lung and brain Hydatid cyst****
- Ectocyst is seen in liver and kidney only

Clinical Features

- MC feature—Hepatomegaly (No pain)
- Jaundice—Hydatid rupture into biliary tree causes jaundice
- Passing of grape like membranes in motion

Investigations

- **IOC to diagnose**—Immunoblast assay**
- **Others**—ELISA, Immune Electrophoresis, Casoni's Intradermal test
- **Radiological IOC**—CECT Abdomen

WHO Classification

- **CE 1:** Unilocular cyst
- **CE 2:** Multiseptated (Honey comb/Rosette like)
- **CE 3:** Floating membrane (water lily sign)
- **CE 4:** Heterogenous cysts with partial calcification
- **CE 5:** Calcified wall

Type 1, 2, 3 are active cysts

Type 4, 5 are inactive and dead cysts

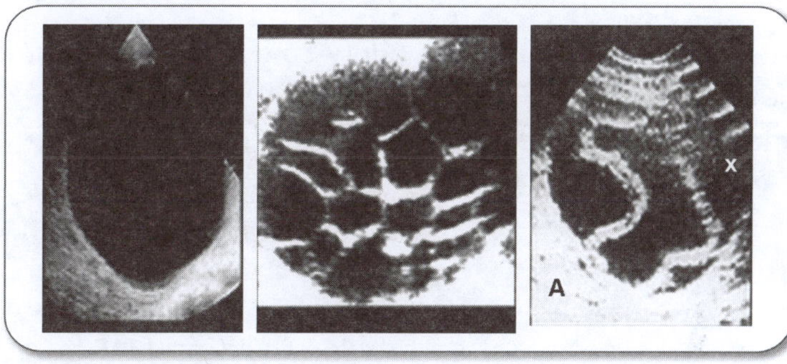

CE 1, 2, 3 hydatid cysts in USG

Complications

- MC is biliary rupture—30%**
- Secondary infections

Management

- T. Albendazole started.
- Under cover of T. Albendazole after 2 weeks we plan for Surgery/PAIR

Surgical Treatment Options

- Partial pericystectomy (leaving part of pericyst there itself)—Surgical best option**

Percutaneous Aspiration, Infusion of Scolicidal agents and Reaspiration (PAIR)

- Given with prophylactic cover of Albendazole.
- Scolicidal agents—**20% hypertonic saline** is used

Contraindications for PAIR

- Superficially located cyst (chance of rupture)
- Honey combing of cysts (multiple thick internal septae)—CE2
- Communication with biliary tree
- Dead or inactive cysts
- Lung/brain cysts

Tumors in Liver

- IOC for SOL liver is CECT abdomen
- IOC for Hemangioma in Liver is MRI**

Benign Liver Tumor

Characters	Hemangioma	Focal nodular hyperplasia	Liver cell adenoma
Incidence	• MC Incidentaloma • MC benign tumor	Second common benign tumor	Rare
Complications	• Rupture/hemorrhage • Giant Hemangioma >5 cm • **Kasabach-Merritt syndrome**—Huge hemangioma consuming platelets and causing Thrombocytopenia+ CCF	Rupture/hemorrhage	Rupture and malignant transformation**
Imaging studies CECT abdomen—Triple phase	• Slow contrast enhancement from periphery to center due to small vessel uptake. Typical nodular peripheral enhancement • MRI – T2 weighted image shows—**Light Bulb sign**	Characteristic central stellate scar seen**	
Treatment	No treatment needed	No treatment needed	Laparotomy and resection**

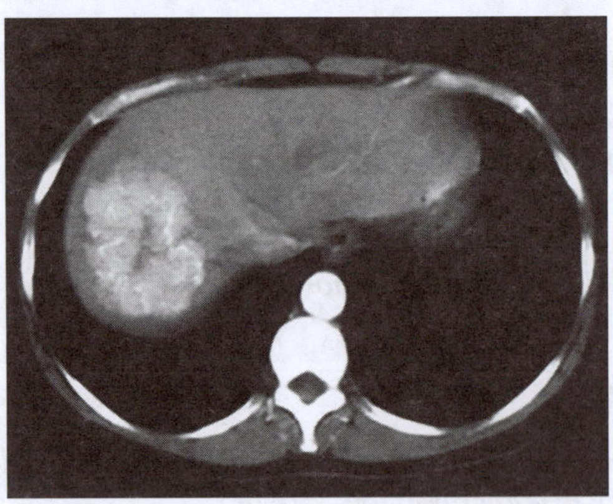

Focal nodular Hyperplasia (FNH)

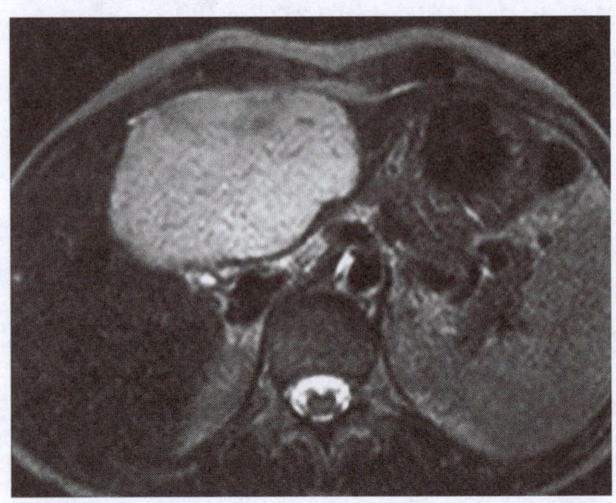

MRI—light bulb sign hemangioma

Malignant Tumors in Liver

- MC malignant tumor is secondary
- MC primary malignant tumor is HCC**

Hepatocellular Cancers

Etiological Factors:

Infections	Cirrhosis	Environmental	Metabolic diseases
HBV HCV	Alcohol Autoimmune Primary biliary	Aflatoxins Pyrrolidone alkaloids Thorotrast Nitrosamines	Hemochromatosis Alpha 1 AT deficiency Wilsons Glycogen storage diseases EHBA

HCC usually arises from Cirrhotic liver background only **except in HBV induced HCC****

Clinical Features:

- K/C/O Cirrhosis sudden decompensation of liver with pain, mass and weight loss all suggest malignancy**
- Paraneoplastic syndromes:
    - MC is Hypercholesterolemia > Hypoglycemia**
    - Hypercalcemia
    - Polycythemia (Erythrocytosis)

Investigations:

Tumor markers:

- AFP >400 ng/mL - Conclusive of HCC
- PIVKA- protein induced vitamin K absence**—Latest tumor marker.

CECT abdomen with triple Phase is Gold standard:

- Rapid contrast enhancement of Tumor in arterial phase**
- Rapid wash out in portal venous phase**

Latest staging system which helps in diagnosis and treatment—Barcelona Clinic Liver Staging (BCLC Staging)

- **Very early stage:** <2 cm size, Single lesion—best treatment is Resection**
- **Early stage:** <3 lesions, <3 cm size all lesion—Resection or Transplant advised.
- Intermediate stage
- Advanced stage—SORAFENIB
- Terminal stage

Liver transplantation: Milan Criteria** of Liver transplant in Cirrhotic liver

- <5 cm single lesion
- <3 lesions all 1–3 cm each
- No Extrahepatic spread seen

Ablative therapies:

- Percutaneous Ethanol Injection (PEI)
- Percutaneous Acetic acid injection
- Percutaneous Thermal Ablations; RFA, Cryoablation**

Interventional Procedures:

- **TACE (Transarterial chemo embolization):** Into hepatic artery we can inject Chemotherapy—Loaded with Lipoidal sodium, which carries chemotherapy to tumor.
- **TARE (Transarterial radio embolization)**

Metastasis to Liver

- **MC primary for Liver mets:** Colorectal cancer
- **MC primary from Extra abdominal:** Breast
- **Mets with good prognosis:** NET mets** >CRC mets
- Resection is approved for CRC and NET mets only so far.

GALLBLADDER AND BILIARY SYSTEM

Calot's triangle	Hepatocystic triangle
Formed between	Formed between
• Inferior—Cystic duct and GB	• Inferior—Cystic duct and GB
• Medial—Common hepatic duct	• Medial—Common hepatic duct
• Above—Cystic artery	• Above—Inferior surface of liver

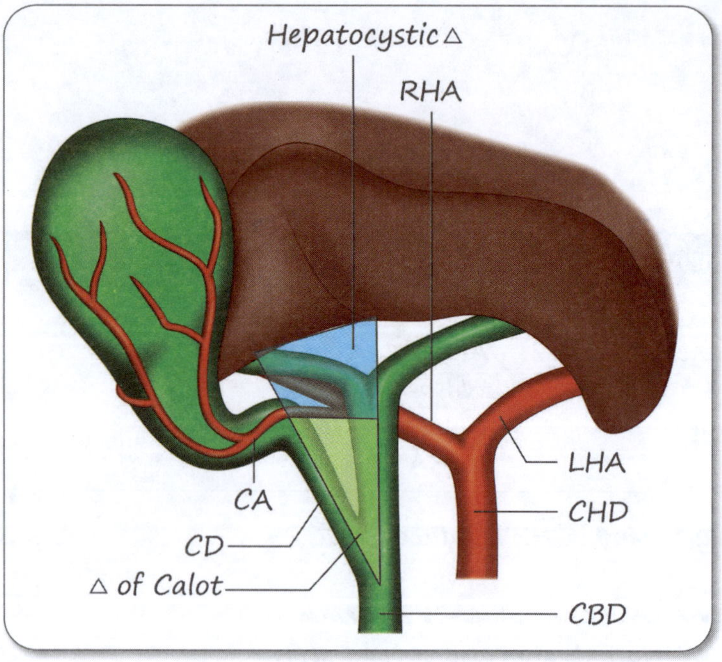

Calot Vs Hepatocystic triangle

- **Node seen in Calot's triangle:** Lund Node, also known as Mascagni Node**

Right Hepatic artery taking a Tortuous course and running in Calot's triangle is known as Caterpillar Turn or Moynihan's Hump**

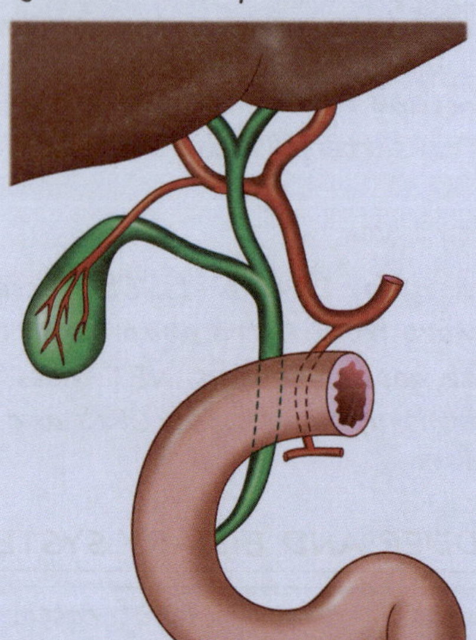

Moynihan's hump

Endoscopic Retrograde Cholangiopancreatography (ERCP)

- Done with the help of side viewing scopy.
- We cut the sphincter at 11 O'clock or 1 O'clock position known as Sphincterotomy.
- The SOD pressure falls down and SOD will be always relaxed and opened.
- The contrast is passed inside the biliary and pancreatic system studied.
- We will keep a stent inside the bile duct known as Double Pig tail or DJ stent.

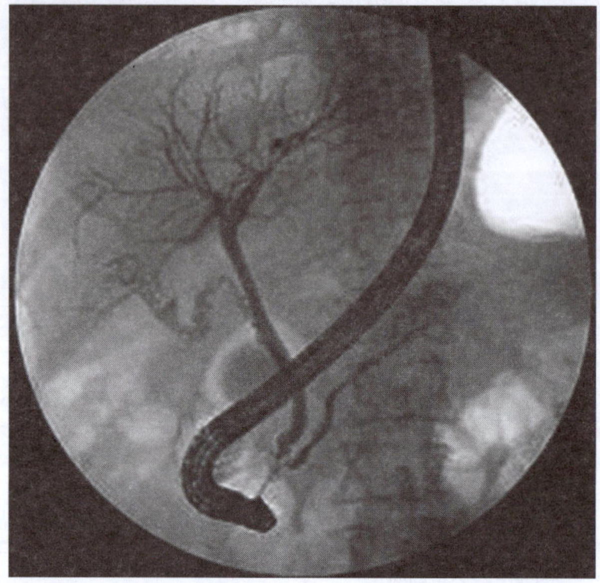

Normal ERCP

Indications for ERCP	Complications
• Sphincterotomy—SOD dyskinesia • Stone removal • Self-expanding metallic stent for growth in bile duct • Biopsy • Pancreas Divisum—Minor duct papillotomy • Gallstone pancreatitis	• Most common – ERCP—induced Pancreatitis** for overall • MC complication is SEPSIS if done for Cholangitis cases. • Cholangitis • Bleeding • Perforation of Duodenum • Mortality**—0.1%

Magnetic Resonance Cholangio Pancreatography (MRCP)

- Noninvasive
- Has replaced ERCP in diagnostic purposes.
- IOC for BD stones, BD malignancy and pancreatic duct pathologies.
- No contrast is used; bile and pancreatic juice act as contrast

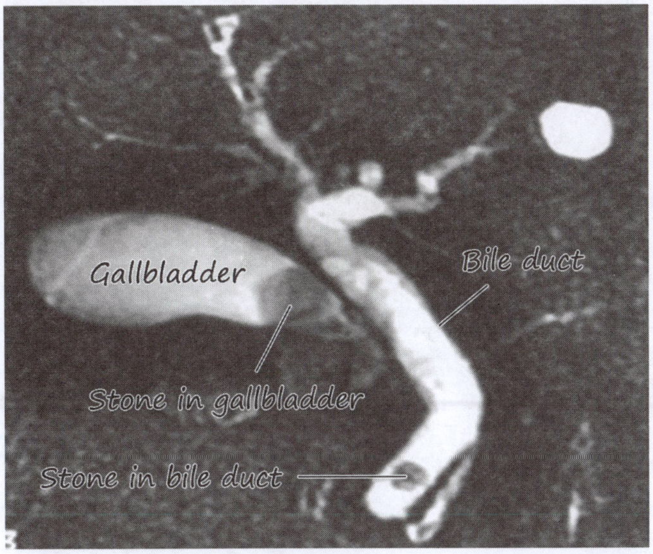

MRCP

Hydroxy Imino Diacetic Acid (HIDA Scan)

It is a radio tracer substance injected into blood stream taken up by liver and excreted into bile duct without metabolization. On the way, it gets concentrated in gallbladder.

Applications:

- Detects physiology of bile flow
- Detects bile leak
- Gold Standard for Acute Cholecystitis**—Non-visualization of gallbladder.

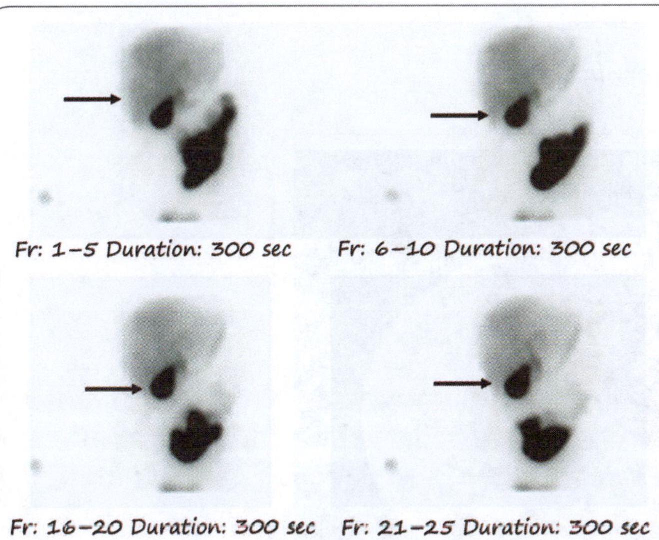

HIDA scan

Protocol for Biliary Pathology

- 1st Investigation done—USG abdomen
- Based on pathology in USG abdomen, we have so many other investigations as choices.

Findings in USG	Salient Points
Gallstones are diagnosed	• Posterior acoustic shadow • 95% sensitive • Mercedes Benz and Seagull sign are seen
Acute cholecystitis	• Shows thickened gallbladder wall >3 mm** • IOC is USG abdomen • Gold Standard is HIDA scan*
CBD stone	• IOC is MRCP** • Gold Standard is ERCP as we can remove the stone via this procedure.

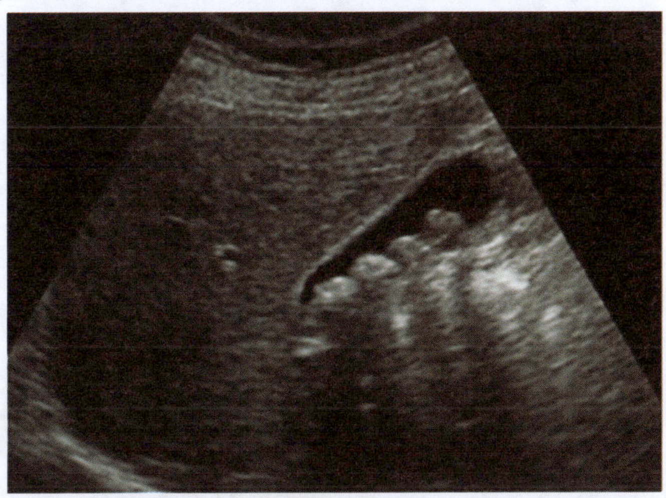

USG shows gallstones
(Note posterior acoustic shadows)

X-ray Abdomen in Bile system

- 10% Gallstones are radio opaque
- Porcelain GB—Calcified GB—Premalignant—Surgery Advised.
- Air in Biliary system is known as Pneumobilia**

One liners for Exam:
- Moynihan's Hump—Caterpillar turn of RHA
- Valves of Heister—Cystic duct and neck valve
- Phrygian cap—MC anomaly of GB, Fundus of GB folded upon itself.
- Mercedes Benz Sign or Seagull Sign is air in Gallstones
- **Meniscus sign**—Feature of CBD
- **Cholesterolosis:** Strawberry Gallbladder; contains multiple cholesterol stones seen

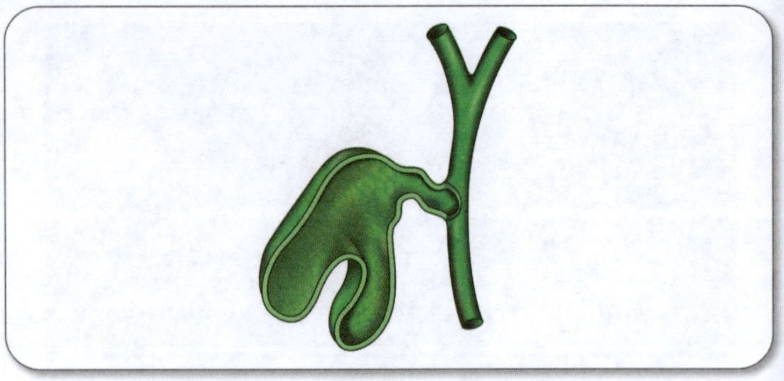

Phrygian cap anomaly in GB

Gall stones

Types of Gallstones

Cholesterol	• MC type of stone in western countries • Golden yellow color • Hard stones	Composed of **Cholesterol Monohydrate crystals**** 15% of these stones are radio opaque
Mixed	• MC type of stone in world • **Cholesterol component is more than 30%****	Contains both pigment and cholesterol together
Pigment	• Black and brown pigment stones • Brown pigment is most common type in Asians and Indians • Black stone is most common type in children • **In pigment stone Cholesterol Component is <30%****	Brown pigment stone is composed of: • Ca. Palmitate • Ca. Stearate • Ca. Bilirubinate

Obese lady with Gallstone:
Saint's Triad—Gallstones + Diverticulosis colon + Hiatus hernia

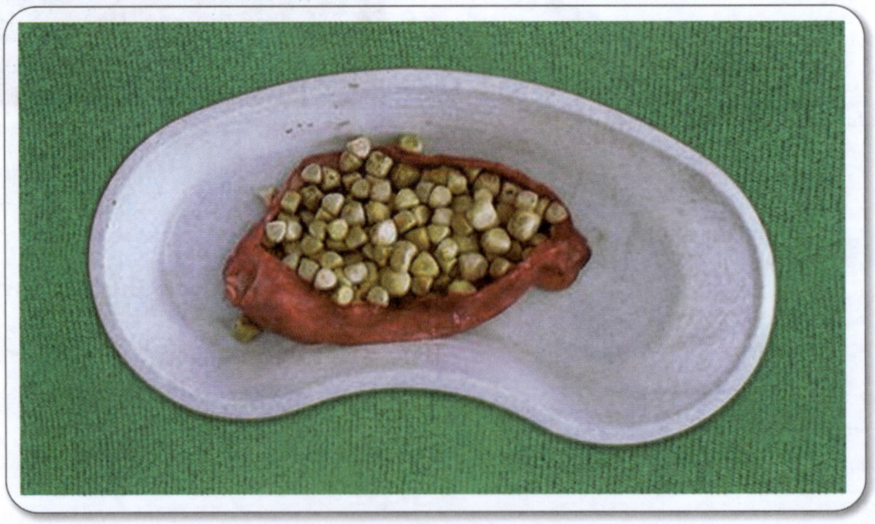

Multiple cholesterol stones in an obese female

Brown pigment	Black pigment

• **Common in Asia***
• **Always radiolucent stone**
• Due to bile stasis and infection**
• **MC stone in infection**—*E. coli**, Ascaris and Clonorchis sinensis
• MC in presence of FB, clips, stents, parasites**
• MC type of stone seen in Hepatolithiasis (Oriental Cholangiohepatitis)—intra hepatic stone.
• Primary bile duct stone formation** (Formed in bile duct itself)—MC primary bile duct stone is Brown Stone.
• **Patient coming with CBD stone after cholecystectomy:**
  ○ <2 years: Retained stone
  ○ >2 years: Recurrent stone
  ○ **MC recurrent stone is brown stone**
	MC in hemolytic states
	• Hereditary spherocytosis, sickle cell disease
	• Heart valves [mechanical]
	• Liver cirrhosis
	• Gilbert's syndrome
	• Cystic fibrosis
	• Ileal resection

Clinical Features of Gallstones

- Mostly asymptomatic
- MC symptom—**Biliary Colicky**** (Pain after eating fatty foods)—Misnomer—it is not a typical colicky pain. The pain increases gradually after food intake and gets relieved once the stone in cystic duct passes out or falls inside the GB. Usually pain starts after 45 minutes. Surgery advised for such cases.

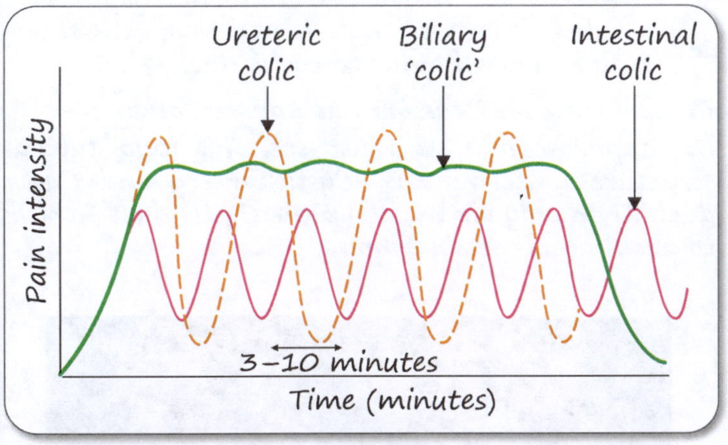

Complications of Gallstones

- Acute Cholecystitis—MC complication
- Chronic Cholecystitis
- Stone impaction at neck of GB/Cystic duct—Mucocele, Empyema and Perforation.
- Stone near Hartman's pouch or neck and compressing CBD—Mirizzi Syndrome
- GB can adhere to adjacent bowel and result in Cholecystoduodenal fistula—Gallstone ileus**
- Cancer GB—0.5%
- CBD entry of stone—Cholangitis, Gallstone pancreatitis

Acute Cholecystitis

- C/F—Pain in right hypochondrium
- **Murphy's sign:** Tenderness in 9th costal cartilage on deep breath. Done in sitting position
- **Moynihan's method:** Patient lies down and the tenderness elicited by palpation using thumb.
- Boas sign—Sign of Hyperesthesia**
- IOC—USG abdomen
- Gold standard—HIDA scan shows nonvisualization of GB.

Tokyo Guideline of Acute Cholecystitis

Mild cholecystitis grade 1	Moderate cholecystitis grade 2	Severe cholecystitis grade 3
Only clinical features seen	• Clinical features+ • Elevated WBC count+ (>18000) • Palpable Mass+ • Gangrene+ • Localized features only	• Signs of organ failure++ • Renal • Respiratory • Hypotension • Altered sensorium
Advised lap cholecystectomy	Immediate surgery by lap or open cholecystectomy	Treatment is urgent percutaneous cholecystectomy

Management:

- Nil oral
- IVF
- Ryles tube aspiration
- Higher antibiotics
- Early or Interval Cholecystectomy
- Early Cholecystectomy (Bailey says in 72 hours; other books say up to 7 days)—Mostly followed. The only problem is more chances of conversion from lap to open method.
- Interval cholecystectomy or delayed one is done after 6 weeks.

Mirizzi Syndrome

- Stone in Hartman's or Neck causing compression of CBD
- Causes Obstructive Jaundice

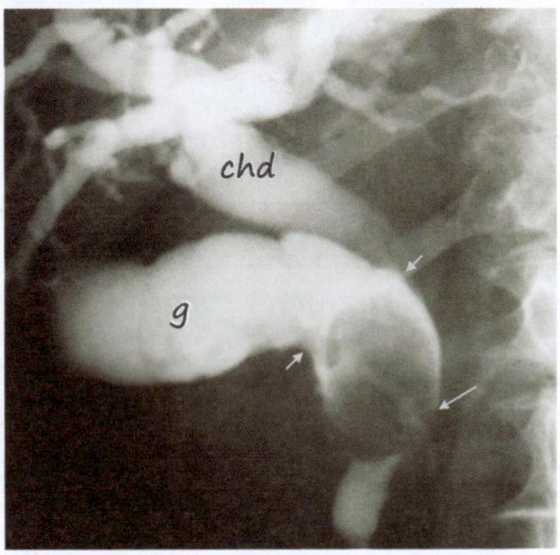

Mirizzi syndrome

Gallstone Ileus

- Inflamed GB adhered with duodenum; huge stone passes from GB to duodenum in the fistula. (usual size >3 cm stone)
- Can cause obstruction in duodenum—Bouveret Syndrome
- Can cause obstruction in terminal ileum—Intestinal obstruction—Gallstone Ileus
- Triad: **Rigler's Triad:**
    - Tumbling obstruction of bowel (motion passed due to movement of stone and there is tumbling obstruction)
    - Fistula between GB and bowel
    - Pneumobilia

Treatment:

- **Unstable patients**—Enterotomy and stone removal
- **Stable patients**—Along with enterotomy and stone removal, GB is removed and fistula is closed

Gallbladder Cancer

- Incidence = <0.5%
- Risk increased—stone >2.5 cm size, Stone + polyp, Family history

Management of Gallstones

Medical treatment:

- Useful only for cholesterol gallstones not for pigment stones*
- Mechanism is by inhibiting HMG-CoA reductase in cholesterol synthesis, thus decrease cholesterol super saturation or by giving Ursodeoxycholic acid (UDCA) and increasing bile salts.

Useful only in**

- Radiolucent
- Size <15 mm
- Functioning gallbladder
- Nonacute symptoms

Surgical treatment:

- Lap or Open Cholecystectomy (MC done is Laparoscopic method)
- 1st Lap Cholecystectomy done by Erich Muhe
- 4 Ports needed—Primary port at umbilicus and three secondary ports along Right Hypochondrium (Epigastrium, MCL and Anterior Axillary Line)
- **Two methods:**
    i. **Antegrade method**—From calot's triangle to fundus (MC done method)
    ii. **Retrograde method**—Fundus first Approach* when calot's triangle is not clear, dissection done from fundus to cystic duct.

Critical view of Strassberg at Laparoscopy:

On Laparoscopy, we must see only two tubular structures entering GB—Cystic artery and Cystic duct. Then only we must clip the Cystic duct—this is to avoid accidentally clipping CBD

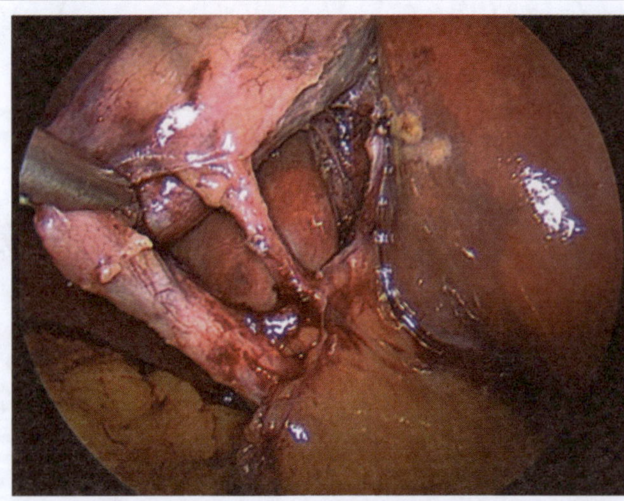

Bile Duct Injury—Protocol

- Post-cholecystectomy patient—C/O Abdominal pain + Fever
- O/E—Severe tenderness in right hypochondrium and increased Pulse rate – **Suspect Bile duct injury**
- **Incidence—0.3–0.8% in Lap and 0.1–0.2% in Open Surgery**
- 1st done investigation is USG abdomen. USG abdomen shows collection in RIF known as **Bilioma**
- Immediately Percutaneous drainage of Bilioma done
- PCD draining bile and gradually gets reduced in two more weeks
- After two weeks, we must do the **IOC for Bile duct injury—ERCP****

  ERCP shows—Strasberg classification for Bile duct injury and leak:
  - **Type A:** Cystic duct leak, or leak from ducts of Luschka
  - **Type B:** Aberrant duct clipped
  - **Type C:** Aberrant duct cut
  - **Type D:** Lateral injury
  - **Type E:** Transection of CBD

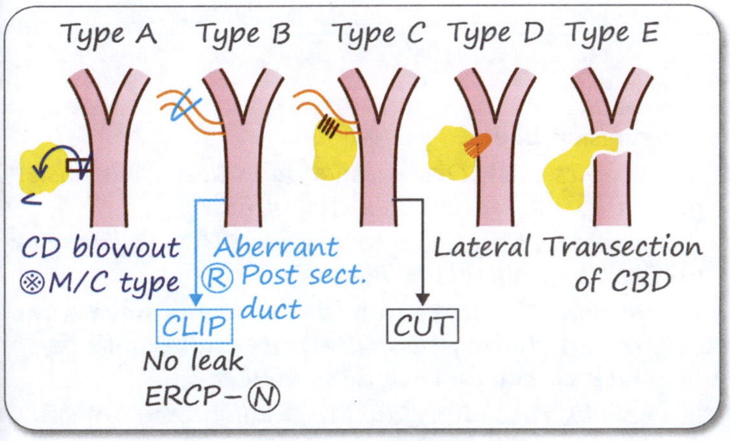

Strasberg classification

After 8-12 weeks, the injuries will heal with strictures; IOC for bile duct strictures is MRCP*

Classification of Bile duct strictures in MRCP—Bismuth classification

- **Type 1:** Low common hepatic duct stricture; stump >2 cm
- **Type 2:** Proximal stricture; stump <2 cm
- **Type 3:** Hilar stricture; confluence intact
- **Type 4:** Destructed confluence; right and left ducts separated
- **Type 5:** Involvement of right aberrant sectoral duct alone or along with stricture at CHD.

Gold Standard treatment of bile duct stricture—**Hepatico Jejunostomy**

CBD Stones

Incidence—6–12% of GB stones*

Primary CBD stone	Secondary CBD stone
• Formed in bile duct itself • Usually they are brown pigment** stones (soft and earthy) • MC in Asian population* • Usually due to foreign bodies, stasis and infection.	• Formed in gallbladder and enters CBD by migration • MC in western countries. • Cholesterol stones

Extra Edge:

- ERCP is the diagnostic and therapeutic treatment of choice*
- A dilated CBD >8 mm strongly suggests Gallstones*
- Increased Serum Bilirubin, SGOT/SGPT and Alkaline Phosphatase implies presence of CBD obstruction.

Cholangitis

Infection and inflammation of biliary tract is known as cholangitis.

Etiological Factors:

- CBD stone (MC cause)
- ERCP
- Benign and malignant strictures
- Parasites

MC Organisms—*E. coli***, Klebsiella, Streptococcal Faecalis, Bacteroides

Clinical Features: MC presentation—Fever with chills and rigors*

Charcot's Triad*

CBD stone causing cholangitis

- Pain
- Jaundice
- Rigors

  Mortality is 10%

Reynolds Pentad*

Includes Charcot triad + Septic shock + Mental status changes

Treatment of Cholangitis:

- Immediately start IV Fluids and Broad Spectrum Antibiotics.
- Urgent Biliary Decompression is the priority in management of Cholangitis if they do not respond to antibiotics.
- Mortality—50%

CBD stone with no cholangitis

- **Treatment of Choice is**
  - ERCP + Sphincterotomy + removal of stones and stenting followed by Lap cholecystectomy (Two stage procedure)
  - Laparoscopic removal of CBD + Cholecystectomy (Single stage procedure)
  - Open Cholecystectomy + CBD exploration and removal of stone
- Most commonly followed procedure is ERCP followed by Lap cholecystectomy**

CBD Exploration:

- Opening the bile duct vertically and removal of stone.
- If CBD <12 mm; T tube and closure
- If CBD >12 mm; Choledochoduodenostomy

ERCP Contraindications:

- CBD stone >1.5 cm
- Multiple impacted stones
- Ampullary stenosis
- More proximal stone

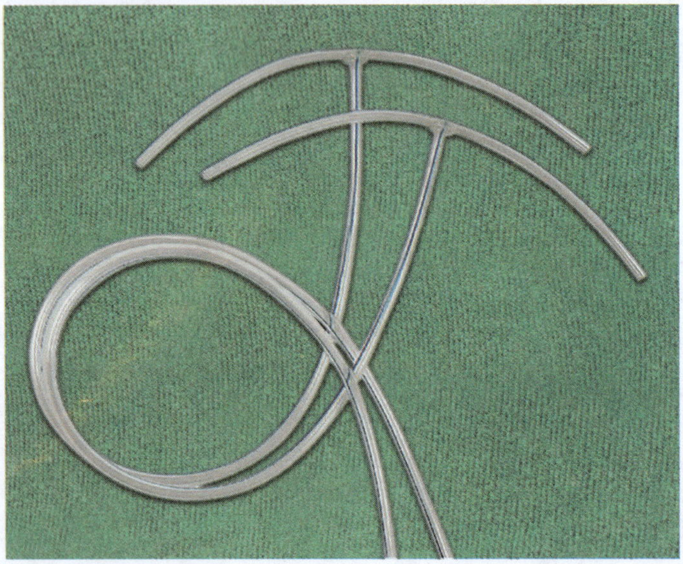

T tube

Removal of T Tube:

- After doing T tube Cholangiogram—usually done on 7/8th POD
- If T tube cholangiogram is normal—Remove the T tube on 10–14 days and discharge

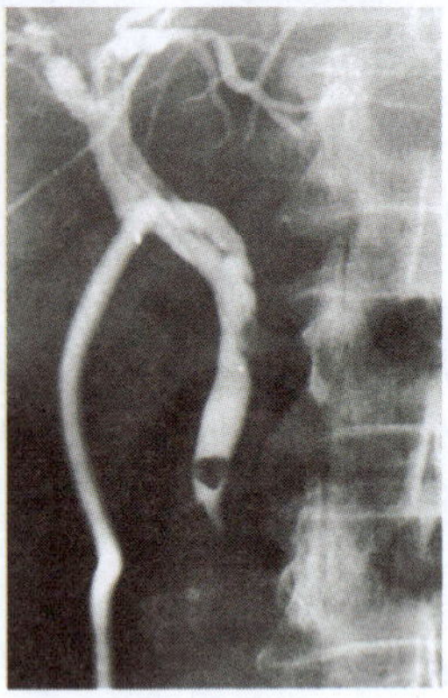

T tube cholangiogram shows missed stone

Retained or missed stone (<2 years)	Recurrent stones (>2 years)—Brown Pigment stone
ERCP and Sphincterotomy and balloon clearance	• The recurrent stones are usually bigger (>2 cm size) and usually not feasible for ERCP. • Choledochotomy and stone removal followed by CHOLEDOCHO DUODENOSTOMY**

Extra mile

Courvoisier Law:

In patients with Obstructive Jaundice: Courvoisier gave a law based on Palpatory finding.

If the obstruction is due to stone in CBD, Gallbladder will not be palpable (Figure A)

- **Reason:** The stone in bile duct would have come from a cholecystitis GB, so its wall would be so thick to get further distended.

If the obstruction is due to malignancy in CBD, Gallbladder will be palpable (Figure B)

- **Reason:** The gallbladder here is a normal GB so it will get distended to the maximum size once the bile duct gets obstructed.

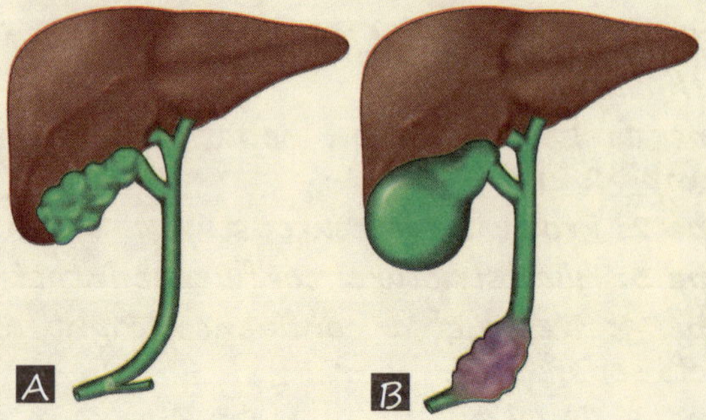

Miscellaneous Lesions

Choledochal cyst	Extra hepatic biliary atresia
Abnormal dilatation of bile duct is known as Choledochal cyst. MC in infants, female	Inside the liver bile duct is normal Once outside the liver the bile ducts are atretic* • MC in newborn • Equal in male and female
Clinical features: Triad of: • Pain • Jaundice • Mass	**C/F:** • Obstructive jaundice • Itching • Cholangitis
Complications: • Stones • Cirrhosis • PV thrombosis • Cholangitis • Malignancy risk—in bile duct, pancreas, liver or GB. MC on posterior wall of cyst	**Complications:** • Cholangitis • Liver cirrhosis—Secondary biliary type

Todani or Alonso Classification:
• **Type 1:** Fusiform dilatation
• **Type 2:** Diverticulum type
• **Type 3:** Ampullary level diverticulum, choledochocele
• **Type 4:**
  ○ 4a—All ducts intra and extra hepatic dilated
  ○ 4b—Extra hepatic dilatation
• **Type 5:** (Caroli's disease)
  ○ Intrahepatic dilatation
	Types of EHBA:
	• **Type 1:** Common bile duct level atresia—GB enlarged
	• **Type 2:** Atresia at CHD, no GB enlarged
	• **Type 3:** At porta hepatis level—90% MC type

Investigations: IOC - MRCP Caroli's Disease—Shows a sign on CECT abdomen; **Central Dot sign****—Portal vein radicle appears like that	**IOC—Liver Biopsy is Gold standard now** (Old answer was percutaneous cholangiography) **USG abdomen**—Triangular cord sign seen.
Management: It needs to be resected as there is malignancy risk • **Type 1 and 2:** Resect the cyst and do Hepaticojejunostomy • **Type 3:** Transduodenal sphincteroplasty • **Type 4 and 5:** Liver transplantation	**Management:** 1st Line—Kasai procedure "Portoenterostomy" Bridging procedure for liver transplant which is Gold standard treatment

Images

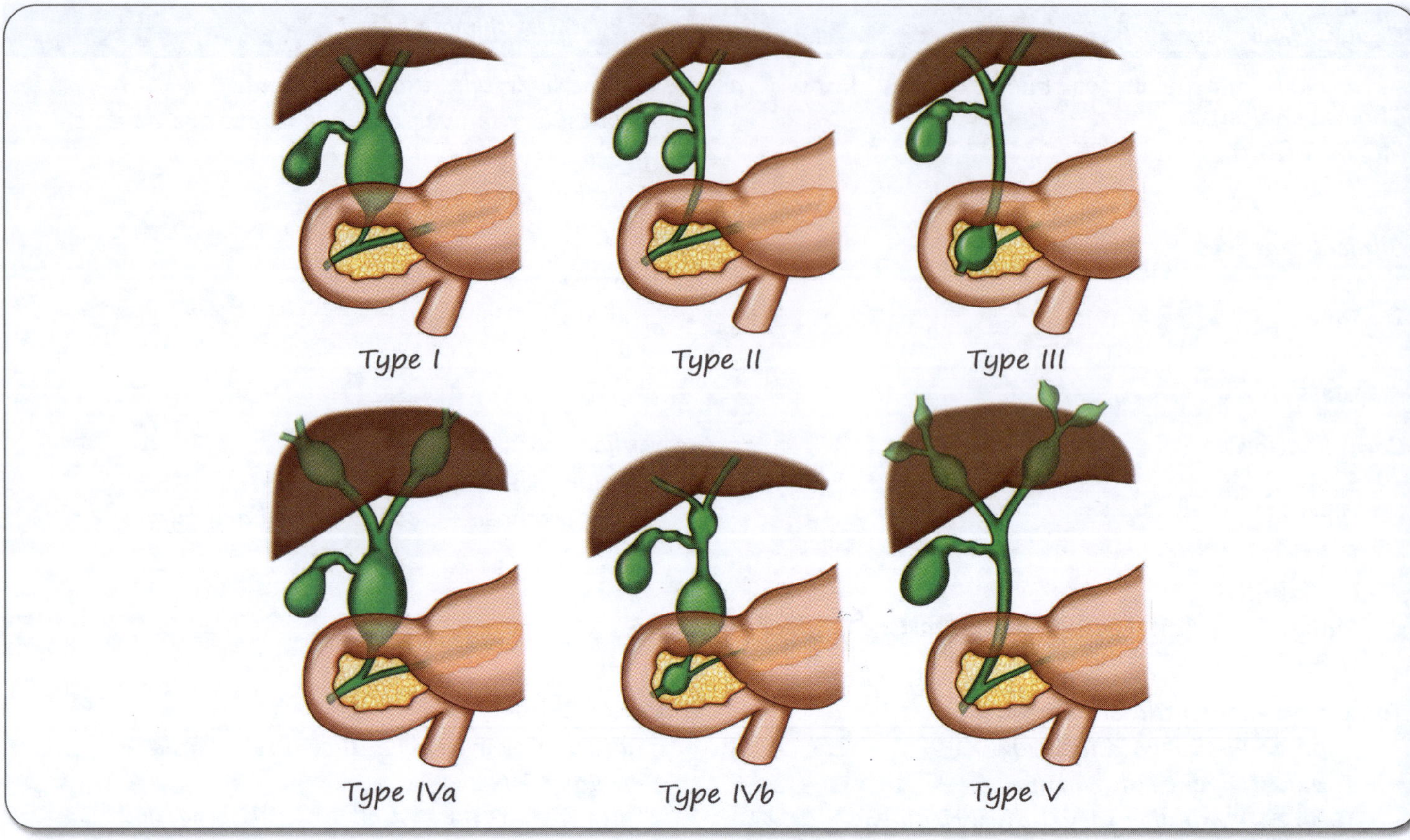

Todani classification

Cancer Gallbladder and Bile Duct

- MC site of malignancy in biliary system—Gallbladder
- In bile duct cancer common at bifurcation—Klatskin Tumor**

Clinical Features

- GB malignancy is associated with stones in 90% cases and mimics symptoms of gallstones.
- Pain, jaundice and weight loss.
- As per Courvoisier law, the GB may be palpable in GB cancer and distal bile duct cancer.

Gallbladder Cancers

Predisposing Factors:

- **MC—Gallstones**
  - 0.5% of gallstones lead to cancer
  - 95% of cancer GB will have stones**
  - Incidence is 10% if stone size 3 cm or more.
- Polyps >10 mm
- Typhoid carriers
- Estrogen
- Clonorchis sinensis
- Ulcerative colitis
- Choledochal cyst
- Primary sclerosing cholangitis
- Carcinogens; nitrosamines, rubber and dyes and chemicals.

Investigations:

- USG usually shows gallstones or gallstones with polyps or a mass lesion is usually the 1st done investigation.
- IOC – CECT abdomen with triple phase contrast
- Tumor Marker—CEA

Management and Staging:

TNM staging	Procedure
T1a—Tumor into lamina propria	Laparoscopic/simple cholecystectomy is enough
T1b—Tumor into Muscle layer	If Perineural invasion, vascular invasion, LN or margins are not involved, laparoscopic cholecystectomy is enough. If above are positive—we do extended Cholecystectomy • Liver resected with a margin of 2 cm • Bile duct is removed if Cystic Duct margin +ve • Nodes removed—pericholedochal nodes, periportal nodes, Celiac nodes, hilar and retro duodenal nodes.
T2—Tumor into perimuscular connective tissue	Radical Cholecystectomy: • Remove segments—4b + 5 • Remove all nodes mentioned already
T3—Serosal perforation and/or direct invasion of the liver or any other single extrahepatic organ	• Radical cholecystectomy—4b + 5 or • Extended right hepatectomy—4a + 4b + 5, 6, 7, 8 or • Central (Taj Mahal) hepatectomy—4b + 5 + 8
T4—Invades main PV or HA or two or more extrahepatic organs	Inoperable cancer

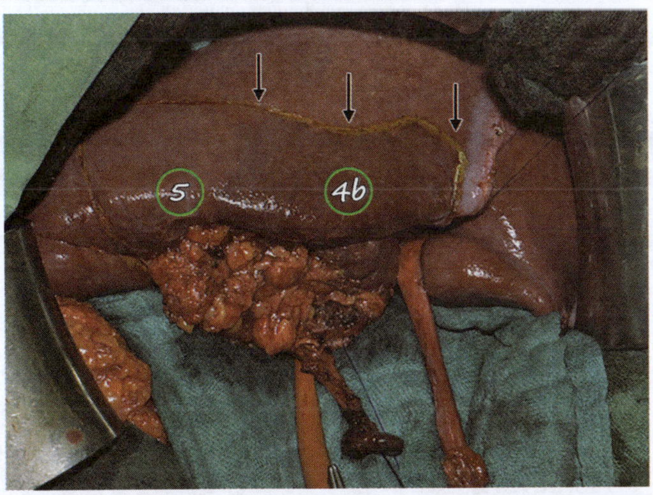

Radical cholecystectomy for cancer gallbladder

Extra mile

- Median Survival of Unresectable cases—2–4 months only*
- Gemcitabine + Cisplatin is used for Unresectable cases.

Bile Duct Cancer

- IOC for staging—MRCP + MRA
- Tumor marker—CA 19–9 and CEA

Bismuth Corlette Classification of Bile Duct Cancers

- **Type 1:** At common hepatic duct only
- **Type 2:** Involving confluence without involvement of secondary ducts
- **Type 3a:** Involving right secondary intrahepatic ducts
- **Type 3b:** Involving left secondary intrahepatic ducts
- **Type 4:** Involves secondary ducts on both sides.

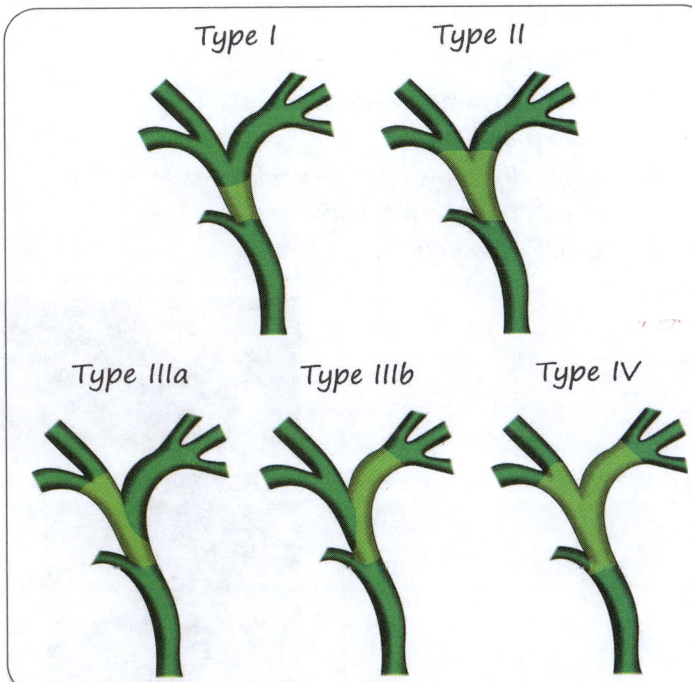

Bismuth Corlette classification of Hilar cancers

PANCREAS

Differences between Annular Pancreas and Pancreas Divisum

Annular pancreas	Pancreas divisum
• Ventral and dorsal bud encircle the pancreas like a ring** • C/F—Gastric outlet obstruction • Associated with Down's Syndrome, Duodenal atresia • IOC – CECT abdomen • ERCP will show absence of ventral bud. • **Treatment:** Duodeno Duodenostomy (Bailey) or Duodenojejunostomy** Resection not needed.	• Minor duct is draining the major part of pancreas. • Hence, there will be recurrent pancreatitis. • IOC—ERCP >MRCP • Treatment—Minor duct sphinterotomy** 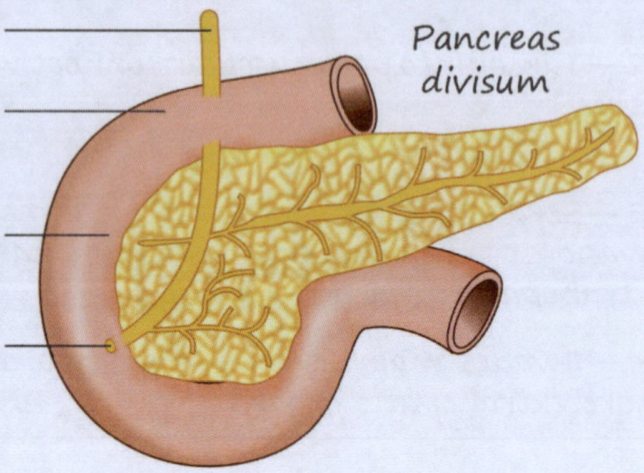

Acute Pancreatitis

Etiology of Pancreatitis

(GET- SMASHED- I)

- G - Gallstones (MC cause in adults)
- E - Ethanol
- T - Trauma (MC cause in children)
- S - Steroids
- M - Mumps
- A - Autoimmune (PAN, SLE, etc.)
- S - Scorpion venom
- H - Hyperlipidemia, Hypercalcemia, Hyperparathyroidism
- E - ERCP, Emboli
- D - Drugs (Azathioprine, Thiazides, Furosemide, Tetracyclines, 6- Mercaptopurine, etc.)
- I - Infections (Coxsackie, CMV, Echovirus)

Symptoms:	Signs
• Pain radiating to back • Nausea • Vomiting • Sudden abdominal pain with partial relief on leaning forward [Mohammedan prayer sign]**	• Grey-Turner's sign—hemorrhagic pigmentation around the flanks* • Cullen's sign—pigmentation around umbilicus* • Fox Sign**—Inguinal Ecchymosis

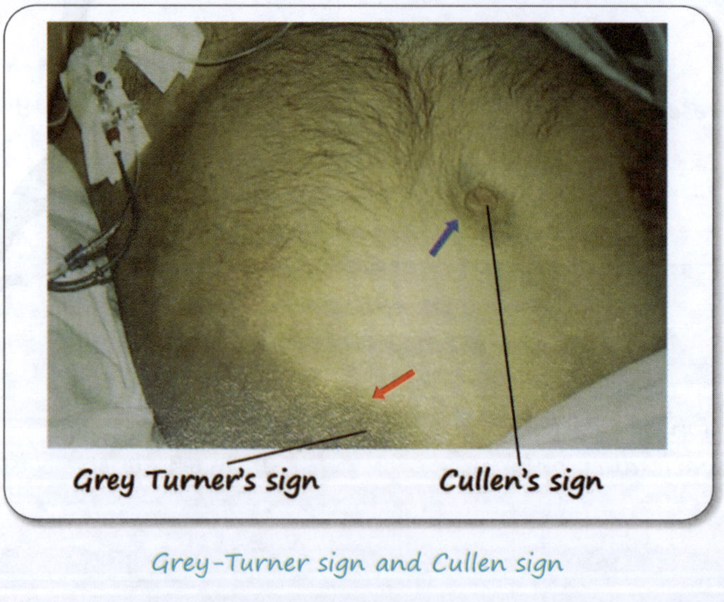

Grey-Turner sign and Cullen sign

X-ray Abdomen Erect Findings

- Gasless abdomen**
- Colon cut off sign**
- Ground glass appearance
- Sentinel loop sign
- Renal halo sign

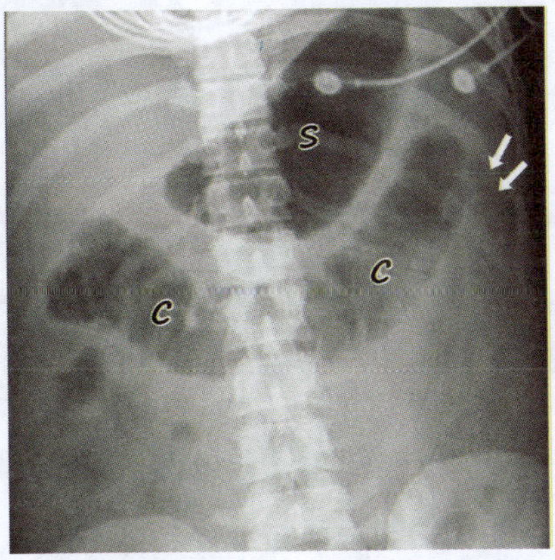

Colon cut off sign

Investigations

- **Serum amylase:** Four times increased than normal, not specific. It can be elevated in other GI pathologies—perforation, obstruction, diverticulitis, mesenteric ischemia.
- Serum amylase usually becomes normal 3 days after attack.
- Most sensitive and specific test- Serum Lipase**
- CRP: >150 implies severe AP.
- Radiological IOC—CECT abdomen with oral and IV contrast (usually advised after 72 hours)—Balthazar Score or CTSI (CT Severity Index).

Scoring Systems in Acute pancreatitis

BISAP Score:

- B – Blood Urea Nitrogen
- I – Impaired Mental status
- S – SIRS
- A – Age >60 years
- P – Pleural effusion

Ranson Score: (Mnemonic – LAGAW BUCHOW)

On admission	Within 48 hours
L – LDH >350 u/L	B – Base deficit >4 mmol/L
A – AST >250 units	U – Blood Urea N2 >5 mg/dL
G – Glucose >200 mg/dL or >1.1 mmol/L	C – Calcium <2.0 mmol/L
A – Age >55 years	H – Hematocrit fall >10%
W – WBC Count >16000/mm^3	O – Arterial O_2 saturation PaO_2 <60 mm Hg
	W – Water sequestration >61

CT Severity Index (old Name Balthazar)

Pancreas inflammation	Necrosis
Normal – 0	<30% necrosis – 2
Focal/diffuse enlargement – 1	30–50% necrosis – 4
Intrinsic changes – 2	>50% necrosis – 6
Single fluid collection – 3	
Multiple fluid collection – 4	

CTSI score	Morbidity	Mortality
Mild: 0–3	8%	3%
Moderate: 4–6	35%	6%
Severe: 7–10	92%	17%

Revised Atlanta Classification:

Organ failure	Local complications	Systemic complications
Shock: SBP <90 mm Hg	Necrosis	DIC
ARDS: PaO_2 <60 mm Hg	Pseudocyst	Metabolic disturbances
ARF: Se. creatinine >2 mg	Abscess	Fibrinogen level decreasing
GI bleed >500 mL/day		

RAC Classification takes into account all the above:

- **Mild:** No local complication or organ failure (only amylase increased)
- **Moderate:** Organ Failure +, but it is transient and it resolves in 48 hours** + Local/Systemic Complications but no persistent organ failure (in 48 hours patient recovers).
- **Severe: >48 hours:** There is persistent organ failure + Local or systemic complications.

Complications of Acute Pancreatitis

- Release of Trypsinogen which will activate all the enzymes from pancreas and does Autodigestion and results in list of complications:

Local complications

- **<4 weeks:** Acute pancreatic fluid collection (APFC)
- **>4 weeks:** Pseudocyst
- **<4 weeks:** Acute Necrotic fluid collection (Necrotic material also seen)
- **>4 weeks:** Walled off pancreatic necrosis (WOPN)
- **MC complication – Infection (Pancreatic abscess)**—MC cause of late death and MC local complication causing death.
- Pancreatic ascites
- Pancreaticopleural fistula
- Pleural effusion
- Splenic vein thrombosis
- Splenic artery aneurysm (false aneurysm caused by Elastase enzyme)
- Colonic gangrene or perforation

Pseudocyst of Pancreas

- Follows acute or chronic pancreatitis
- MC site is lesser sac. (But can happen anywhere inside abdomen)
- MC near body and tail of pancreas**

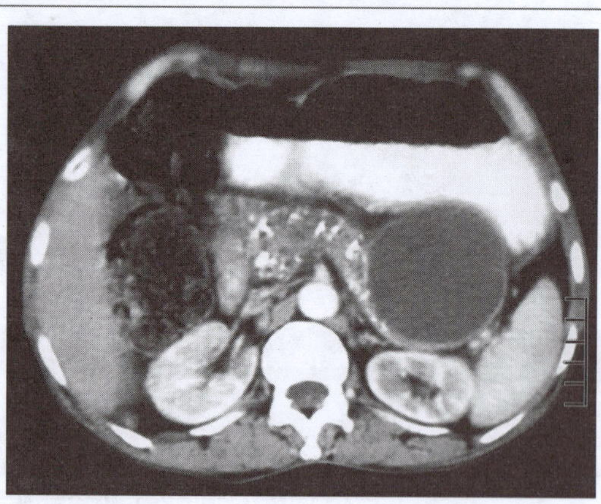

Pseudocyst in tail of pancreas in a chronic pancreatitis

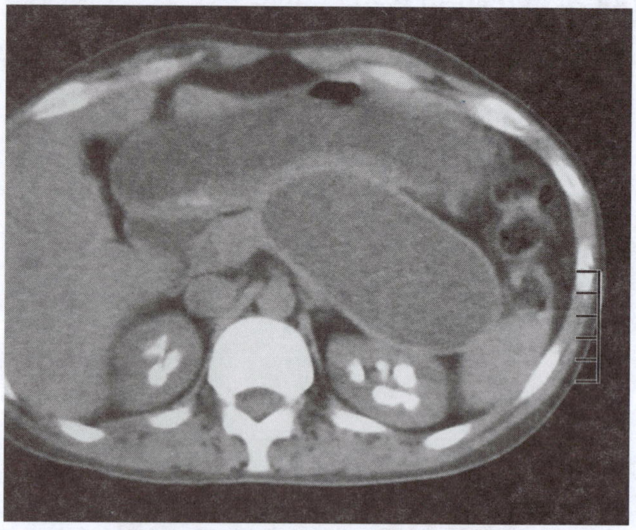

Pseudocyst in pancreas following acute pancreatitis

- C/F—Presents after 4 weeks with persistent pain and epigastric fullness and vomiting and early satiety**
- Persistent elevation of Serum Amylase
- IOC – CECT abdomen;
- EUS guided Fluid analysis shows—Increased amylase and Normal CEA (To differentiate from Cystic Neoplasm)

Management

- Surgery advised for Symptomatic pseudocysts only and for complications.
- Old Rule: Rule of 6: Surgery done if cyst >6 weeks, >6 cm diameter or thickness 6 mm wall.

Complications in Pseudocyst

- MC complication—Infection (Pancreatic abscess)
- Rupture into abdominal cavity causes pancreatic ascites
- Rupture into Thoracic cavity—Pancreaticopleural fistula
- Bleeding (Known as Hemosuccus Pancreaticus**)

Surgical Treatment

- **Internal drainage:** Cystojejunostomy > Cysto-gastrostomy or Cystoduodenostomy
- Cystogastrostomy done by open method, Endoscopic method or laparoscopic method
- Infected Pseudocyst—External drainage done

Extra Edge

- MC cause of death in these cases in MODS-Multiple organ dysfunction syndrome.
- Mortality in first 2 weeks—MODS
- Mortality after 2 weeks—Septic Complications

Chronic Pancreatitis

Chronic pancreatitis is a triad made of:

- Endocrine loss: >90% lost results in Diabetes
- Exocrine loss: >90% lost results in Steatorrhea
- Strictures and stones—Severe Pain Epigastric region radiating to back; pain is not due to enzymes; it is due to Ductal Hypertension.

TIGAR—O Classification of Etiology

- T - Toxic (Alcohol)—MC causes
- I - Idiopathic/Tropical—Unknown cause; Eating Casava Root fibers in Kerala
- G - Genetic-PRSS gene mutation, SPINK-1 gene mutation, CFTR gene mutation
- A - Autoimmune
- R - Recurrent Acute Pancreatitis (like in Pancreas Divisum)
- O - Obstructive

Clinical Features

- Pain abdomen; severe recurrent pain; addicted to Opioids
- Diabetes—responds only to Insulin
- Steatorrhea

Investigations

- **Tests for steatorrhea:**
  - Fecal measurement of Elastase: <100: severe deficiency; >200 is normal
  - Fecal fat excretion (on 100 g fat given): >7 g/day in stools is steatorrhea
- IOC to diagnose established Chronic Pancreatitis: CECT abdomen—stricture, stones and atrophy
- Gold standard to diagnose early cases of Chronic Pancreatitis: ERCP—Chain of lakes appearance seen**
- Recent Gold standard to diagnose early cases of Chronic Pancreatitis: EUS
- ERCP Criteria—Known as CAMBRIDGE Criteria**
- EUS criteria—Known as Rosemont Criteria**

Management

Pain management:

- Analgesics is given initially
- Celiac plexus Block using Absolute Alcohol**- Laparoscopic or CECT guided method
- Thoracoscopic Sphlanchinectomy also available

Surgical Management:

Drainage procedures	Resection + drainage procedures (Hybrid procedures)	Resection procedure
Dilated duct: >7 mm diameter: Modified Puestow procedure-Lateral Pancreaticojejunostomy procedure	Frey's Procedure—Head coring along with Lateral Pancreaticojejunostomy	Presence of head mass duodenum preserving pancreatic head resection (DPPHR) • Beger's Procedure • Bern's Modification

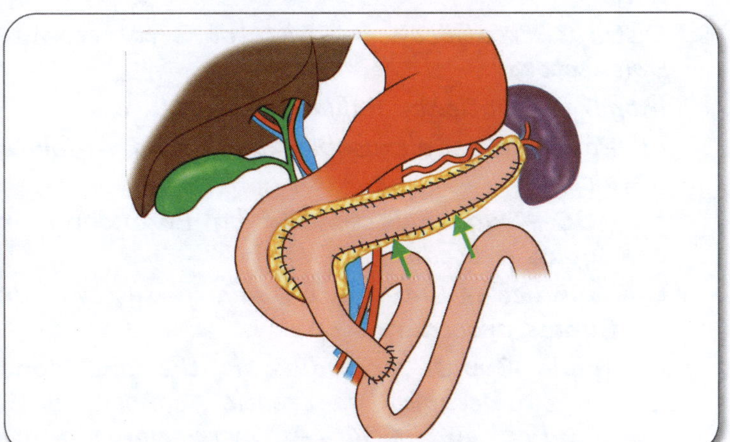

Modified puestow operation

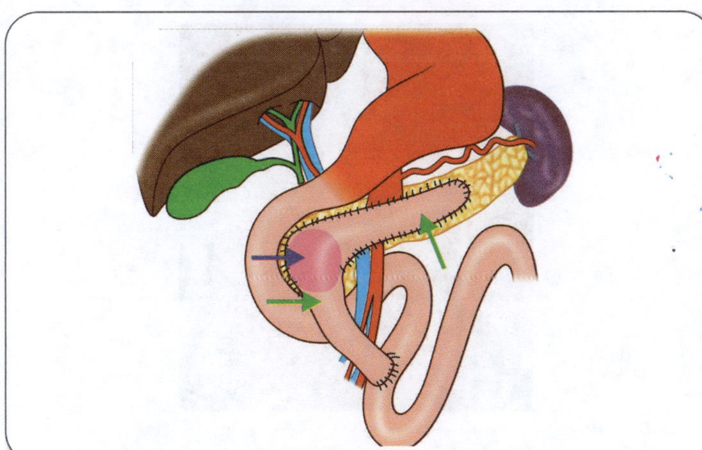

Frey procedure (head coring)

Tumors in Pancreas

Adenocarcinoma of Pancreas

Location of the Cancer in Pancreas:

- Tumor within 2 cm of ampulla is known as Periampullary cancers
- Head of pancreas—Most common site
- Body and tail.

Periampullary cancers	Pancreatic head cancers	Body and tail
• C/F- Painless intermittent jaundice due to sloughing out of tumor • Early presentation and hence has good prognosis • 60% are operable	• C/F- Pain abdomen+ Jaundice • Late diagnosis • Only 10% operable • 90% are inoperable	• Worst prognosis • Presents with mets in 100% cases

Hereditary Risk Factors:

- PRSS1 and SPINK 1 gene mutation- Familial pancreatitis
- STK11- Peutz Jeghers – 100 fold increased risk (Highest risk of all)
- Familial Atypical Mole and Malignant Melanoma Syndrome
- CFTR mutation
- BRCA-2 mutation
- MLH- 1 mutation - Lynch syndrome
- FAP- Familial adenomatous polyposis

K-ras is the most common and the earliest mutation to occur in pancreatic cancers** and is associated with 95% of pancreatic cancers*

Clinical Features:

- Pain abdomen—Head tumors
- Painless intermittent Jaundice—Periampullary cancers
- Vomiting—MC cause is due to external compression of duodenum by tumor**
- Courvoisier's Law—Gallbladder is enlarged in pancreatic cancers.

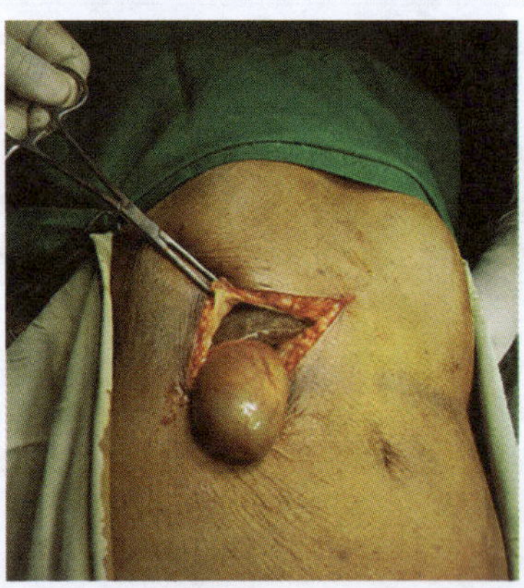

Periampullary cancer with GB enlarged

Investigations:

- CECT abdomen is the IOC for staging
- Tumor Marker—CA – 19–9**
- ERCP/MRCP—Double duct sign seen*

Management of Pancreatic Cancer:

- Resectable cancer in Head of pancreas/ Periampullary cancer is Whipple's operation is done.
- Distal pancreatic cancers-Distal pancreatectomy+ Splenectomy
- Inoperable patients: Palliative procedures
  - Pain; Celiac plexus blockade using Absolute alcohol
  - GOO—Duodenal stenting by Endoscopy or Bypass procedures
  - Jaundice—SEMS into biliary system or Bypass procedures
  - Triple Bypass procedure is the one done for inoperable pancreatic cancer with jaundice and GOO – Gastrojejunostomy+ Cholecystojejunostomy + Jejunojejunostomy

Operable cancers: Whipple's Procedure

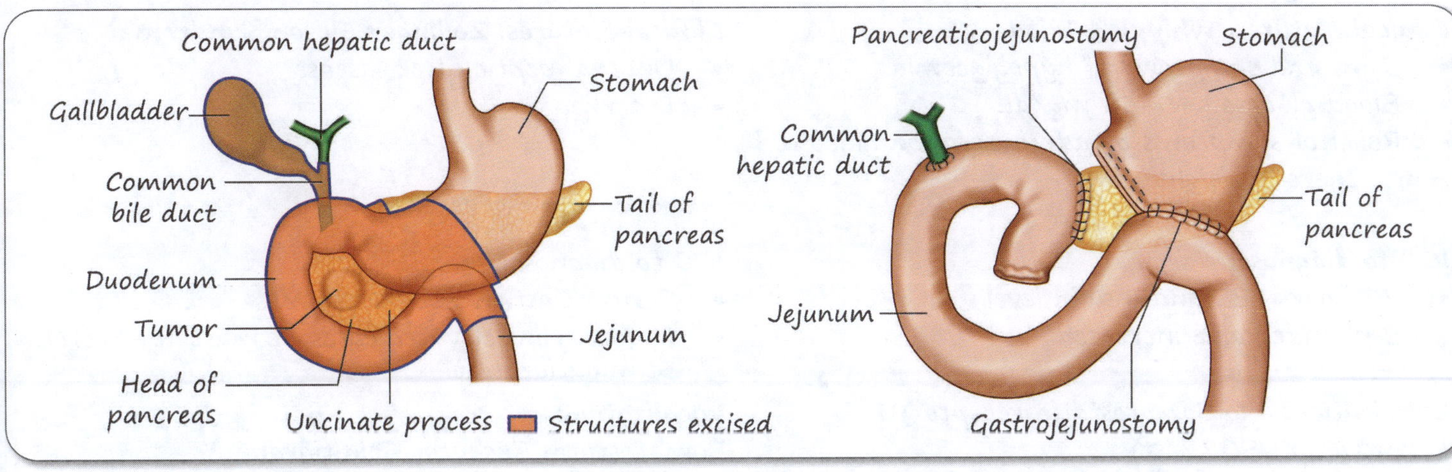

- The most important step in this operation—Pancreaticojejunostomy**

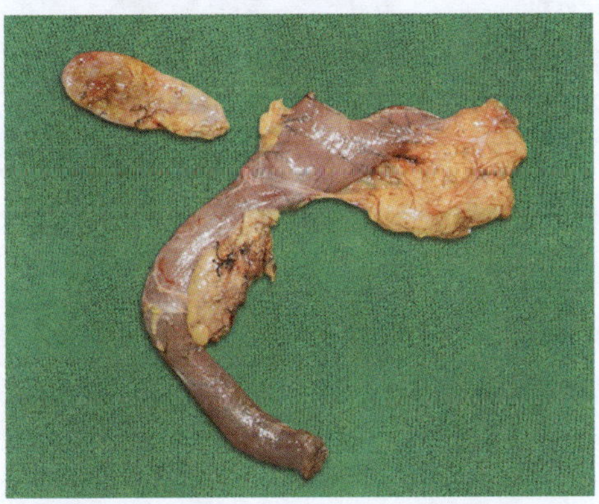

Whipple specimen

Complications of Whipple's Operation:

- **Delayed gastric emptying**—increased Ryles tube aspirate or vomiting—**Incidence 18%**
- **MC cause of death**—PJ anastomosis leak**
- **Pancreatic fistula:** Drain kept after Whipple's operation shows fluids which is having increased amylase content.
- **Bleeding**

Endocrine Tumors of Pancreas

- **MC NET of pancreas:** Pancreatic Polypeptidomas (PPomas)—Nonfunctional
- **MC Functional NET:** Insulinoma in sporadic**; Gastrinoma in MEN-1 Syndrome**

Insulinoma	Gastrinoma
MC NET	MC NET in MEN-1 Syndrome
MC site = Equal in H = B = T	**MC in Passaro triangle** • Junction of CD/CBD • Neck of pancreas • 2/3rd part duodenum 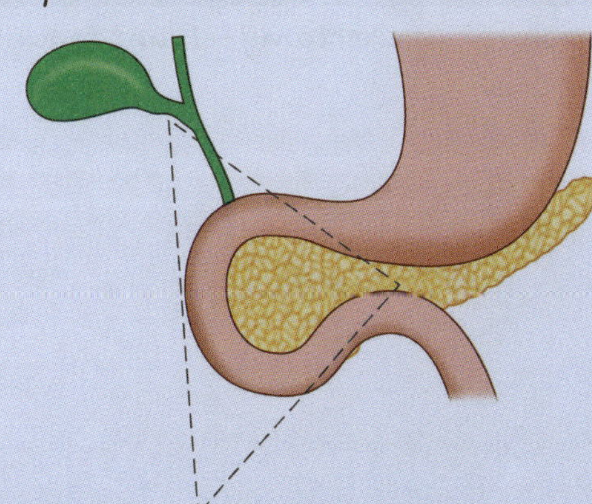 MC site – Duodenum > Pancreas

Contd...

Mostly benign	Mostly malignant
Clinical features: Whipple's Triad • Signs and symptoms of hypoglycemia • Blood glucose <40-50 mg/dL • Relief of symptoms by administration glucose Hence there is weight gain.	**Clinical features: Zollinger Ellison Syndrome** • Unusual peptic ulcer disease • Diarrhea
IOC to diagnose: • 72 hours FBS and Insulin level • C peptide value increased	**IOC to diagnose:** • Serum Gastrin >1000 pg/mL • In borderline elevated cases we must do - Secretin Stimulation test**
Localization: (No Somatostatin receptor) • Intra op USG (Best) • Endo USG • Selective Arteriography venous sampling of blood	**Localization:** Somatostatin Receptor Scinitigraphy**
Management: Enucleation is enough as this is a Benign tumor**	**Management:** Malignancy and hence radical resection needed. • Whipple's is TOC for head tumors • Distal Pancreatectomy for tail and body cases

Other NET

- **Glucagonoma:**
  - Presents with Diabetes+ Dermatitis
  - Dermatitis- Necrolytic migratory erythema**
  - MC in Head*
  - Mostly malignant
- **VIPoma:**
  - Also known as Verner Morrison Syndrome/WDHA syndrome/Pancreatic cholera
  - WDHA syndrome—Watery Diarrhea + Hypokalemia + Achlorrhydria
  - MC site is tail**

SPLEEN

Indications for Splenectomy

Emergency splenectomy	Elective splenectomy
MC indication for splenectomy—Blunt trauma	Idiopathic thrombocytopenic purpura is the MC Elective indication
	During some other surgery: • D2 Lymphadenectomy • Gastric cancer + Spleen infiltration • Pancreatic Tail neoplasm
	Hemolytic Anemias • Sickle cell • Auto immune • Hereditary spherocytosis
	Multiple Abscess in Spleen
	Tumors in Spleen

Methods

- Open method
- HALS—Hand Assisted Laparoscopic Surgery. Hand port used to remove the specimen finally
- Laparoscopic method

Complications of Splenectomy

Immediate complications	Intermediate complications	Delayed complications
• Hemorrhage • Gastric distension • Hematemesis	• MC complication overall is Left Lung Atelectasis** • Pancreatic fistula • Gastric fistula • Subphrenic abscess	• Thromboembolic manifests • OPSI • PV thrombosis

Opportunistic Postsplenectomy Infections

- MC after splenectomy for Hematological causes > trauma causes
- **Bacterial infection****—Inability to remove capsulated bacteria—Streptococcal Pneumonia, H. Influenza and meningococcal
- Parasitic Infection—Babesia and malaria
- Viral Infection—Not increased

Hematological Effects:

- Increased Platelet Counts can cause Thrombotic manifests (if count >10 lacs; Antiplatelet drugs like ASPIRIN started)
- Increased WBC counts

Peripheral Smear after Splenectomy:

- **Howel jolly bodies**—Nonfunctional nucleus
- **Heinz Bodies**—Denatured Hemoglobin
- **Pappenheimer bodies**—Iron particles in RBC
- Target cells

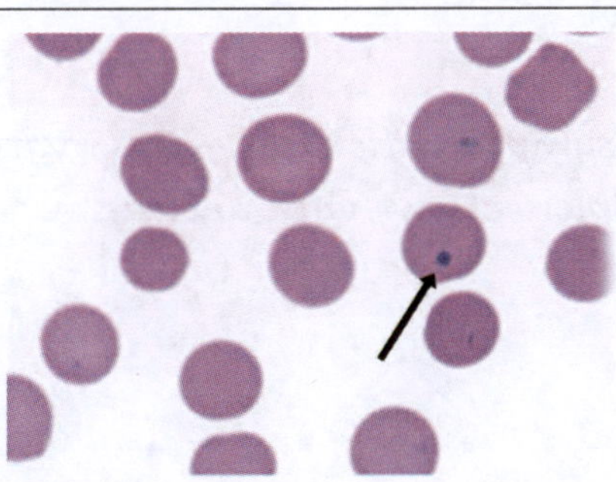

Howel jolly bodies- non functional nucleus

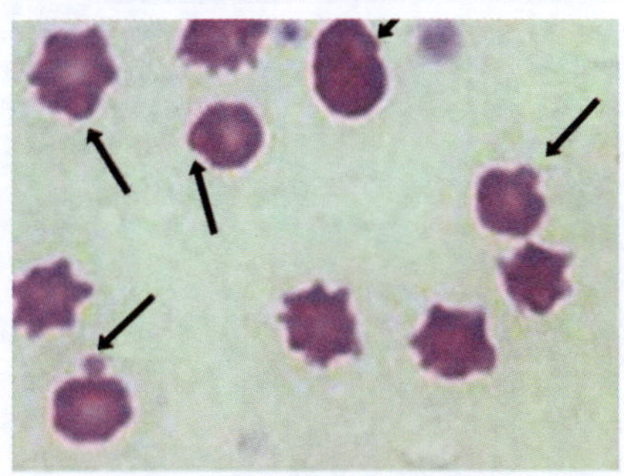

Heinz bodies- denatured Hb

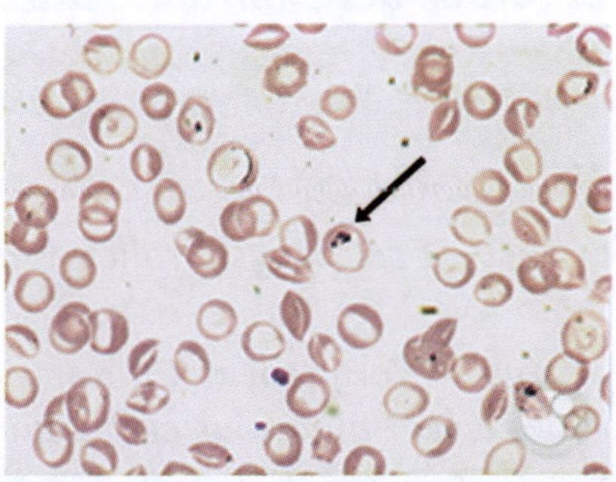

Pappenheimer bodies- iron particles

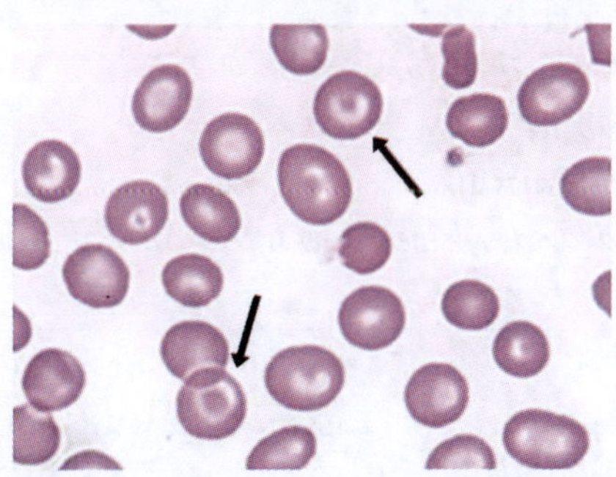

Target cells

Prevention of OPSI:

Three vaccines are given:

- Pneumococcal vaccine
- Meningococcal vaccine
- H. Influenza vaccine
- These vaccines should be ideally given 10–12 weeks prior to elective splenectomy** and at least 14 days prior to surgery.
- If the patient did not receive these vaccines before surgery such as in emergency surgery, vaccine should be given 14 days after splenectomy or upon discharge (to improve compliance) whichever comes first

Vaccination Chart (Latest)

	Pneumococcal	Meningococcal	H. Influenza
Adults	PCV13 PCV 23, 8 weeks later	MenACWY conjugate or polysaccharide and MenB series once	Hib one dose
Booster	PCV 23 at every 5 years	MenACWY every 5 years once	No Booster

Ectopic Spleen: (Splenunculi = Accessory Spleen)

- MC reason is due to embryological non-fusion or incomplete fusion during 5th week of IUL
- Incidence = 10–30%

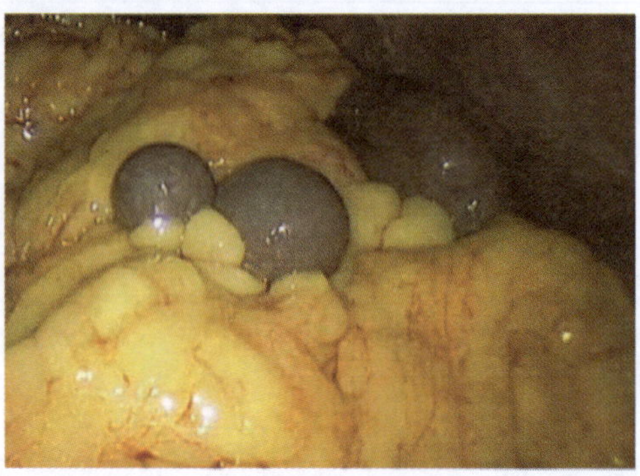

Ectopic spleen

- **It is seen along the Dorsal Mesogastrium:**
  - Splenic Hilum (MC)
  - Tail of Pancreas (2nd MC)
  - Splenocolic ligament
  - Presacral
  - Renal
  - Left side scrotum
- **Properties of Ectopic spleen:**
  - Multiple usually
  - Always have capsule
  - Contains red and white pulp like normal spleen
  - MC to go for torsion**

Splenosis

- Rupture of spleen and its distribution all along the abdominal cavities
- Seen anywhere in abdominal cavity (DD-Ectopic spleen in Dorsal mesogastrium only)

Splenic Artery Aneurysm

- Incidence <1%
- Old age: MC in females
- Solitary
- MC cause- Arteriosclerosis**
- Other etiology: Sepsis and pancreatitis**
- Usually asymptomatic, may rupture suddenly**
- Rupture risk is increased in:
  - Young females
  - Pregnancy (2nd and 3rd trimester)
  - Absence of Calcification
  - Hypertension
  - Size >1.5 cm
- **Management:**
  - Up to 2 cm (Asymptomatic cases)—Observation
- **Indications for Splenectomy with aneurysm:**
  - Symptomatic
  - >2 cm
  - Pregnancy
  - Young age
- Angioembolization can be done for unfit cases.

Splenic Cyst

- MC cyst in spleen—Hydatid Cyst
- MC nonparasitic cyst—Pseudocyst following a Trauma**
- MC cause of true cyst—Congenital Epidermoid Cyst; Rare <10% (Lined by Squamous epithelium). Fluid analysis shows CEA, CA 19–9 +ve. But they are benign**. Partial splenectomy done and leave 25% of spleen to prevent OPSI.

KIDNEY AND URETER

Renal Stones

Types of Stones

Calcium Oxalate (Calcium Oxalate Monohydrate and Dihydrate)

- Also known as mulberry stone due to the appearance
- Most common (MC) type of stone overall
- MC stone to cause hematuria

Triple Phosphate

- Also known as struvite stone
- Staghorn stone due the shape of the stone
- Also known as Jack stone
- MC in infection (associated organism—Proteus)
- MC stone in alkaline urine**

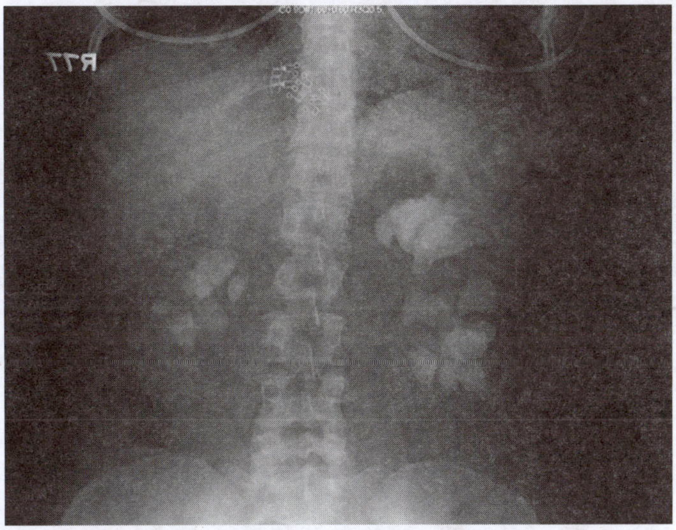

Staghorn calculi

Cystine

- Hard stone
- Associated with cystinuria

Uric Acid

- Radiolucent stone
- Associated with hyperuricemia in gout, cancer

Rare Stones

- Indinavir (HIV patients)—radiolucent
- Xanthine (in xanthine oxidase deficient patients)—radiolucent

Urinary crystals

Image	Description
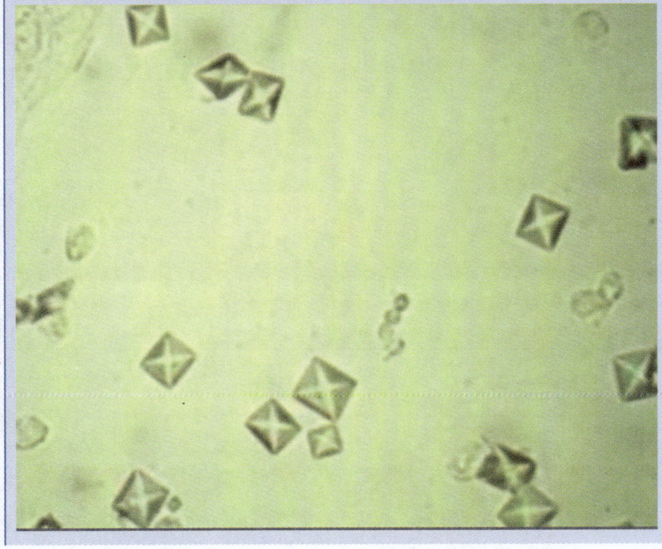	**Calcium oxalate:** • Bipyramidal shape/Envelope-shaped • MC type of crystals in urine

Contd...

Image	Description
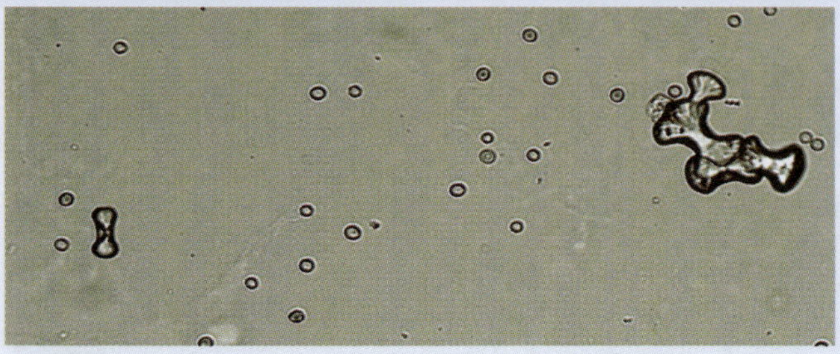	**Calcium oxalate monohydrate:** Dumbbell-shaped or Hourglass-shaped crystals
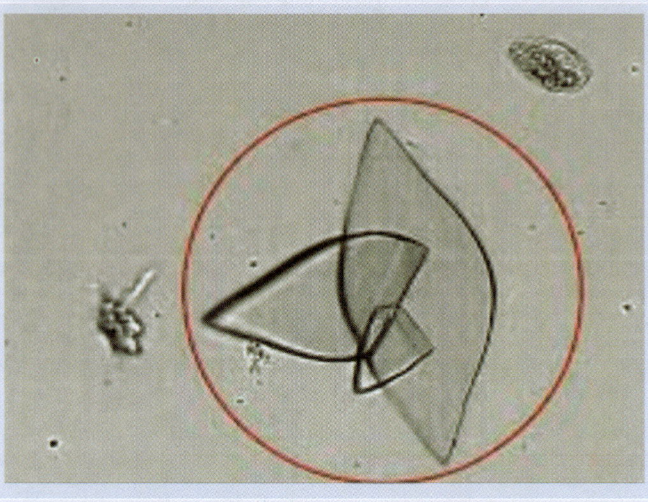	**Uric acid crystals:** • Multifaceted • Irregular plates • Rosettes like
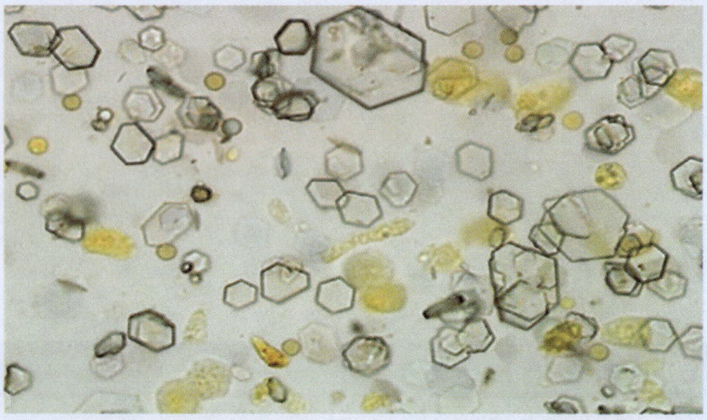	**Cystine crystals:** • Hexagonal • Benzene ring like
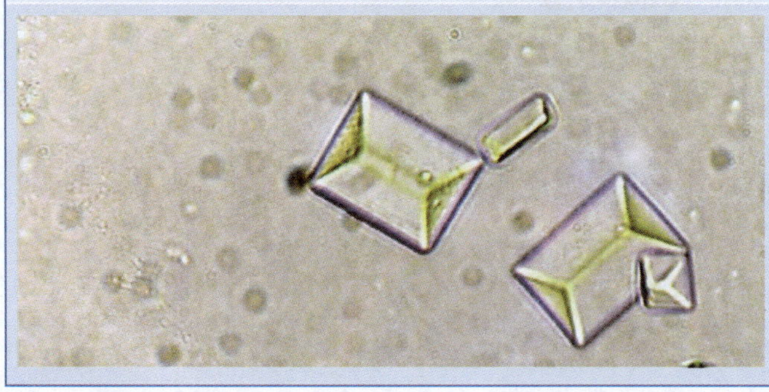	Struvite: Coffin lid shape

Management

Extracorporeal Shock Wave Lithotripsy (ESWL)

Indications:

- <1.5 cm size
- Mainly done for stone in kidney, pelvis, upper ureter

Contraindications:

- Absolute—pregnancy, bleeding diathesis
- **Relative:**
    - Obstruction/distally
    - Infection

Complications:

- Hematuria
- Incomplete clearance
- If stone >1.5 cm, a rare complication known as steinstrasse (Stone street)** happens.

Percutaneous Nephrolithotomy (PCNL)

Indications:

- Stone >2 cm
- Infected
- Obstructed
- Cysteine
- Failed ESWL

- Procedure:
- Transcostal approach
- Subcostal approach
- We insert a guidewire under fluoroscopic guidance—we dilate the tract and insert the nephroscope via the tract and remove the stone.

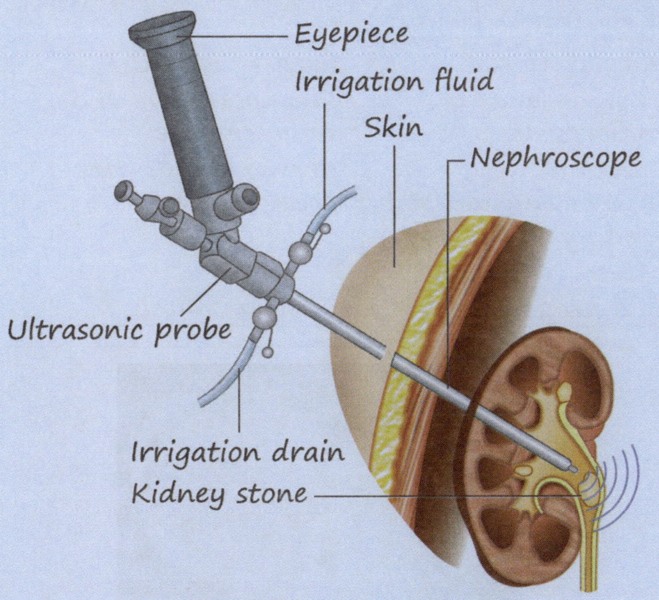

Percutaneous nephrolithotomy

Retrograde Intrarenal Surgery (RIRS)

- For renal pelvis stone
- By retrograde method, we use ureteroscopy to remove intrarenal stones.

Ureteric stone management:

- <5 mm—it will pass
- >5 mm/impacted somewhere—removed by Dormia basket technique.

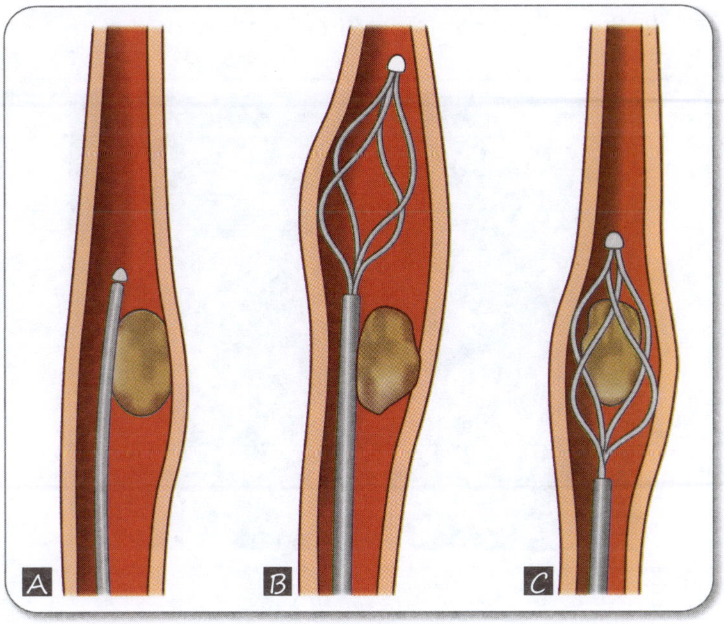

Dormia basket removal

Renal Cell Carcinoma or Grawitz Tumor or Hypernephroma

- Also known as clear cell adenocarcinoma
- MC site—upper pole
- Origin—proximal convoluted tubule
- MC in 50–60 years
- MC in men 2:1 ratio
- MC malignant neoplasm
- MC arises from proximal convoluted tubule**
- MC presentation—renal cell carcinoma (RCC) triad
    - Hematuria (MC symptom)
    - Pain
    - Loin mass

Pathology

Clear cell type	Papillary type	Chromophobe type	Medullary type
• Most common type • MC type • Von Hippel-Lindau (VHL) gene mutation • 3p mutation**	MC in PCKD patients on dialysis	Best prognosis	Associated with sickle cell trait

Clinical Features

- Earliest and MC feature—Hematuria[**]
- Mass can grow inside renal vein—it can grow up to right atrium—it is still operable.
- Young male patient can present with left side varicocele which is irreducible on lying down[**]
- Hematogenous metastasis—pulsatile skull secondaries and cannonball secondaries can develop.
- IOC to diagnose is by CECT abdomen.

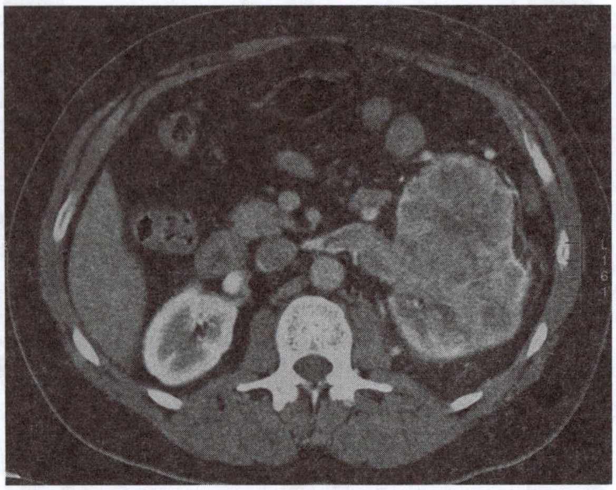

Left side renal cell carcinoma

Paraneoplastic syndrome in:

- Increased ESR (MC)[**]
- Hypertension (2nd MC)
- Anemia (3rd MC)
- Hypercalcemia (5%)
- Polycythemia (3%)
- Stauffer's syndrome—nonmetastatic liver enzyme elevation[**]

Grading and Scoring Systems

- Fuhrman: Nuclear grading system
- Leibovich score: Histological scoring

Radical nephrectomy	Partial nephrectomy (nephron-sparing procedure)
Structures removed: • Kidney • Adrenal gland • Perinephric pad of fat • Regional nodes • Ureter • Gerota's fascia	**Indications:** • T1—<7 cm (even with normal opposite kidney) • Single functioning kidney • VHL mutation—bilateral RCC[**] cases • Renal failure (DM, HTN)

Renal cell cancer	Wilms tumor
Chromosome 3p mutation	8/11th chromosome mutation
Age: 50–60 years	Age: 1–5 years
MC tumors in adults	MC primary tumor in children
C/F: • Hematuria (MC presentation) • Mass • Pain	C/F: • Hematuria • Mass (MC presentation) • Pyrexia **Associated with:** • **Beckwith-Wiedemann syndrome:** Macroglossia + Visceromegaly + Hyperinsulinemia • **WAGR syndrome:** Wilms, Aniridia, Genitourinary (GU) anomalies and Renal anomalies
MC distant metastasis—lung	MC distant metastasis—lung
No need of preoperative biopsy	Preoperative biopsy is must
Surgery is TOC Chemo—and radioresistant **Sunitinib**[**]—(monoclonal antibody) used for metastatic RCC	Surgery is TOC Chemosensitive and radiosensitive Chemo—vincristine, actinomycin
Bad prognosis	Good prognosis

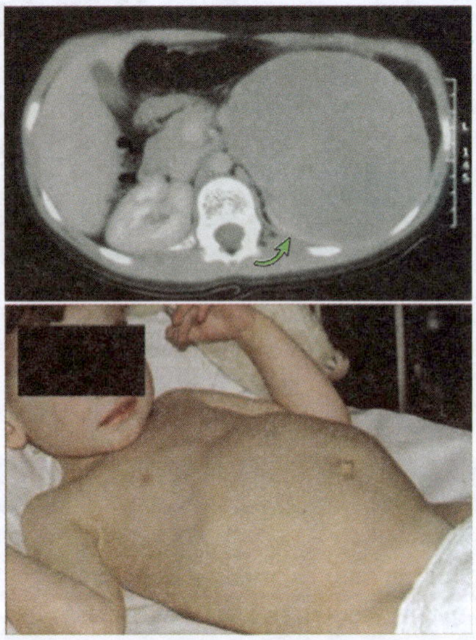

Wilms tumor

Angiomyolipoma

- Hamartoma
- **Associated with 50% of tuberous sclerosis (EPILOA:** Epilepsy + Low Intelligence + Adenoma Sebaceum)
- **This contains:** Blood vessels + Muscles + Fat content inside**
- **IOC:** CT scan (Fat inside lesion)
- **Tumor marker:** HMB-45 +ve
- **Clinical features:**
  - Hematuria
  - Hypertension
  - Mass
  - Pain
  - Anemia
  - Wunderlich syndrome—spontaneous retro-peritoneal hemorrhage—self-limiting
- **Treatment:**
  - <4 cm—no treatment
  - >4 cm—partial nephrectomy
  - Selective embolization

Renal Tuberculosis

- **MC site:** Kidney; other sites: ureter and bladder
- **Route of entry:** Hematogenous route
- **Earliest and MC features of renal tuberculosis** (TB): Increased frequency**
- **O/E of urine in renal TB:** Sterile pyuria** (Bacteria are absent but WBC count is increased)
- ****Early morning urine specimen for 3 days:** Acid-fast bacilli to diagnose TB
- **IOC to diagnose early TB:**
  - **Earliest feature in TB kidney:** Blunting of calyx**
  - **Old modality:** Intravenous pyelogram (IVP)
  - **New modality:** CT pyelogram**
- **Complications of chronic TB:**
  - Cement or putty kidney
  - Golf hole ureter
  - Thimble small bladder
- **Treatment of chronic TB:**
  - Resection and reconstruction (optimum after 6–12 weeks after ATT started)

TRAUMA TO URINARY SYSTEM

Renal trauma:

- MC mechanism: Blunt injury
- Hematuria (ominous sign)
- **IOC:** CECT abdomen

Ureteric injury:

- Usually during surgery
- Ureter can be identified by looking for the—Peristalsis**
- Ureteric injury—repair it end to end by using 3-0 Vicryl**
- Boari flap using the urinary bladder as shown below figure.

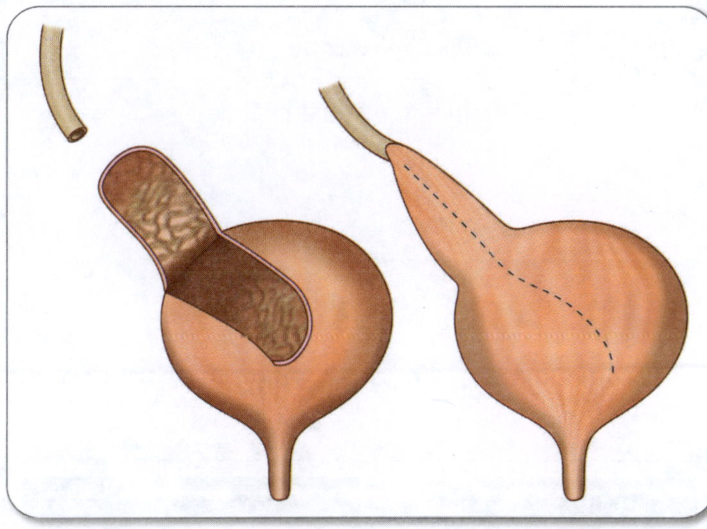

Boari flap operation

Congenital Anomalies and Diseases in Upper Urinary System

Ectopic Ureter

- **MC anomaly of urinary system:** Duplication of renal pelvis and ureters**
- Unilateral > bilateral
- Ectopic ureter arises from upper pole, it runs lateral, outward and joins distal to normal ureter**
- **Ectopic ureter opens into:**
  - **Boys:** Prostatic urethra
  - **Girls:** Distal to external urethral sphincter. Hence, girls will have paradoxical urinary incontinence and continuous dribbling of urine seen.

Weigert-Meyer Rule:

- Upper pole ureter is ectopic ureter and its orifice inserts inferomedially to normal ureter.

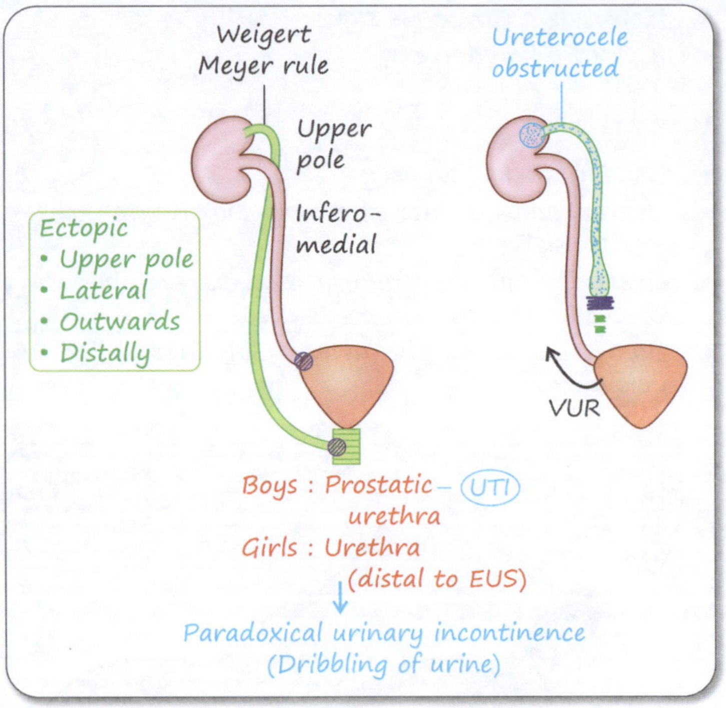

Weigert-Meyer rule

- Ectopic ureter shows drooping lily appearance on IVP.

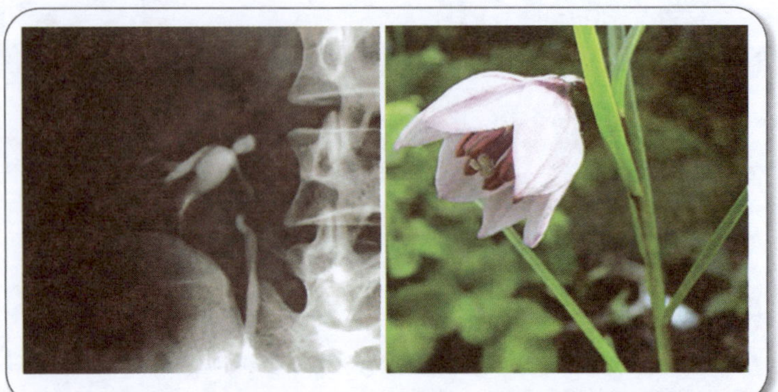

Drooping lily sign on IVP in ectopic ureter

Polycystic Kidney Disease

Autosomal Dominant Polycystic Kidney Disease Adult Type (ADPKD)

Criteria to diagnose ADPKD are based on USG:

- **On USG, one kidney:** 3 cysts
- **B/L kidney:** 2 in each

Clinical features:

- Before 40 years—presentation—hypertension (from 20 years onward)
- kidney failure from 40 years onward
- **End-stage renal failure:** MC in male than female
- Intravenous pyelogram shows spider leg appearance**

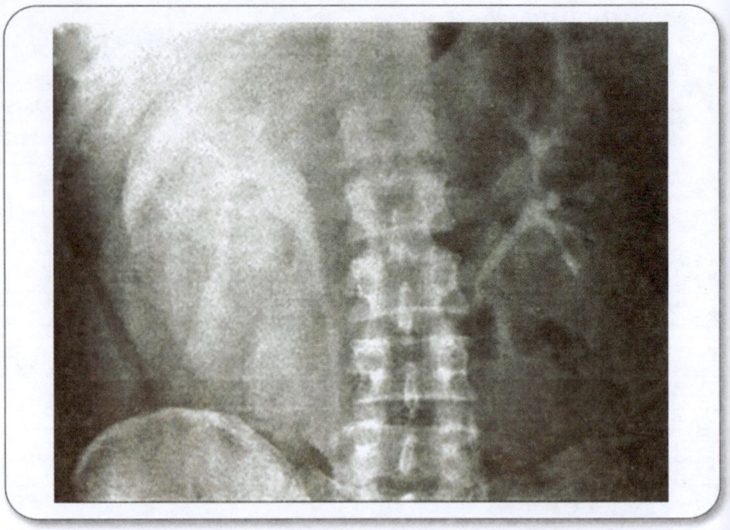

Spider leg appearance on IVP

Associated anomalies:

- Cysts in liver, spleen, pancreas, ovary
- Berry aneurysm
- Mitral valve prolapse syndrome
- Colonic diverticulosis

Treatment:

- **Tolvaptan**
  - Vasopressin receptor antagonist
  - 1st approved drug
  - Increased urine excretion
  - Increase sodium content in the body
- **Treatment of choice:** Renal transplant

Congenital Pelviureteric Junction Obstruction

MC cause of congenital hydronephrosis** is pelviureteric junction (PUJ) obstruction

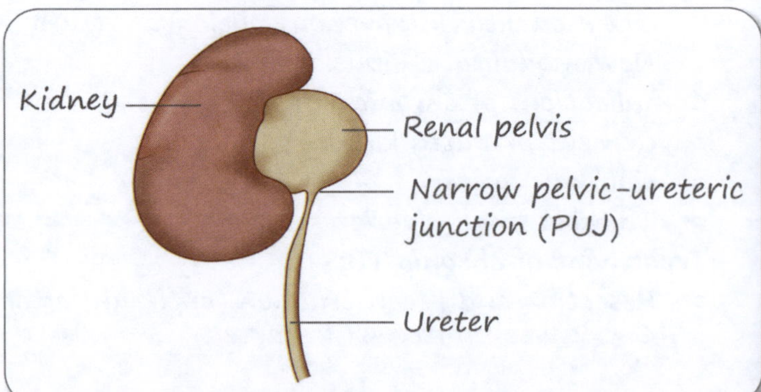

Congenital PUJ obstruction

- **MAG-3 (mercaptoacetyltriglycine scan):** IOC for PUJ obstruction**
- **Treatment:** Anderson-Hynes pyeloplasty operation**

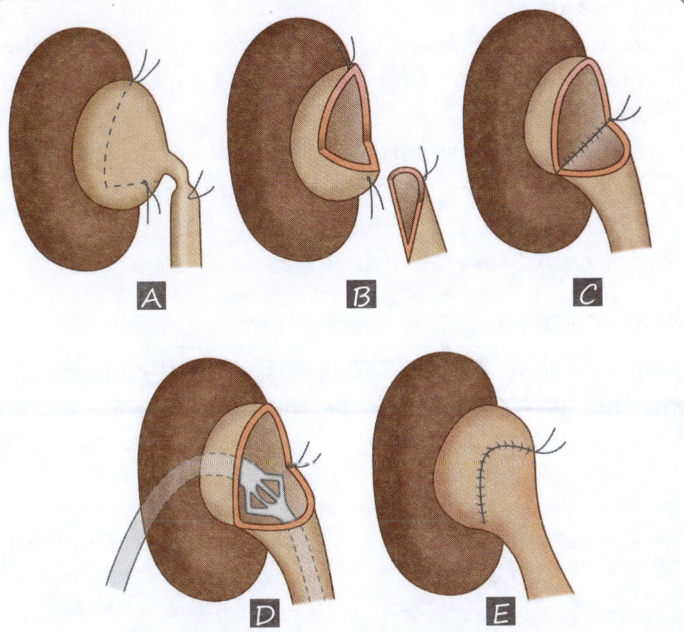

Anderson-Hynes pyeloplasty

Vesicoureteral Reflux

- Congenital—MC in boys
- Acquired—MC in girls
- Main problem is the longitudinal bladder muscle deficiency**
- The urine from the bladder reflux into the ureter on micturition.

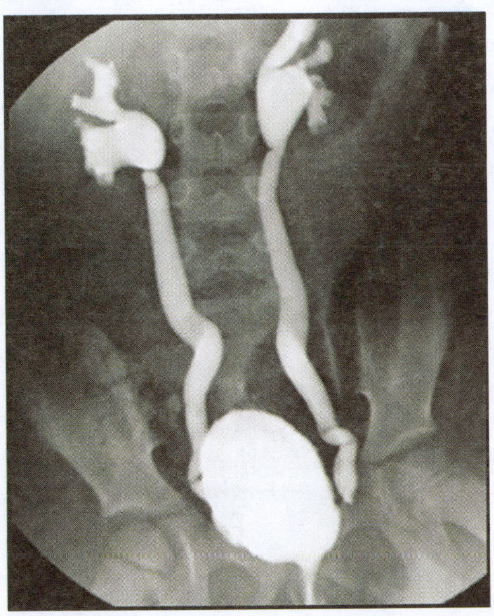

IOC: Micturating cystourethrogram**

Management:

Surgical treatment: Reimplantation of ureter

Horseshoe Kidney

- 1 in 1,000
- MC in men
- Lower pole fusion at L4
- Most of them are asymptomatic
- The isthmus is cut only in one surgery: Abdominal aortic aneurysm surgery
- Blood supply is from Major arteries nearby.
- Pregnancy is not a contraindication—but urinary infection is common for them**
- IVP—flower vase or handshake appearance**

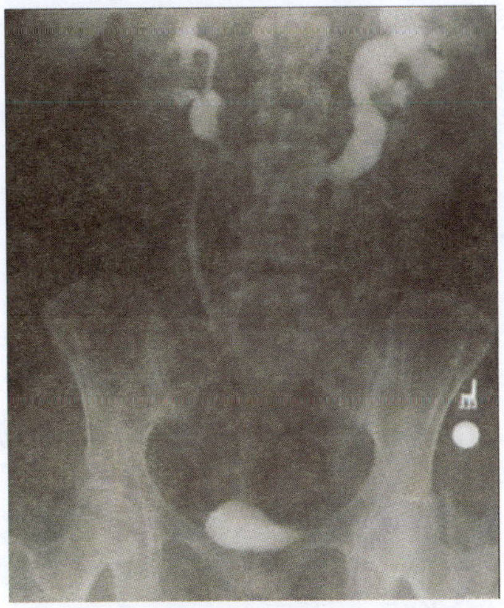

Flower vase appearance in horseshoe kidney

Ureterocele

- IVP—Cobra head appearance
- **Treatment:** Ureteric reimplant

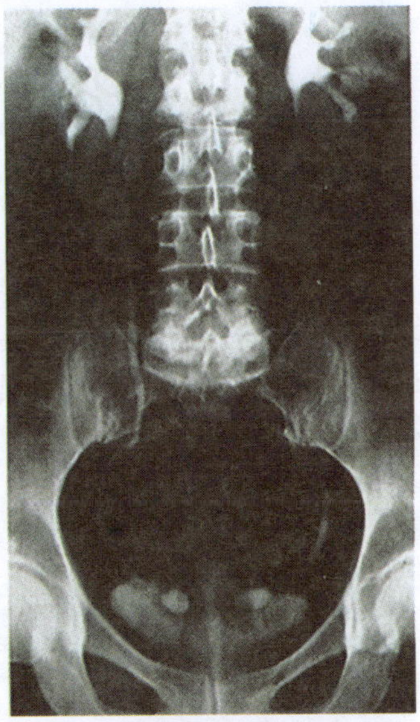

Cobra head deformity on intravenous pyelography

BLADDER, PROSTATE AND URETHRA

Bladder Cancer

- **MC type:** Transitional cell cancer (90%)
- **2nd MC type:** Squamous cell carcinoma (SCC)
- **3rd MC type:** Adenocarcinoma (arises from urachal remnants)

Risk factors:

Transitional cell cancer	Squamous cell cancer

• MC risk factor—smoking
• Schistosomiasis
• Occupational due to Dyes
  ○ Beta-naphthylamine (coal)
  ○ Diaminobiphenyl (aniline)
	• Stones
	• Schistosomiasis
	• Special diseases—diverticular diseases, long-term catheters

- **MC presentation:** Painless terminal hematuria
- **MC site:** Dome and lateral wall of bladder**
- Cancer from anterior wall producing spread to posterior wall is known as **Kissing cancer****

Diagnosis of urinary bladder carcinoma:

- Cystoscopy with transurethral resection is the IOC for obvious lesions.
- Urinary cytology is the IOC for carcinoma in situ—NMP22 and MCM protein in urine.

Treatment:

- **Nonmuscle invasive cancers:** Transurethral resection of bladder tumor and intravesical BCG or mitomycin
- **Muscle Invasive cancers:** Radical cystectomy
- **In situ cancers:** BCG intravesical therapy.

Bladder and Urethral Injuries

Bladder injury:

Intraperitoneal rupture of bladder	Extraperitoneal rupture of bladder
• MC due to direct blow in dome of bladder • Cause uremic peritonitis • Immediate surgery needed	• Cause: fracture of pelvis** • Superficial extravasation of urine with urine extravasated from nipple level to Holden's line level • Catheter inserted immediately • Wait and watch—gradually the injury heals

Urethral injury:

Clinical features of urethral injuries:

- Blood at urethral meatus**
- Retention of bladder

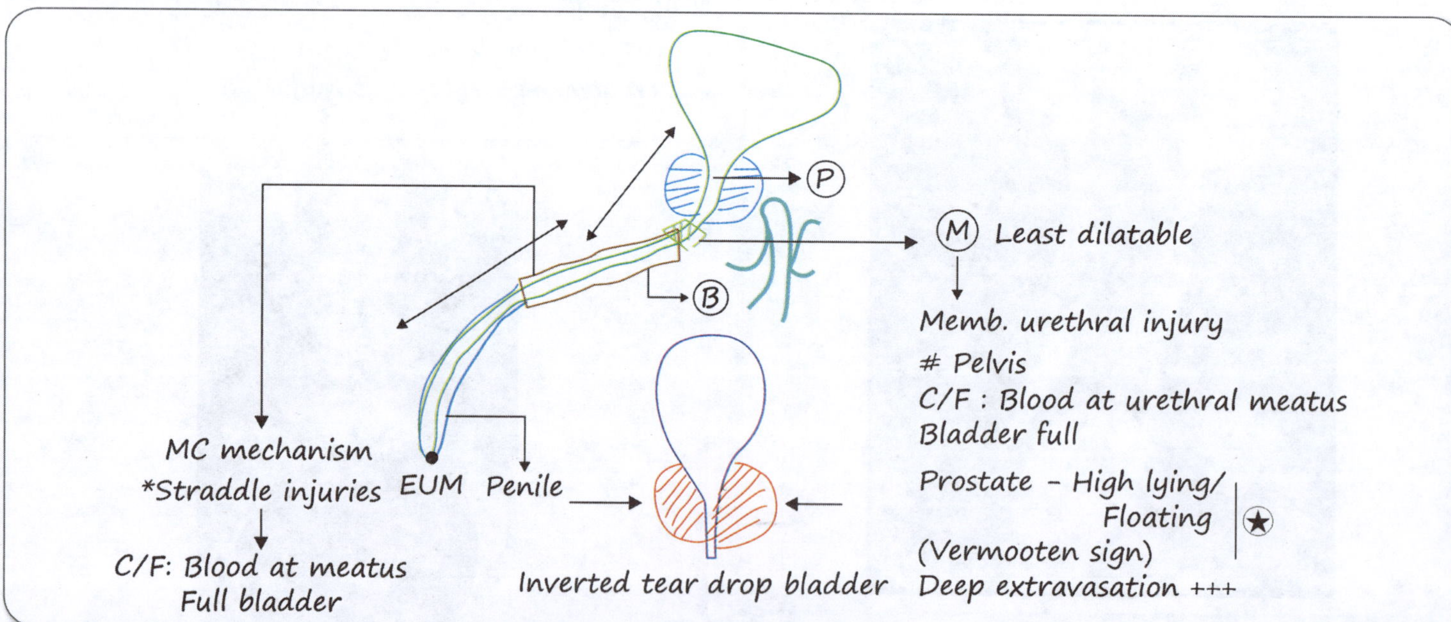

Types of Urethral injury

Membranous urethral injury	Bulbar urethral injury
• Mainly due to fracture pelvis • **Per rectal examination:** Prostate: high lying and floating (**Vermooten sign**)** • The above examination is not advised in latest guidelines of ATLS • Deep extravasation +++ of blood seen • **Bladder shape:** Inverted tear drop	• Mainly due to straddle injury • Typical presentation of urethral injury seen

Steps to be done in urethral injury:**
- Never put Foley's catheter as it will cause more damage of the urethra
- Once bladder is full put suprapubic catheter (SPC)
- Via SPC we can do descending cystourethrogram/ micturating cystourethrogram
- **Other investigations:** Retrograde urethrogram (via Foley's inserted only up to penile urethra and push contrast)
- Repair done after 6 weeks.

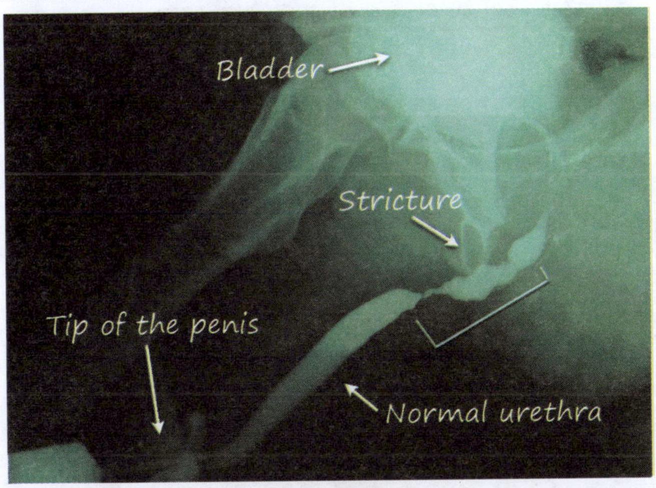

Retrograde urethrogram (RGU) shows urethral stricture

Prostate Anatomy

Basic anatomy: McNeal's three surgical zones
1. Transition zone
2. Central zone
3. Peripheral zone

In benign prostatic hyperplasia (BPH)—transition zone is more involved*

In cancer—peripheral zone is more involved**

Benign Prostatic Hyperplasia

- MC in old age
- Symptoms of BPH are given by bladder outlet obstruction.

Irritative symptoms	Obstructive
• Increased frequency (MC symptom) • Nocturia • Urgency • Hesitancy • Hematuria	• Dribbling • Thin stream urine • Retention

- IOC to detect bladder outlet obstruction: **Uroflowmetry****

Normal Uroflowmetry

Urine flow rate:
- For a voiding volume of >200 mL, a peak flow rate of >15 mL/second is normal*
- Flow rate <10 mL is low

Voiding pressure:
- Voiding pressure at <60 cm H_2O is normal
- Voiding pressure >80 cm H_2O is high

Medical Treatment:
- **Alpha-1A blocker:** Tamsulosin
- **5-alpha reductase inhibitor:** Finasteride

Surgery:
- **Transurethral resection of the prostate (TURP):** Gold standard
- **Open methods:**
  - **Retropubic method:** Millin operation
  - **Transvesical method:** Freyer operation
- **Points to know from TURP procedure:**
  - **Distal limit of TURP:** Verumontanum**
  - **If you go beyond Verumontanum, we can injure the EUS:** Results in incontinency**
  - **If you injure the IUS (MC complication)**:** Retrograde ejaculation
  - **If you injure the bladder neck:** Bladder neck stenosis
- **During surgery:**
  - **Fluid of choice for monopolar diathermy:** 1.5% isotonic glycine**
  - If not available—use distilled water

- NS is not used during surgery using Diathermy currents.
- Postoperative of fluid of choice for washing bladder and irrigation with Three-lumen Foley's catheter—18 G catheter: Normal saline.

- **Immediate postoperative complications:**
  - **Hemorrhage:** Usually arises from Floch arteries—arising from Inferior Vesical arteries**
  - **TUR syndrome:** Patient confused, irrelevant words, if we use distilled water there is high chance of dilutional hyponatremia and water intoxication.

Cancer Prostate

- **Clinical presentation:** Bladder outlet obstruction + back pain
- **Screening protocol:** Digital rectal examination + PSA (combined**)

Prostate-specific antigen:

- **Normal value:** <4 ng/L
- **>10 ng/L:** Localized cancer+
- **>35 ng/L:** Metastatic cancer prostate+

Other values:

- PSA velocity
- PSA density
- **Old tumor marker:** Acid phosphatase

Biopsy methods:

• **TRUS-guided biopsy**	• **Transperineal template biopsy (TPTBP)**
○ Traditional ○ Increased risk of infection ○ Less areas of biopsy possible	○ Detect lesion in anterior aspect of prostate ○ No infection risk is there
Gleason score is used for prostatic cancer from biopsy	

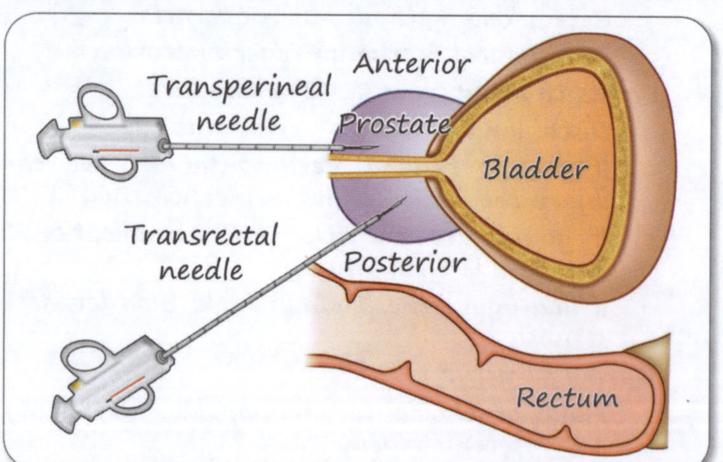

Transperineal biopsy of the prostate

Management:

- **T1, T2:** Radical prostatectomy
  - <70 years
  - Fit for surgery
- >70 years, unfit—T1/T2 prostatic cancer—wait and watch
- **T3, T4, M1:** Androgen ablation (1st step)

Androgen ablation methods:

- **Gold standard method for androgen ablation:** Subscapular orchidectomy or Conventional orchidectomy + testicular prosthesis kept
- **If not willing for orchidectomy:** LHRH agonist like Flutamide; Leuprolide, Goserelin

PENIS AND TESTIS

Hypospadias

- MC congenital anomaly (lower urinary)
- **Features:**
  - Dorsal hood
  - Ventral opening of urethra
  - Ventral chordae

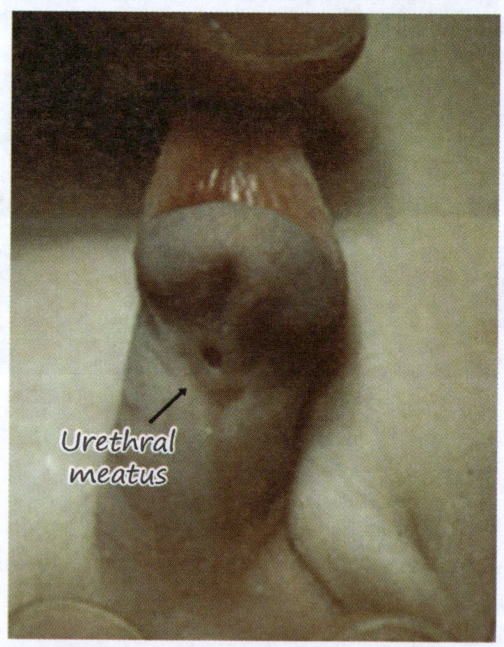

- **Age group for surgery:** Six months to 1 year
- Circumcision is contraindicated.
- **Treatment:** MAGPI (Meatal Advancement and Glanuloplasty Incorporated)
- **Order of reconstruction of MAGPI****
  - Orthoplasty (Penile straightening)
  - Urethroplasty
  - Glanuloplasty
  - Meatoplasty

- Scrotoplasty
- Skin reconstruction and circumcision is done as last step**

Epispadias
- Dorsal opening of urethra
- Rare
- MC associated with Ectopia vesicae (Exstrophy of Bladder)

Phimosis

- Unable to retract the prepuce backward
- Smegma gets collected under prepuce is carcinogenic.

Congenital phimosis	Acquired phimosis
• Physiological adhesions up to 6 years • No need to operate before 6 years • Wait up to 5–6 years	• Inflammation • Diabetes • Balanitis xerotica obliterans (BXO) • Cancer • Trauma • Surgery is done for all acquired cases

- Less than 1 year child with severe Ballooning of prepuce will need surgery as this is causing severe obstruction.
- Less than 1 year children can be operated by a **Hollister/PlastiBell device—suture less method.**

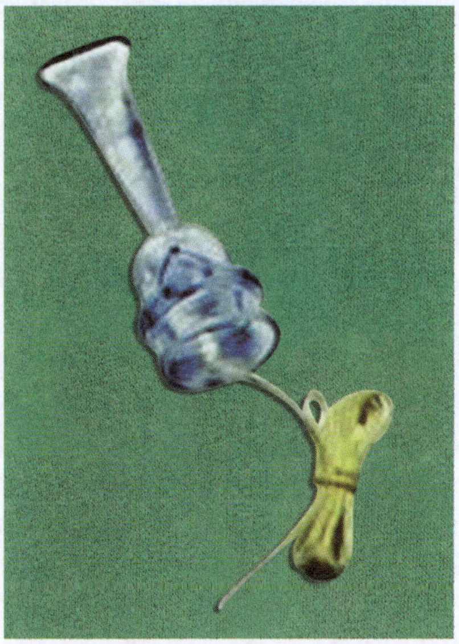

PlastiBell device

Peyronie's Disease

- Peyronie's disease is characterized by: Penile deformity + Palpable penile plaques + Erectile dysfunction + Pain on erection.
- X-ray shows calcified penis.

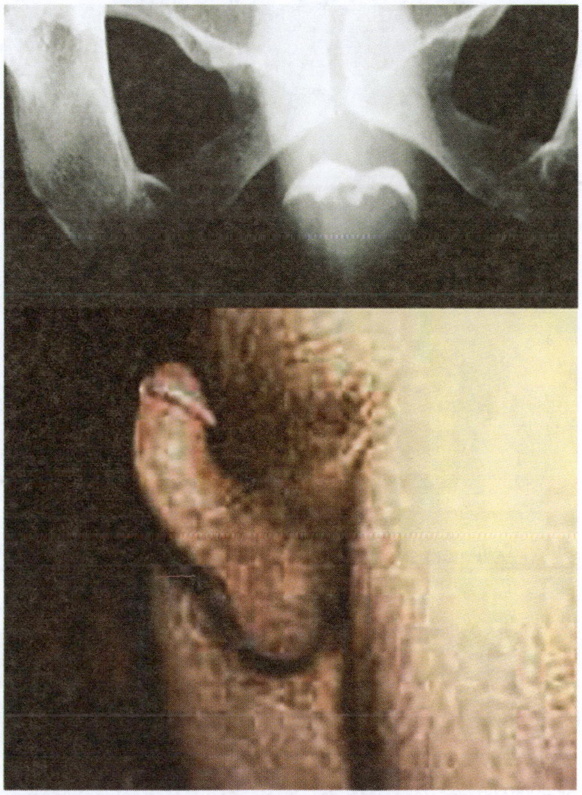

Peyronie's disease

- If the penile deformity is distressing, **Nesbit's operation** can be performed to straighten the penis.

Priapism

- Painful erected penis following sexual activity.
- Two types are there: (1) High flow type and (2) Low flow type.
- Low flow type is due to venous blockage in sickle cell anemia or leukemias and is more dangerous.

Immediate treatment:
- Injection phenylephrine/adrenaline (**should be injected intrapenile within 36 hours)
- **>36 hours:** Shunt operations are done.
  - **Winter:** Distal corpora spongiosum shunt
  - **Gray hack:** Corpora cavernosa with saphenous vein.

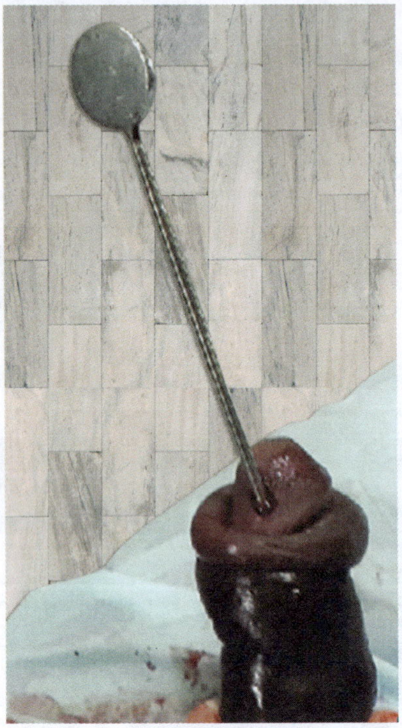

Winter shunt operation for priapism

Posterior Urethral Valve

- Most common of obstructive uropathy in a male child is posterior urethral valve.
- It most commonly lies just distal to the verumontanum or at the verumontanum.
- It occurs only in males.
- Diagnosis is made by:
- Voiding cystourethrogram
- Urethroscopy

Carcinoma Penis

- MC in 4th decade of men.
- **MC type:** SCC; rare type—verrucous carcinoma
- **Common sites:**
  - Glans penis (50%)
  - Preputial skin (20%)
- **Predisposing condition:**
  - **MC:** Smegma**
  - **Other risk factors:**
    - Leukoplakia
    - Balanitis xerotica obliterans
    - Buschke Lowenstein tumor (caused by Human papillomavirus)
- **Cancer in situ of glans:** Erythroplasia of Queyrat**
- **Cancer in situ of shaft of penis:** Bowen's disease

Clinical features:

- Fungating growth
- Foul smelling odor (due to secondary infection)
- **Sentinel node of cancer penis:** Cabanas node** (Superficial inguinal node)

Nonsurgical	Surgical treatment is best

• Radiotherapy
• Interstitial brachytherapy
• 5FU cream
• Mohs micrographic surgery
• Laser excision
	• 2 cm margin is given and after resection at least 2 cm of stump must be available for Sexual activity and passing urine in standing position
	• Usually, partial amputation of penis is done for glans and distal growth
	• **Indications of total amputation:**
	  ○ <2 cm shaft
	  ○ Urethral involvement++

Testicular Cancer

Pathological types:

Germ cell tumors	Sex cord tumors
Seminomas ***Nonseminomas:*** • Choriocarcinoma • Yolk sac • Teratoma • Embryonal cell	Leydig cell tumors Sertoli cell tumors

Seminomas	Nonseminomas
• 4th decade • Highly radiosensitive • LN metastasis > hematogenous metastasis • Good prognosis	• Seen in 30s • Radioresistant • **Tumor markers:** HCG, alpha-fetoprotein (AFP), LDH • Bad prognosis

Predisposing factors:
- **Undescended testis (seminoma):** Please remember even by doing orchidopexy the risk is not reduced; but helps in early diagnosis**
- Klinefelter's syndrome
- Testicular feminization syndrome

Clinical presentation is Painless lump in scrotum**

Investigations for testicular tumors:
- IOC
- **To diagnose:** Biopsy** *via* inguinal canal, Trans-scrotal biopsy is contraindicated**
- **To stage:** MRI**
- **Tumor markers:** HCG, AFP, LDH

Treatment:
- High inguinal orchidectomy
- Nodal secondaries must be managed according to the type of tumor**
- Seminoma is radiosensitive and hence RT given to nodes
- Nonseminoma is not radiosensitive and hence we do retroperitoneal lymph node dissection (RPLND)

Varicocele Testis

- MC in young tall thin males
- C/F: Bag of worms on palpation
- Cough impulse (+)
- Disappears on lying down
- MC in left side**

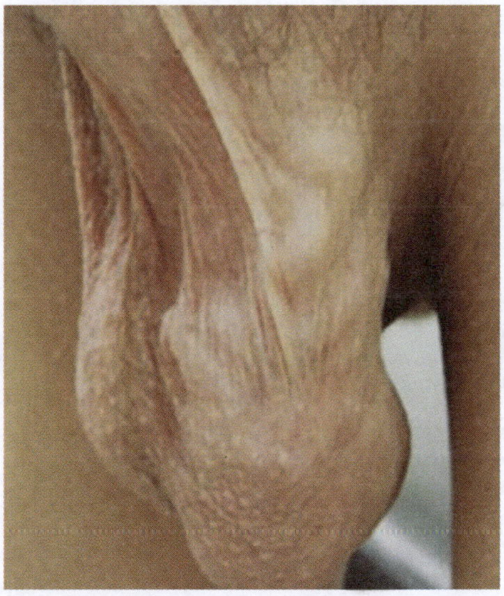

Varicocele testis

- MC cause of infertility in men**
- **Palomo operation:** Retroperitoneal ligation of testicular veins.

Torsion Testis Versus Orchitis

MC anomaly associated is Bell clapper deformity.

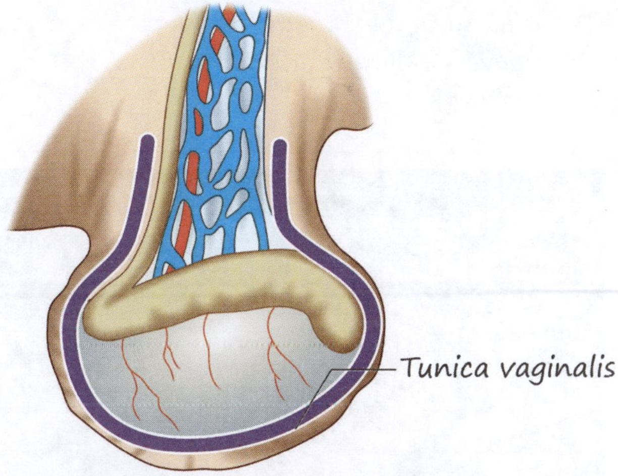

Horizontal lying bell clapper deformity

- **Prehn's sign:**
  - To differentiate between torsion and orchitis
  - **On lifting the testis**
    - If pain increases—suggestive of torsion
    - If pain decrease—orchitis

Management of torsion testis (Surgery done as emergency)
- **<4 hours:** Save testis
- **>4 hours:** Testis would be Gangrenous
- **IOC:** Color Doppler scan**
- **Bilateral exposure is done for Torsion testis always:**
  - Because the pathology for Torsion may be seen in Normal side also.
  - Affected testis removed if gangrenous.
  - Unaffected testis may have pathologies like Bell clapper deformity and hence do orchidopexy using 3-point fixation in the scrotal wall.

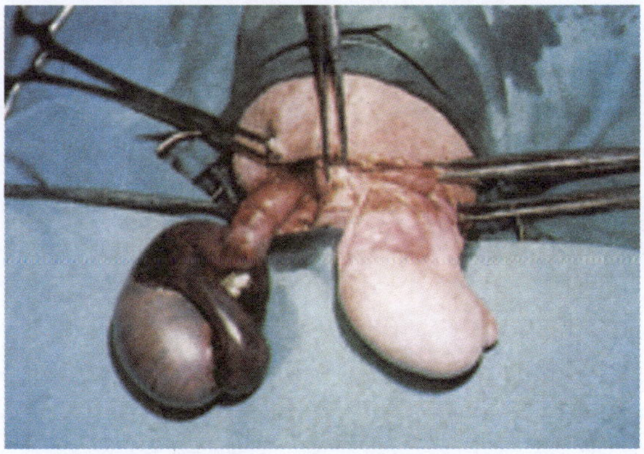

Bilateral exposure for torsion testis by horizontal incision in torsion

Hydrocele

Collection of fluid between tunica vaginalis

Clinical features:
- Transilluminant+
- Get above swelling+
- Fluctuation+

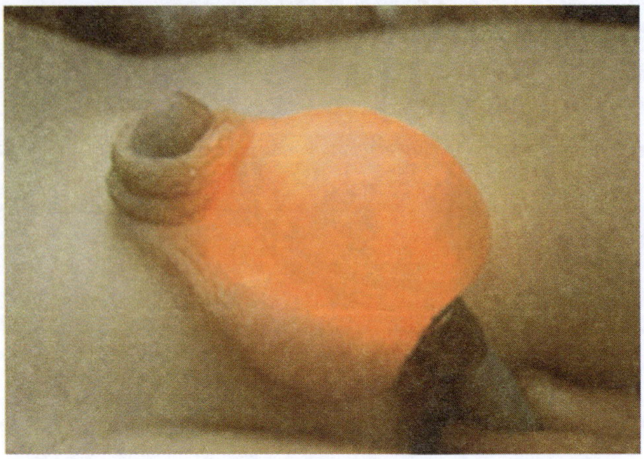

Transilluminant hydrocele

Types of hydrocele based on closure of tunica vaginalis:
- **Vaginal**
  - Confined only to scrotum
  - Get above the swelling+
- **Infantile hydrocele**
  - Fluid collection seen up to superficial ring
  - Get above swelling not possible
- **Congenital hydrocele**
  - Communicating with the peritoneum
  - Reduced on lying down overnight
  - **Inverted ink bottle effect is seen****
- **Encysted hydrocele cord**
  - Decreased movement on traction

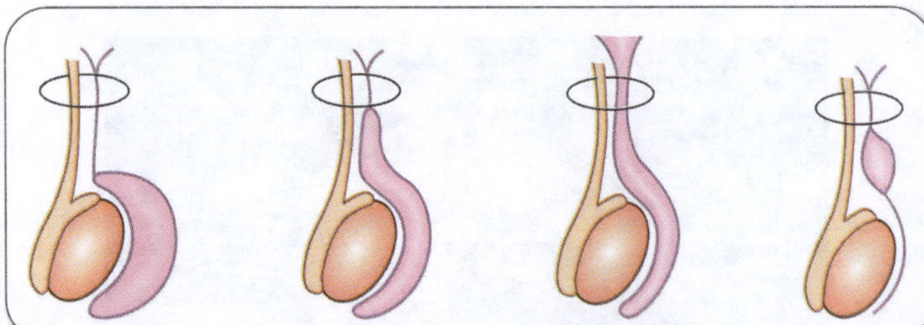

Vaginal-infantile-congenital-encysted hydrocele types in order

Management of hydrocele:
- **Jaboulay's Eversion of sac:** Bigger hydrocele
- **Lord's plication of sac:** Small hydrocele with thin sac

Undescended Testis

- Testis is an organ of lumbar region.
- It descends from Lumbar region to Scrotum.
- The descent is by the Gubernaculum tail.

Gubernaculum has five tails:
1. Pubic tail
2. Perineal tail
3. Femoral tail
4. Inguinal tail—if inguinal tail is taking the dominance, it will reach superficial inguinal pouch **(MC site of ectopic testis)**
5. Gubernaculum tail—normal one reaching scrotum.

Undescended testis	Ectopic testis

• Arrest in normal path
• Underdeveloped
• **Can cause:**
  ○ T: Torsion
  ○ E: Epididymo-orchitis
  ○ S: Sterility
  ○ T: Trauma
  ○ I: Indirect inguinal hernia
  ○ S: Seminoma
• **Scrotum not developed****
	• Deviation from normal path
	• Normal development
	• Can cause trauma as only complication
	• Scrotum normal

Clinical features:
- MC location—inguinal canal
- 70% of it resolve by 2 months
- MC preterm babies
- Right side
- Leydig cell normal, Sertoli cell affected—so secondary sexual characters normal**

Investigations:
- **Gold standard:** Diagnostic laparoscopy
- **Inguinal undescended testis (UDT):** USG is enough (Indirect inguinal hernia is also noted)

Treatment:

Orchidopexy is done between 6 months and 1 year of age.

ANEURYSM

- **MC cause of aneurysm:** Atherosclerosis
- **MC site of aneurysm:** Circle of Willis
- **MC extracranial site of aneurysm:** Abdominal Aorta (Infrarenal AA is MC site)
- **MC peripheral artery aneurysm:** Popliteal artery
- **MC site of visceral artery aneurysm:** Splenic artery
- **MC site of mycotic aneurysm:** Femoral artery (Mycotic aneurysm is a misnomer it is caused by bacteria).

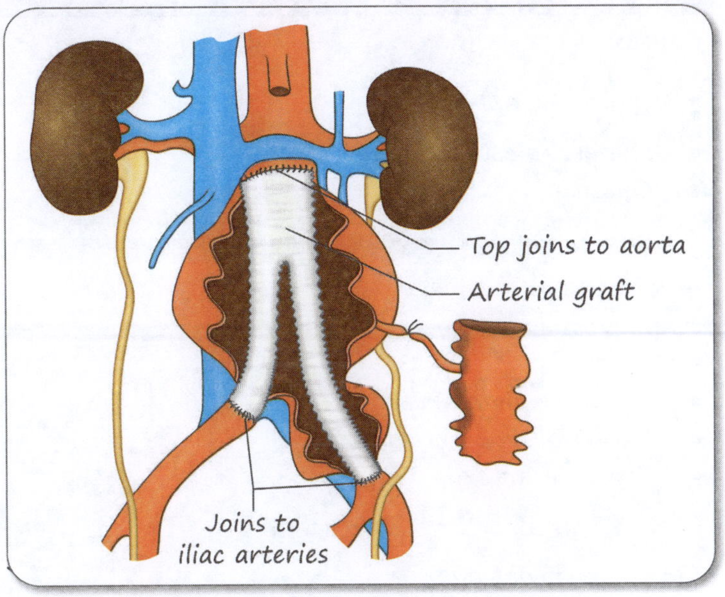

Dacron graft

Classification of Aneurysm

- **True aneurysm:** Contains all the layers of blood vessel
- **False aneurysm:** Lacks 1 or 2 layers of the blood vessel
- **Fusiform aneurysm:** Symmetric dilatation of blood vessel
- **Saccular aneurysm:** Asymmetric dilatation of blood vessel
- **Dissecting aneurysm:** Dissection happens in between the layers of tunica.

Abdominal Aortic Aneurysm

- **MC location:** Infrarenal AA
- **MC presentation:** Back pain

IOC for AAA

CT Angiography**

Indication of Treatment

- Symptomatic patient
- **Asymptomatic patient:** AP diameter >55 mm (until 5.5 cm if patient is asymptomatic follow-up)

Conventional Treatment

- Resect the aneurysm out
- Replace it with dacron pant type graft

Endovascular Aneurysm Repair (EVAR) is the latest treatment:

- A stent is placed inside the blood vessel at the site of aneurysm.
- Blood flows through the stent and the aneurysm collapses.

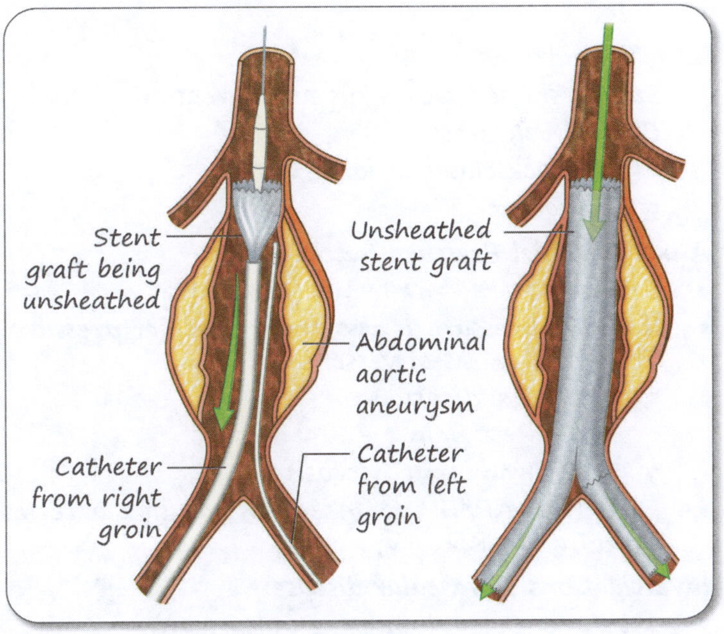

EVAR

CHRONIC LIMB ISCHEMIA

Peripheral Vascular Disease—Atherosclerosis of LL	TAO
Causes: • DM • HTN • Hypercholesterolemia • Obesity	**Cause** Smoking
Thrombus formed in vessel occludes the vessel	Vasospasm occludes the vessel
Involves Major vessels • Aorta • Common iliac artery • External iliac artery • Femoral artery	**Involves** Infrapopliteal arteries
It is U/L or B/L	It is BL symmetrical
Common in old age	Common in young age <50 years**
Males > females	Seen only in males
UL not affected	UL also affected
Adjacent veins and nerves not affected	Adjacent veins and nerves are affected
C/F: Intermittent claudication • **MC site of claudication pain:** Calf** • **MC site of occlusion:** Superficial femoral artery	**C/F:** • Young male with bilateral leg claudication pain. • On CT angiography: symmetric lesion is seen.

Lerich Syndrome:

- Saddle shaped thrombus at bifurcation of aorta.
- **Clinical Features:**
  - Buttock claudication
  - Impotence

Ankle Brachial Pressure Index:

- ABPI = AP/BP = 0.9–1.1 (Normal)
- **If Ankle pressure is less than Brachial pressure:** There is stenosis of vessel seen:
  - **<0.9:** Claudication
  - **<0.5:** Rest pain
  - **<0.3:** Imminent necrosis
- False high AP/BP >1.3 seen in calcified arteries in DM and CKD

Investigations of vascular disease:

- **1st done:** Color doppler (Duplex scan)
  - Noninvasive
  - Repetitive
  - Gold standard: CT Angiography (Road map)

Treatment:

Conventional bypass operation is done using

- Dacron (for aortic bypass and Aortic-femoral bypass. Suture material 3'0 or 4'0 Prolene)
- PTFE (for Ileo femoral artery bypass. Suture material 5'0 Prolene)
- Saphenous vein (for infra femoral bypass)

Angioplasty: Gold standard treatment now

Seldinger needle is passed beyond the block and an Intra-arterial stent is placed

Diagnostic Criteria for TAO

- History of smoking
- Onset should be before 50 years
- Infra popliteal occlusion only
- UL involvement present
- Superficial phlebitis present
- No other risk factors except smoking

TAO—Surgery: Lumbar sympathectomy

- On one side L1, L2 and L3 are cut on the other side L2 and L3 are cut.
- L1 on one side is preserved to prevent retrograde ejaculations.

Indications of lumbar sympathectomy**

- Rest pain
- Ulcer
- Gangrene

Contraindications for lumbar sympathectomy

- Intermittent claudication
- ABPI >0.3
- Diabetic patients

RAYNAUD DISEASE

- Due to unknown cause
- If it happens due to Scleroderma SLE, it is called Raynaud's phenomenon
- Vasospasm is due to:
- Cold exposure
- Continuous vibrations

Phenomenon Seen

- **W-B-C:** Initially limb color is white later blue and then crimson red
- **White:** Due to spasm of both arteries and veins
- **Blue (cyanotic phase):** Here arteries are still in spasm and veins and capillaries open
- **Crimson red:** Arteries open in an extensive way, veins already in opened state.

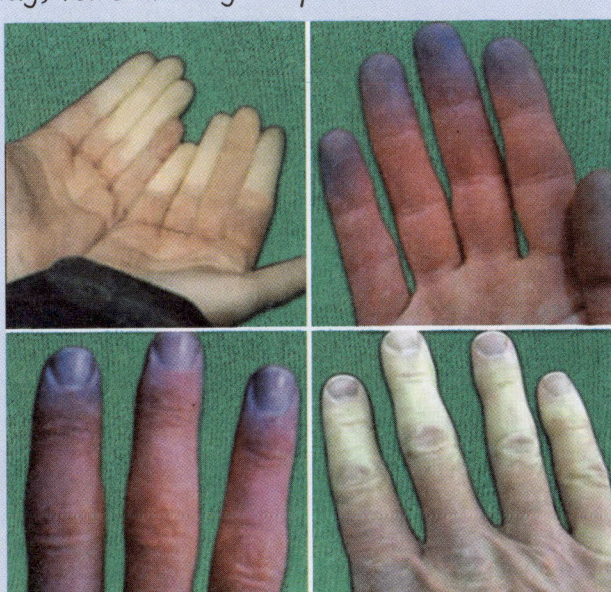

Treatment

- Calcium channel blockers
- Avoid cold

VARICOSE VEINS

CEAP Classification of Varicose Veins

Clinical Classification**

- C1: Telangiectasia/reticular veins
- C2: Varicose veins
- C3: Edema in legs
- C4a: Pigmentation, eczema
- C4b: Lipodermatosclerosis or Atrophic Blanche
- C5: Healed venous ulcer
- C6: Active venous ulcer

Clinical class is further characterized whether patient is Symptomatic(S) or Asymptomatic(A)

Etiological Classification

- **Ep:** Primary
- **Ec:** Congenital
- **Es:** Secondary

Anatomical Classification

- **As:** Superficial veins
- **Ap:** Perforators
- **Ad:** Deep veins

Pathological Classification

- **Pr:** Reflux
- **Po:** Obstructive
- **Pro:** Reflux + obstruction

Risk Factors

- Family history
- Long standing job
- DVT
- Defective valves
- Mass in abdomen
- Pregnancy
- Congenital syndrome: **Klippel Trenaunay Syndrome**
  - Port wine stain
  - Lateral varicose veins
  - Limb lengthening

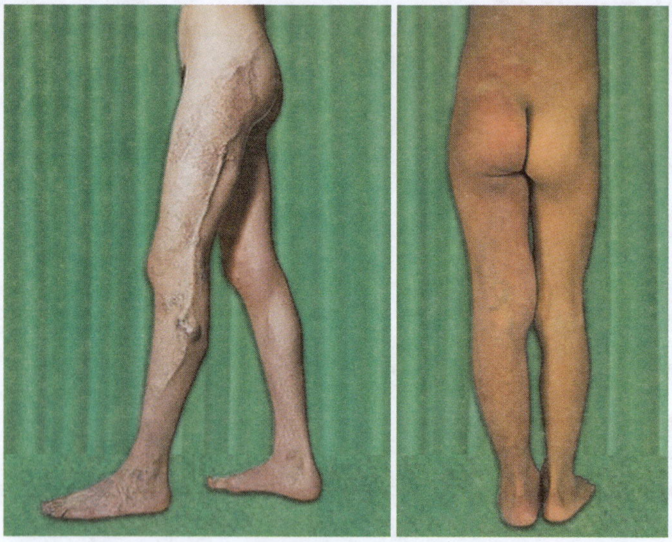

Klippel trenaunay syndrome

Complications of Varicose Veins

- Inverted Champagne bottle leg due to Lipo-dermatosclerosis*
- Venous ulcer on medial malleolus

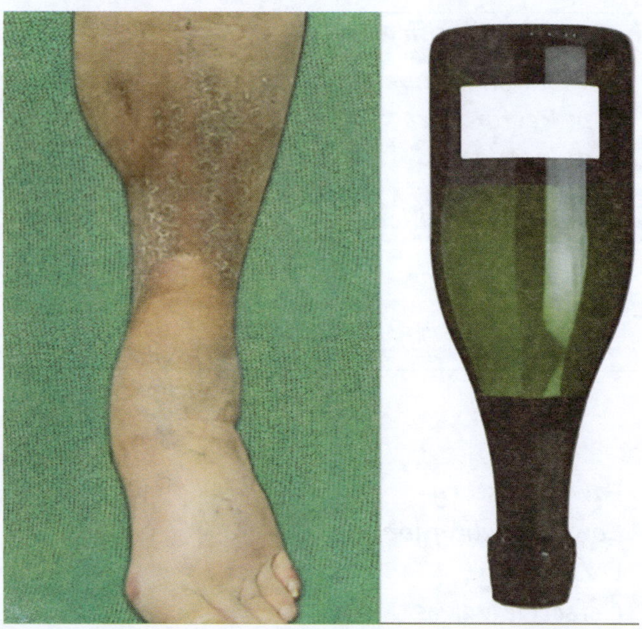

LDS with inverted Champagne Bottle appearance

- **IOC: Color doppler (Duplex scan)**
  - Normal flow blue color
  - **Reflex red color:** Incompetence
  - **Mickey Mouse Sign: Face Femoral Vein, Lateral ear: Femoral Artery, Medial ear: GSA**
  - Duplex scan is done to: R/O DVT and to mark the perforators

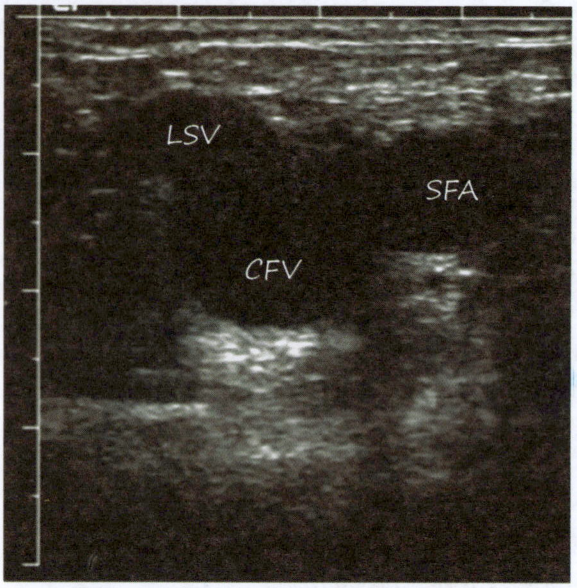

Mickey mouse sign

Surgical Management of Varicose Veins

Conventional Treatment

- Trendelenburg Operation + Stripping of Varicose veins
- **Perforator incompetence:**
  - Subfascial ligation of Cockett and Dodd (can be done in LDS)
  - Subfascial Endoscopic Perforator Surgery (SEPS):
    - Perforators are clipped below the fascia on visualizing through an endoscope.

Recent Advances

- Trivex system
- Foam sclerotherapy
  - By using USG, dilated veins are sclerosed by Tessari method, Sodium tetradecyl sulfate is commonly used.

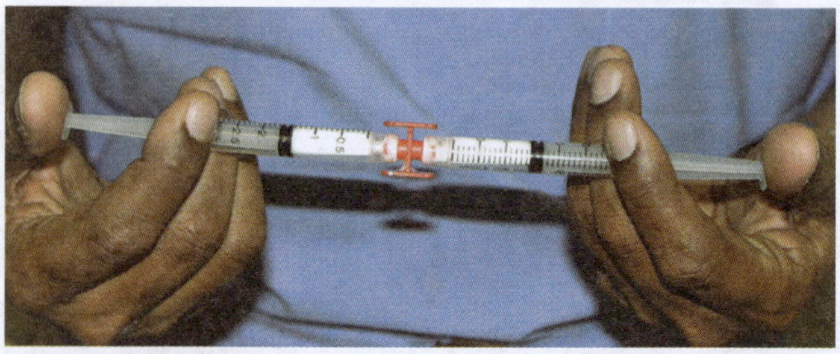

Tessari method of FOAM sclerotherapy

- Endovenous Laser Ablation (EVLA)
- Radio Frequency Ablation

LUNG TUMORS

Benign	Malignant
• **MC:** Pulmonary Hamartoma • Pulmonary hamartoma • MC in males • **X-ray:** Popcorn calcification • MC located peripherally	• Bronchogenic cancers • Malignant mesothelioma (it arises from pleura)

Bronchogenic Cancer

- MC primary malignant tumor in mediastinum
- MC seen in Lung Hilum
- MC visceral cancer
- MC cause of death due to cancer

Pathological Types

Small cell cancer (Oat cell)	Non-small cell cancer
	• Adeno cancer • SCC • Large cell cancer • Broncho alveolar cancer (it spreads by air, satellite lesions are present)
• High risk of metastasis present • Poor prognosis • Response to chemotherapy is excellent	• Less risk of metastasis • Good prognosis • No response to chemotherapy
	• MC type Adenocarcinoma • MC type among smokers is SCC • Undifferentiated type is large cell cancer
Increased paraneoplastic syndromes are present**	Low risk of producing Paraneoplastic syndromes
Usually centrally located**	Peripherally located (SCC is centrally located)**
High chances of metastasis • Brain • Bone • Liver • Adrenal	Less risk of metastasis

MC location of tumor is right lung upper lobe**

C/F of Lung Cancer

- MC is cough
- Dyspnea
- Chest pain
- Hemoptysis (Source of hemoptysis is bronchial artery)**
- Malignant pleural effusion
- Clubbing is present (resolves after tumor excision)
- Hoarseness + (RLN involvement)
- SVC obstruction (SCC)

Pancoast Tumor

- A tumor located at the apex of lung
- Causes destruction of 1st and 2nd ribs
- Causes atrophy of hand muscles
- Causes Horner's syndrome
  - Ptosis
  - Miosis
  - Anhidrosis

It is usually SCC**

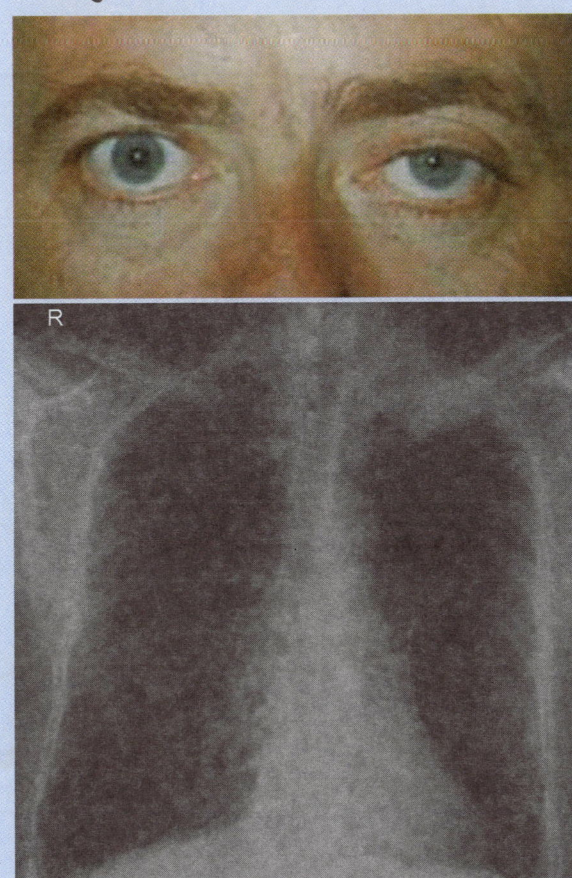

Squamous Cell Cancer of Lung

- **MC cancer in India:** SCC
- **MC among smoking males:** SCC
- **Pancoast tumor is:** SCC
- **Usually centrally located****

- It can form cavity inside the tumor
- It has the best prognosis
- **PNS:** It produces ectopic PTH—Hypercalcemia, Hypophosphatemia and Clubbing**
- **Treatment:** Surgical excision of tumor

Adenocancer

- MC type worldwide
- MC in females
- MC peripherally located
- It produces lung to lung mets
- Good prognosis (not as good as SCC)
- Noguchi Classification was used in olden days (now TNM is used)
- **PNS:** DIC, Hypertrophic pulmonary osteo-arthropathy and migratory thrombophlebitis (Trousseau's syndrome)

Small Cell/Oat Cell Cancer

- Most aggressive cancer
- Worst prognosis
- Responds to CT and RT
- MC type causing extrathoracic metastasis
- PNS MC: Produces
- Ectopic ADH – SIADH—Hyponatremia
- Ectopic ACTH—Hypocalcemia and Cushing syndrome
- Myasthenic eaton lambert syndrome
- Cerebellar degeneration

Paraneoplastic syndrome (Nonmetastatic complication)

Small cell cancer	Squamous cell cancer	Large cell cancer	Adenocarcinoma
• Excess ADH secretion causes SIADH and hyponatremia • Ectopic ACTH causes hypokalemia and Cushing syndrome • Myasthenic Eaton—Lambert syndrome	• Ectopic PTH production causes: Hypercalcemia and hypo phosphatemia • Clubbing in all non-small cell cancer	• Galactorrhea in females • Gynecomastia in males	• Hypertrophic pulmonary osteoarthropathy • DIC • Migratory thrombophlebitis (Trousseau's syndrome)

ACUTE CORONARY ISCHEMIA

Blood Supply to Heart

- **Left coronary artery:** It gives two branches, Left anterior descending artery that runs in the anterior interventricular groove and Left circumflex artery that runs in AV Septum.
- **Right coronary artery:** It gives Right circumflex artery that ends as Posterior descending coronary artery in 90% and in 10% LCA gives Posterior descending artery.

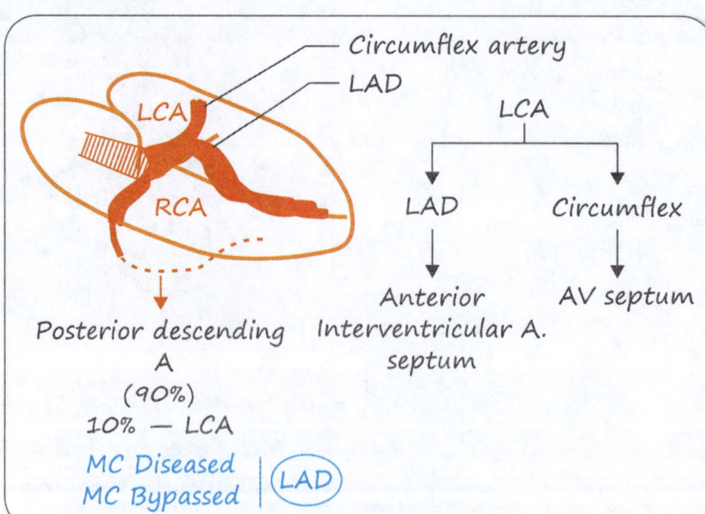

Blood supply to heart

Three Vessels that Supply Blood to Heart

- Lt anterior descending (LAD) artery
- Lt circumflex artery
- Posterior descending coronary artery
- **MC diseased artery:** Lt anterior descending artery
- **MC bypassed artery:** Lt anterior descending artery.

IOC for Coronary Occlusion

Selective coronary angiography

CABG Indications:

- >50% stenosis of Lt coronary artery
- >70% stenosis of anterior interventricular artery
- Triple vessel disease
- Poor ventricular function

Chronic Stable Angina:

- PTCA (Percutaneous Transluminal Coronary Angioplasty) > CABG

Treatment

Bypass Operation

Commonly used vessels

- Long saphenous vein
- Lt internal mammary artery (LIMA)

Long saphenous vein	LIMA (Lt internal mammary artery)
MC used vein	For LCA and LAD bypass we use only LIMA
10 years patency 60%	10 years patency is 90%
Other veins • Short saphenous vein • Cephalic vein	**Other arteries** • Rt internal mammary artery • Radial artery (Allen test is done before taking radial artery)
	Wound infection in diabetic patients

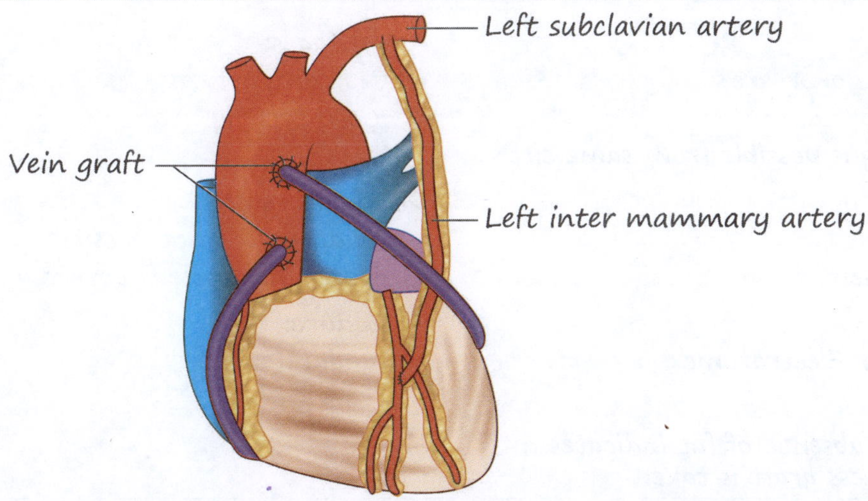

Prognosis

- 95% living at 1 year after operation
- 90% after 5 years
- 75% after 10 years

11. PLASTIC SURGERY AND RECONSTRUCTIVE SURGERY

Skin Graft		Flaps	
Graft is a piece of tissue without its own blood supply		Flap is a tissue carrying its own blood vessel • Pedicle flap • Free flap: Micro vascular anastomosis needed	
Partial thickness graft Involves epidermis + part of dermis	**Full thickness graft** Involves epidermis + full dermis	**Axial pattern flap** Contains named blood vessel	**Random pattern flap** Leash of unnamed blood vessel supply

SKIN GRAFT: SURVIVAL

- **First 48 hours:** Plasma Imbibition
- **48 hours—5 days:** Inosculation (alignment of blood vessels)
- **>5 days:** Revascularization

Absolute contraindication for skin grafting—Beta hemolytic streptococci present on wound.

Partial thickness graft (Also called Thiersch graft)	Full thickness graft (Also known as Wolf graft)
Donor site: • Thigh • Back	**Donor site:** Behind ear
Advantages: • No need to cover donor area • Wider areas can be taken • Repeated grafting is possible from same site	**Advantages:** • No contracture • Cosmetically good
Disadvantages: • Cosmetically ugly • Contractures present	**Disadvantages:** • Wider areas not possible • Donor area needs coverage
Procedure: Using Humby knife or Electrotome	**Procedure:** Manually done
At donor site: Punctuate spots and absence of fat indicates a proper partial thickness graft is taken	

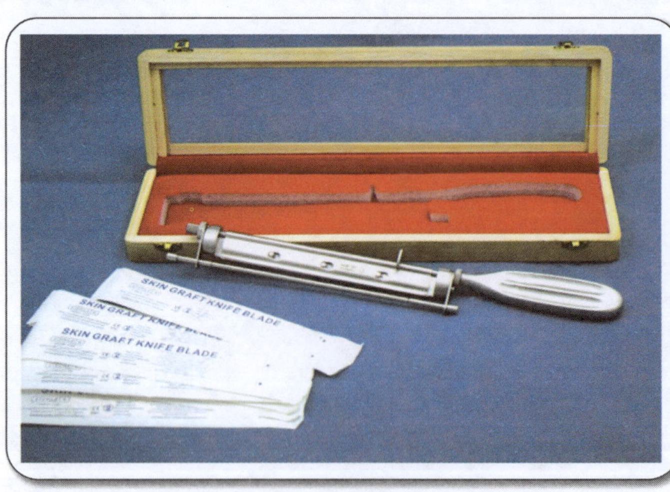

Humby knife for SSG

MESHING: SPLIT SKIN GRAFT

- Size of the graft can be increased
- It helps to drain any fluid

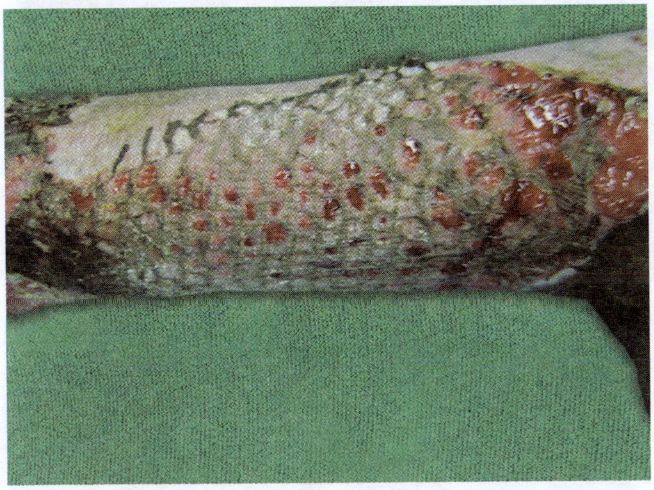

Partial thickness split skin graft

- Delto pectoral (DP) flap based on Internal Mammary artery
- TRAM flap based on superior epigastric artery or Inferior epigastric artery
- DIEP flap (Deep inferior epigastric artery free flap) based on inferior epigastric artery
- PMMC and DP flap used in Oral cavity reconstruction
- TRAM and DIEP flap is used in breast reconstruction

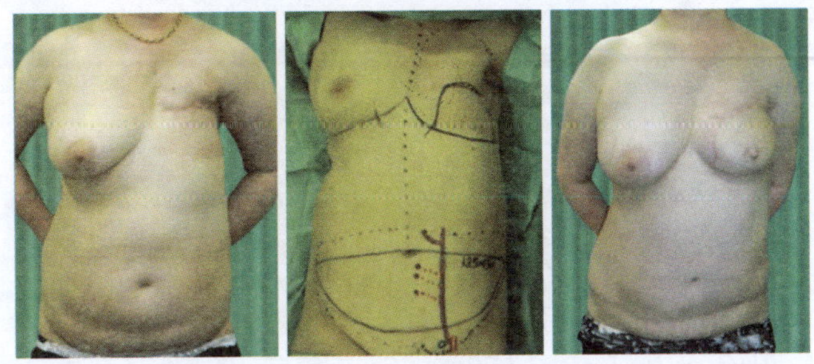

DIEP flap (Free flap)

Indications of Flap

Axial pattern flap (Based on a named blood vessel)

- PMMC flap based on Thoraco acromian artery

Random Pattern Flap

- It is based on dermal and subdermal plexus
- Accepted length: Width ratio = 3:1

Types

Types of random pattern flaps	Figures corresponding
Transposition flap: Flap rotated about a pivot point into adjacent defect	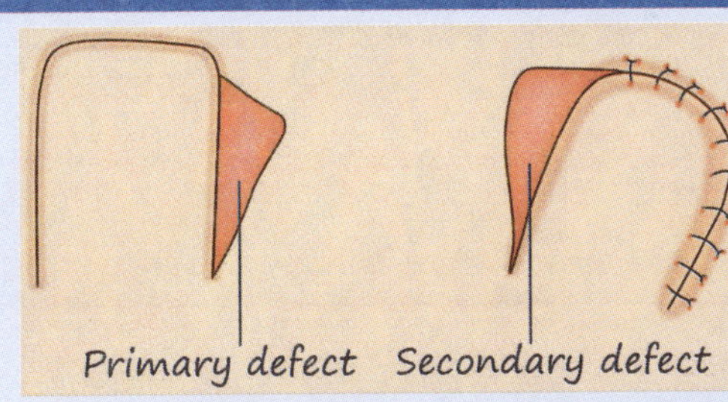
Z plasty: A type of transposition flap, 1.7 times elongation of wound happens in 60° angulation. Used mainly for burns contracture.	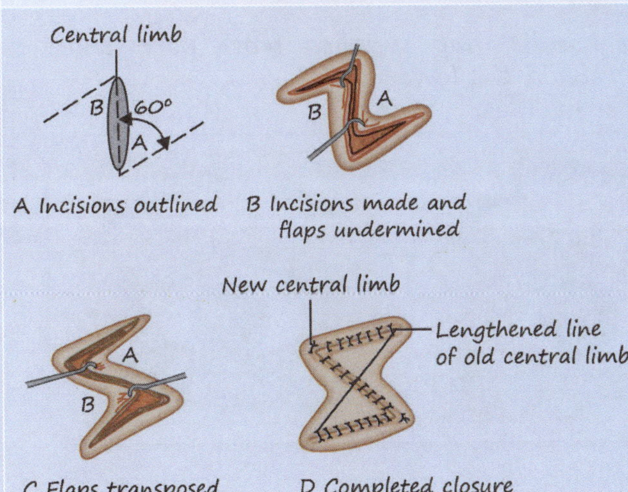

Contd...

Rhomboidal flap (Limberg flap):
A type of transposition flap, it can be used in any place. Very commonly used in pilonidal sinus surgery.

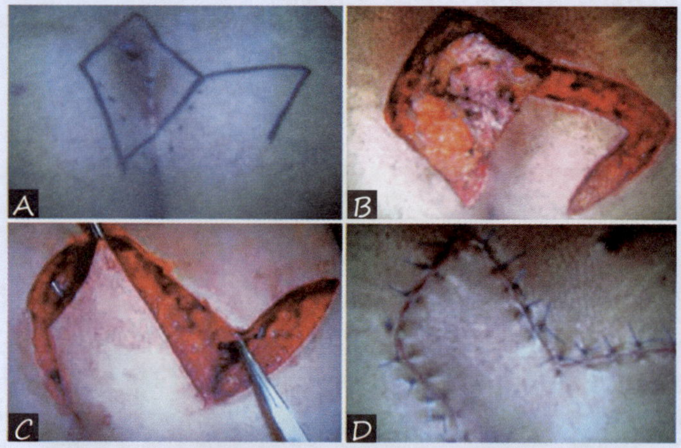

Advancement flap:
- Burow's triangle is made and the flap slides forward or backward.
- Common variants include rectangular advancement flap, V-Y advancement flap and Abbes flap (to reconstruct lip cancer after resection).

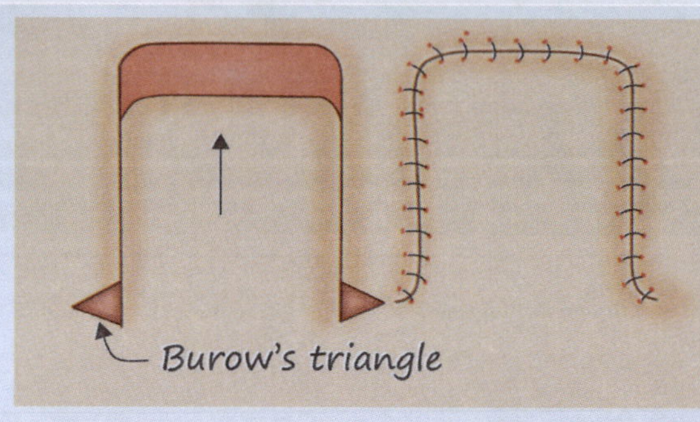

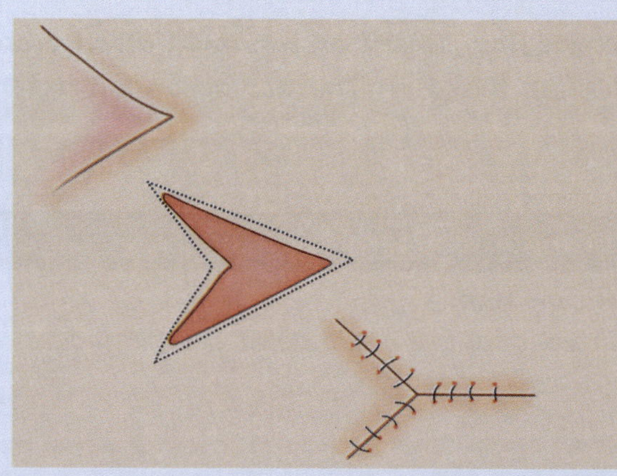

Bipedicle Flap

A 'bucket-handle' flap supplied from both ends. Usedul to rebuild the lower eyelid.

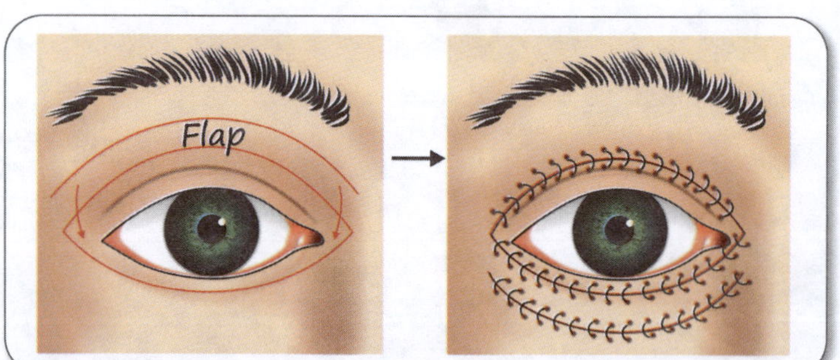

Order of anastomosis of cut limb/digit:
- B – Bone
- E – Extensor tendon
- F – Flexor tendon
- A – Artery followed by vein
- N – Nerve
- S – Skin

ENDOCRINE SURGERY

MEN-1 (Wermer Syndrome)

- Autosomal dominant
- Male and female = Equally affected
- Manifests from age of 5 years**
    - **3P's affected**
        1. **Parathyroid hyperplasia**
        2. **Pituitary adenoma (Prolactinoma MC)**
        3. **Pancreas NET (Gastrinomas MC)**

MEN-2A (Sipple syndrome)	MEN-2B
• Medullary thyroid cancer: 100% • Pheochromocytoma: 40–50% • Parathyroid adenoma/hyperplasia: 20% • Hirschsprung disease** • Cutaneous lichen amyloidosis	• Medullary carcinoma thyroid: 100% • Pheochromocytoma: 40% • Intestinal ganglioneuroma • Mucosal neuromas in lips: 100% • Megacolon: 100% • Marfanoid features • Ganglioneuromas in intestines • Esophageal dysmotility

Hyperparathyroidism

- **Primary:** Due to intrinsic abnormality
- **Secondary:** Physiological increased secretion in response to lowered calcium.

Primary Hyperparathyroidism

- 5th–6th decade, MC in females (3:1 ratio)
- Most are asymptomatic
- MC presentation is **kidney stones** (15–20%)
- 40% patients will have **hypercalciuria****

Etiology:

- MC cause is **solitary adenoma****
- Multigland disease (hyperplasia)—15%—associated with MEN syndromes.

Clinical features:

Salt and pepper skull appearance**

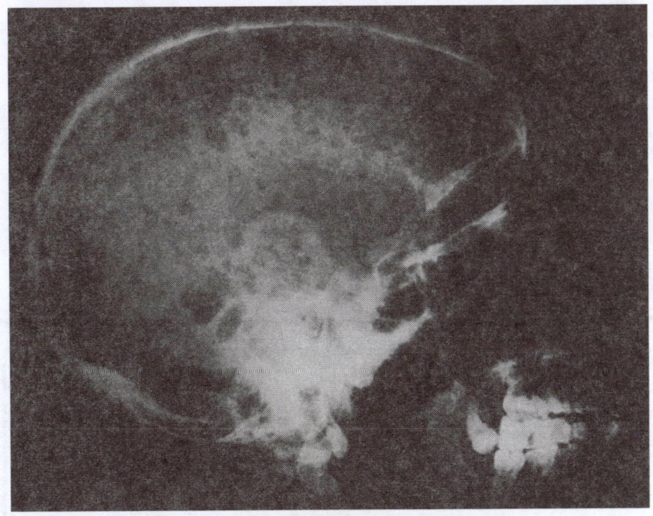

Salt and pepper skull appearance

- **Brown tumor:**
    - Brown tumor, also known as osteitis fibrosa cystica and rarely as osteoclastoma
    - Excess osteoclast activity resulting in subperiosteal bone resorption.

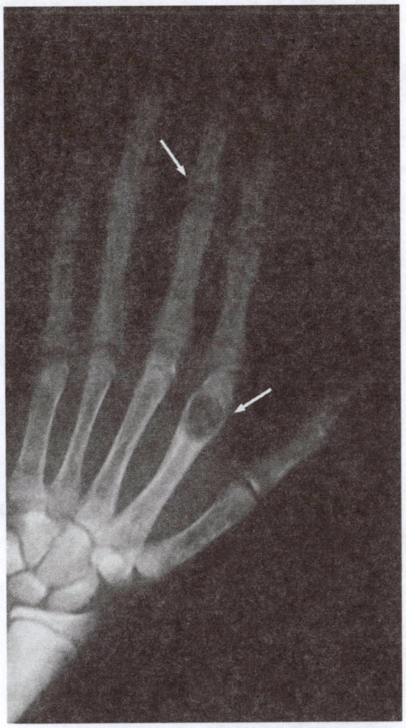

Brown tumor

Mnemonic for features of Hyperparathyroidism: Bones-Stones-Abdominal groans-Psychic moans

Diagnosis:

- Elevated total and ionized calcium levels
- Increased PTH levels
- Low serum phosphate
- Elevated alkaline phosphatase

Localization studies:

Sestamibi nuclear scan is the most accurate and reliable method to localize the adenoma**

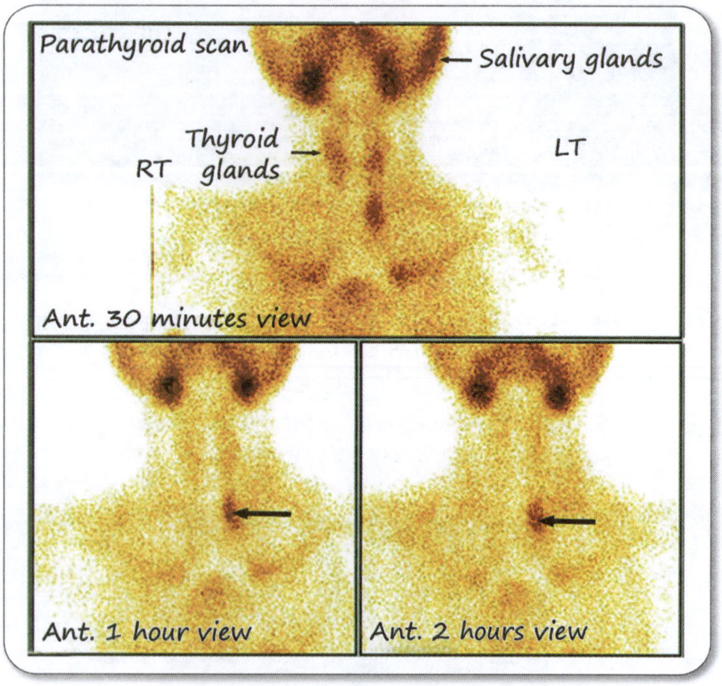

Sestamibi Nuclear scan—to localize the adenoma

Surgical options:

- Focused minimally invasive parathyroidectomy (MIP)—by an incision less than 3 cm in neck, or
- Bilateral neck exploration operation with removal of all 4 glands or 3 and half glands.

Indications for Bilateral Neck Exploration

MIAMI criteria

- Drop in PTH to normal range and to less than half of the maximum per operative PTH at 10 minutes appears to accurately predict the Single gland disease.
- If no such drop is detected suspect Multiglandular disease or Hyperplasia and plan bilateral cervical neck exploration.

Pheochromocytoma

Catecholamine producing tumor from adrenal medulla and sympathetic chain.

- **Extra-adrenal pheochromocytomas:** MC site is para-aortic region (75%).
- **"10% tumor" is the other name of pheochromocytoma:**
  - 10% extra-adrenal (closer to 15%)
  - 10% occur in children
  - 10% familial (closer to 20%)
  - 10% bilateral or multiple (more if familial)
  - 10% recur (more if extra-adrenal)
  - 10% malignant
  - 10% discovered incidentally

Syndromes associated with pheochromocytoma:

- MEN-2A and 2B
- Familial paraganglioma syndrome
- Von Hippel-Lindau syndrome
- Sturge-Weber syndrome
- Neurofibromatosis type 1

Clinical features:

- **The 5P's:**

i.	Pressure (HTN)	90%—MC manifestation
ii.	Pain (Headache)	80%
iii.	Perspiration	71%
iv.	Palpitation	64%
v.	Pallor	42%

- **The classical triad seen in >50% cases: pain (headache), perspiration, palpitation**

Hormones produced by each site:

- Most pheochromocytomas produce **NA >Adrenaline***
- Extra-adrenal pheochromocytomas will **secrete only Noradrenaline***

Investigations for pheochromocytoma:

- **Screening investigation** is 24 hours urinary VMA, urinary catecholamines like metanephrines, normetanephrines.
- **Plasma metanephrine is IOC to diagnose.**
- **IOC to localize the tumor is MRI**** for adrenal, extra-adrenal pheochromocytoma in pregnancy (Even for ectopic IOC is MRI).
- **Iodine-123 MIBG (metaiodobenzylguanidine) scan** is used only for metastatic and multiple extra-adrenal tumors.
- **But now FDG PET and DOPA PET have more sensitivity to detect mets****

Preoperative preparation:
- **Phenoxybenzamine (alpha-blocker):** 20–160 mg daily until patient develops postural hypotension.
- **Propranolol (beta-blocker):** For patients with tachycardia and arrhythmias (Must be started after complete alpha-blockade happened)
- Surgical management of choice is Laparoscopic adrenalectomy**
- **Anesthesia of choice:** Enflurane or Isoflurane** (Do not use Halothane**)

PEDIATRIC SURGERY

<table>
<tr><th colspan="2">Omphalocele or exomphalos</th><th>Gastroschisis</th></tr>
<tr><td colspan="2">It is a congenital defect in anterior abdominal wall with bowel protruding outward with covering membrane (peritoneal covering)</td><td>It is a congenital defect in the abdominal wall with bowel protruding out in angry looking manner with no covering membrane</td></tr>
<tr><td colspan="2">Umbilical cord attached to the summit of the membrane</td><td>Umbilical cord attaches to left of the defect**</td></tr>
<tr><td colspan="2">CVS anomalies: Septal defects seen in 20–40%</td><td>It can be associated with intestinal atresia [Most common (MC) cause for short bowel syndrome in children]</td></tr>
<tr><td>Major
• Defect <5 cm
• Small bowel protrudes
• Can wait and watch
• Good prognosis
• Strapping</td><td>Minor
• Defect >5 cm
• Small bowel, liver
• Difficult to close abdomen wall
• Poor prognosis
• Surgical closure</td><td>• Size of defect <4 cm
• Immediate closure</td></tr>
<tr><td colspan="2">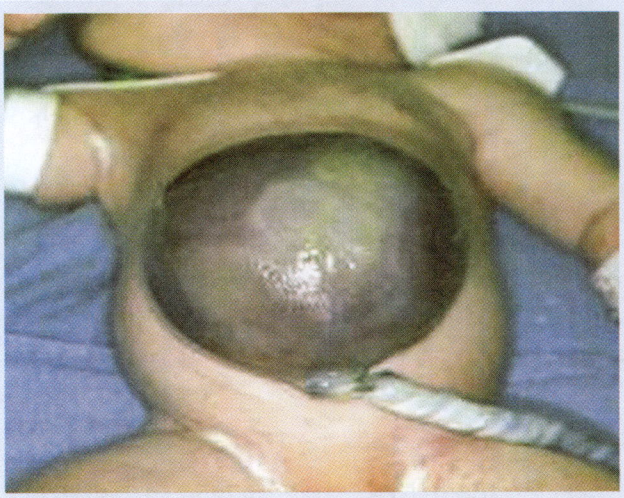</td><td>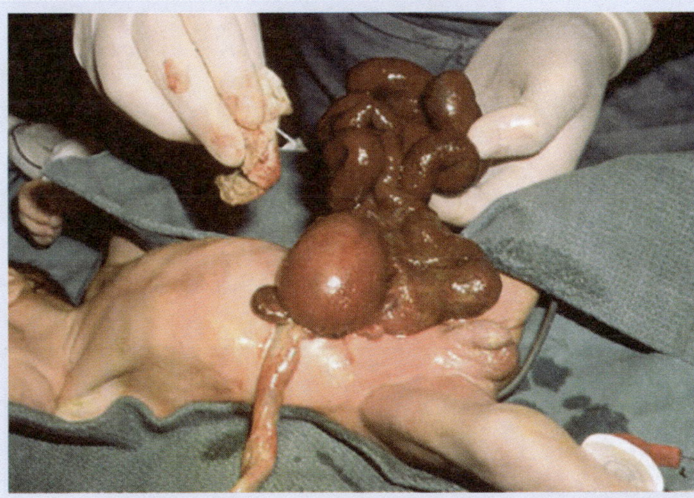</td></tr>
</table>

Congenital Diaphragmatic Hernia

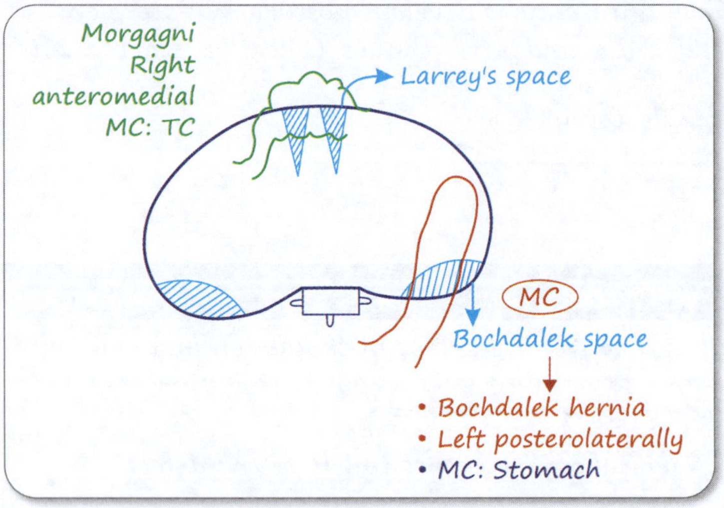

Congenital diaphragmatic hernia

Bochdalek hernia	Morgagni hernia
Herniation through Bochdalek space	Herniation through Larrey space
MC on left posterolateral side	Seen MC on right side anteromedially
MC content is stomach	MC content is transverse colon

- **C/F of congenital diaphragmatic hernia:** Difficulty in breathing (Bag and mask ventilation is contra-indicated); intubate the baby immediately
- **X-ray chest:** Bowel contents present in the chest
- **Ryle's tube:** Present in the chest
- **Prognosis depends on:** Pulmonary hypoplasia
- **In 24–48 hours, lung expands honeymoon phase:** Transabdominal repair of the hernia.

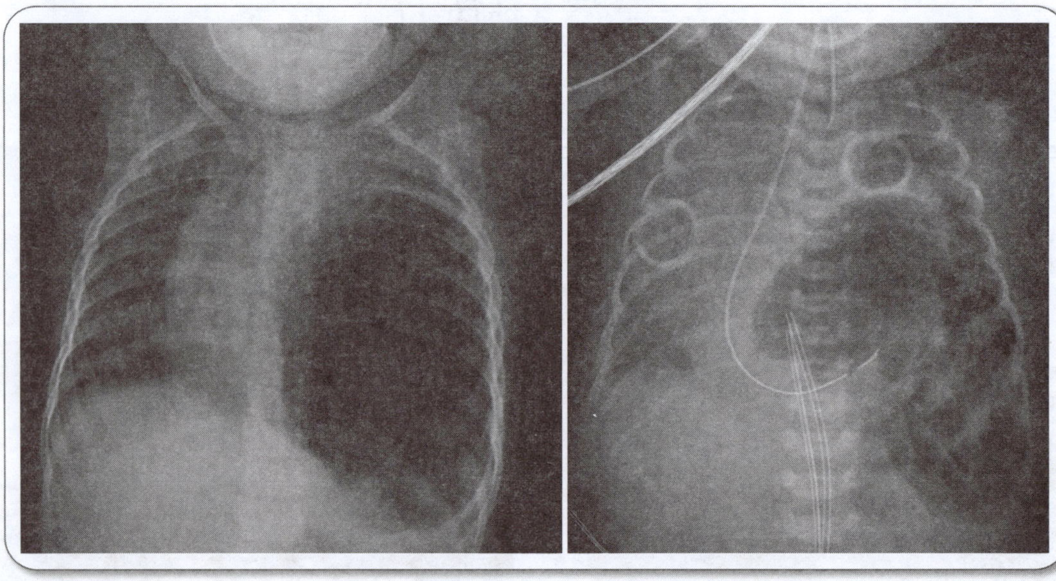

Bochdalek hernia with stomach inside left side chest. Note the Ryle's tube inside the chest on 2nd film

Pediatric Oncology

- **MC cancer in childhood:** Leukemia
- **MC solid tumor or 2nd MC cancer of childhood:** Brain tumor (Astrocytoma grade I or Pilocytic astrocytoma)
- **MC abdominal tumor or MC extracranial solid tumor:** Neuroblastoma > Wilms tumor
- **MC malignancy in <1 year child:** Neuroblastoma
- **MC soft tissue sarcoma in children:** Rhabdomyosarcoma
- **MC renal tumor in childhood:** Congenital mesoblastic nephroma > Wilms tumor
- **MC pediatric tumor producing mets:** Neuroblastoma (Mets to long bones)

NEUROSURGERY

Berry Aneurysm

- Berry aneurysm that leads to subarachnoid hemorrhage (SAH) is seen in 10–15/lakh population.
- **C/F:** Thunderclap headache + LOC (sudden).

Predisposing factors:

- Females
- Hypertension patients
- Smokers
- Cocaine
- Family H/o berry aneurysm
- ADPKD

- Marfan syndrome
- Ehlers-Danlos syndrome
- Fibromuscular dysplasia

Site of berry aneurysm:
- **MC:** Anterior communicating artery
- **2nd common:** Middle cerebral artery
- **3rd common:** Posterior cerebral artery
- **Least common:** Basilar tip

Clinical features:
- 10–15% die on spot
- 1/3rd hospitalized people die
- 1/3rd develop neurological deficit
- 1/3rd recover

- **Clinical grading of SAH: Hunt and Hess scale**
- **Fisher grading on SAH based on CT scan**

Complications:
- Most common cause of death after reaching hospital: **Rebleeding**
- **Terson syndrome:** Combination of SAH and vitreous hemorrhage (in 10–20% cases)

Management:
- **Medical: Delayed ischemic neurological deficit (3–10 days) should be prevented (due to vasospasm)**
- Oral Nimodipine
- **Triple H therapy****
  H: Hypervolemia
  H: Hypertension
  H: Hemodilution
- Surgical clipping and coiling of aneurysms

Brain Tumors

Metastatic Brain Tumors

- **MC brain tumor:** Mets from Lungs 40% > Breast 15% > Melanoma 10% > Renal 10%
- **MC brain tumor in females:** Mets from Breast cancer**
- **MC brain tumor in Males/overall:** Mets from Lungs cancer (Small cell cancer)
- **IOC for brain mets:** MRI with gadolinium contrast

Management of brain mets:
- **DOC:** Steroids
- **Single met (up to 3):** operated
- Whole brain RT can be given
- Stereotactic radiosurgery can be done with Gamma knife or Cyberknife.

MC primary tumor of brain:
- **Children:** Grade I Astrocytoma (Pilocytic)
- **Adults:** Grade IV Astrocytoma (Glioblastoma multiforme)

Brain tumors arising from glial cells:
- **Astrocytes:** Astrocytoma
- **Oligodendrocytes:** Oligodendroglioma
- **Ependymal cells:** Ependymoma

Other brain tumors:
- **Meningioma:**
  - Tumor arising from meninges
  - 2nd MC tumor
  - It is the MC extra-axial tumor (Vestibular schwannoma is other axial tumor)

Astrocytoma
- **Grade 1:** Pilocytic astrocytoma
- **Grade 2:** Diffuse astrocytoma
- **Grade 3:** Anaplastic astrocytoma
- **Grade 4:** Glioblastoma multiforme
- **Grade 1 and 2:** Low grade tumors/Benign tumors
- **Grade 3 and 4:** High grade tumors/Malignant tumors
- **Grade 4** is high grade and can extend into opposite hemisphere also and hence known as **Butterfly tumors****

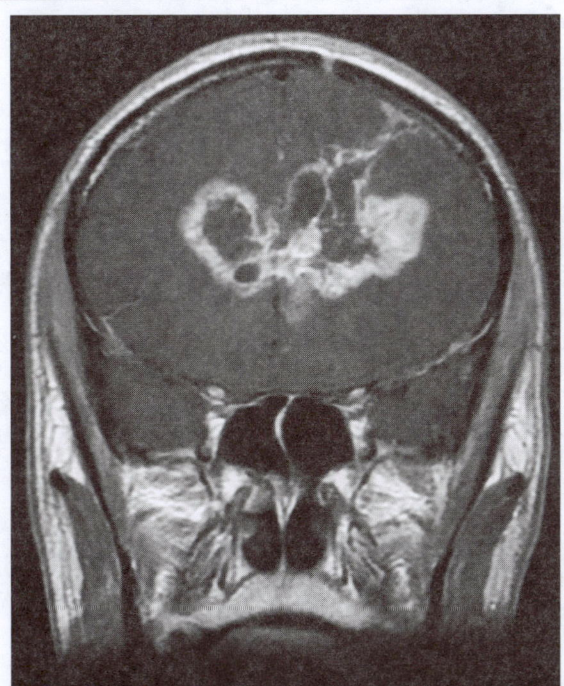

Glioblastoma (GBM)—butterfly shaped

Oligodendroglioma

Calcifications + in the tumor

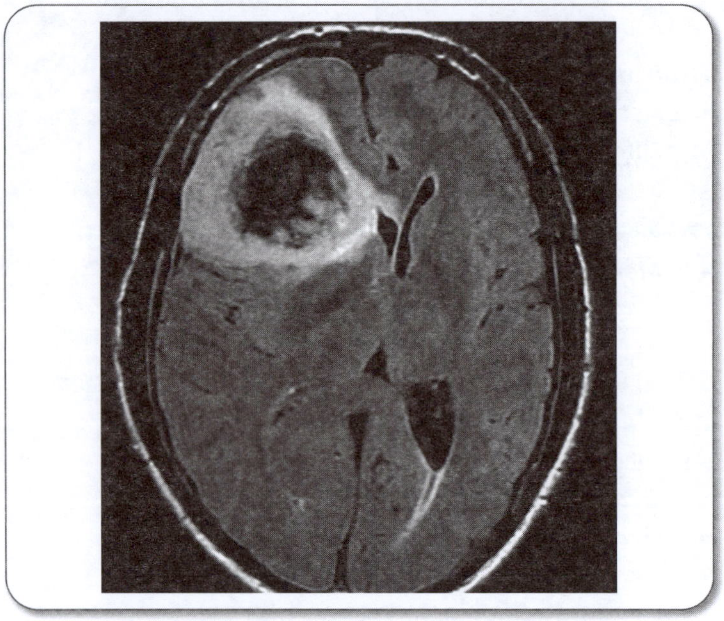

Calcifications in oligodendroglioma

Histopathological examination (HPE):

- Fried egg appearance
- Chicken wire blood vessels
- Microcalcifications

Medulloblastoma

- Neuroendocrine tumor of brain
- Associated with turcot syndrome
- 3–4 years of children
- MC location: Infratentorial or Cerebellum
- Drop mets into the CSF is seen
- Most radiosensitive tumor among the brain tumors
- Since it has Drop mets into CSF: Craniospinal irradiation is advised
- Chang's staging is used for Medulloblastoma

Meningioma

- Tumor arises from meninges
- Calcifications present
- Meningiomas are associated with NF1 and NF2
- MC in females
- On HPE, psammoma bodies seen (due to dystrophic calcification)
- Good prognosis
- Recurrence is predicted by Simpson grading system**

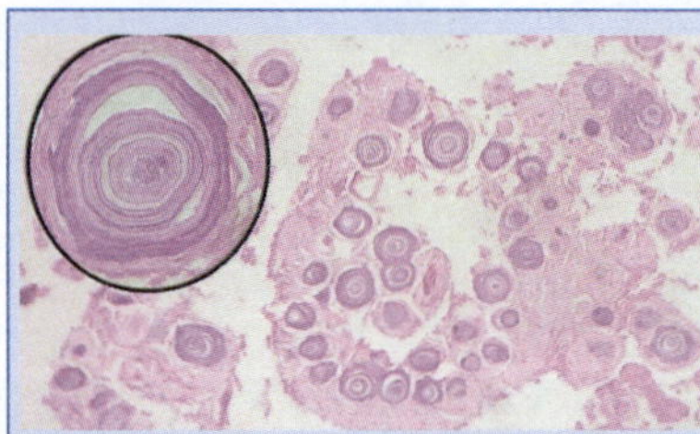

Psammoma bodies:

- Papillary cancer of thyroid
- Papillary variant of RCC
- Serous cystadenoma ovary
- Meningioma
- Prolactinoma

Craniopharyngioma

- It arises from **Rathke's pouch.**
- Classical finding: **Suprasellar calcification + Polyuria.**
- Seen in children.

Neural Tube Defect

- It can be due to genetic or folic acid deficiency or drugs (Trimethoprim, Phenytoin and Pheno-barbitone, Sodium valproate)

Types of defects:

- Spina bifida occulta
- **Spina bifida aperta:**
  - **Meningocele:** Sac of meninges (Dura + Arachnoid)
  - **Meningomyelocele:** Sac of meninges (Dura + Arachnoid) containing Spinal cord or Nerves

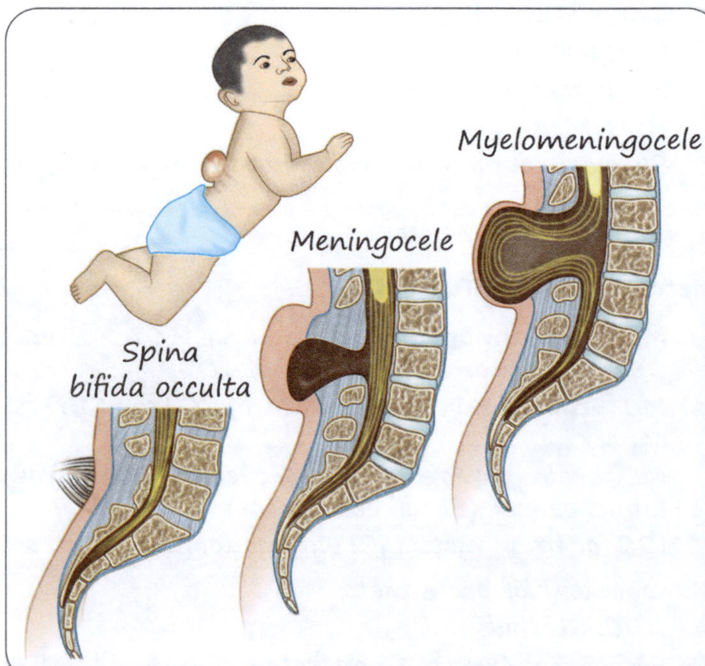

Spina bifida

Spina Bifida Occulta

- Congenital absence of spinous process without exposure of meninges or neural tissue
- Tuft of hair
- No neurological abnormality
- IOC: X-ray

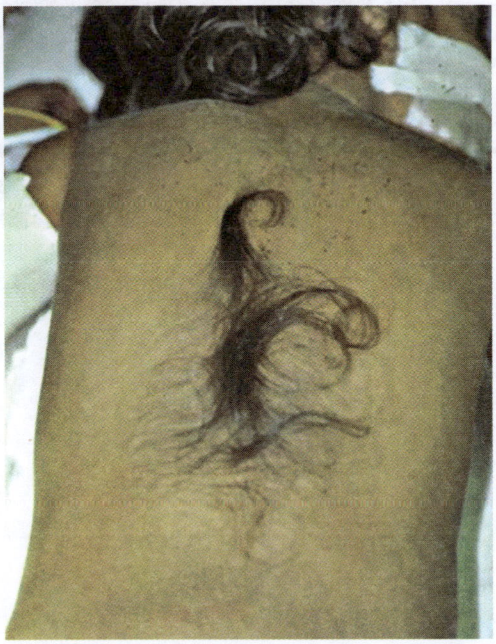

Spina bifida occulta

Meningocele

- Sac of meninges (Dura + Arachnoid) covered by skin
- If not covered by skin continuous CSF leak is present
- **MC location:** Lumbar region
- **C/E:** Transillumination +ve, Fluctuation +ve
- **X-ray:** Opened vertebra

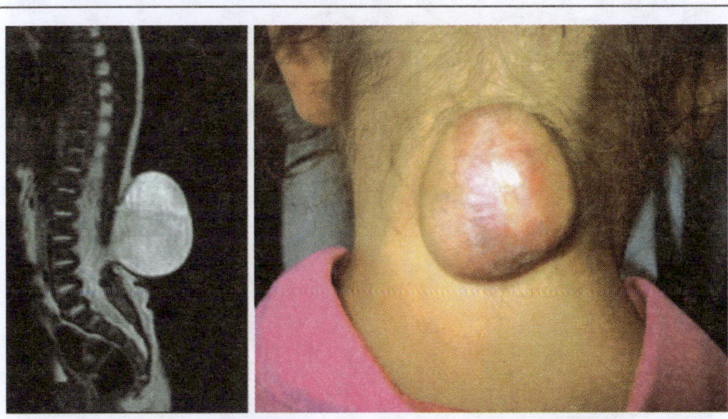

Meningocele

Meningomyelocele

- Sac of meninges (Dura + Arachnoid) containing spinal cord or nerves
- MC location—seen in lumbosacral region

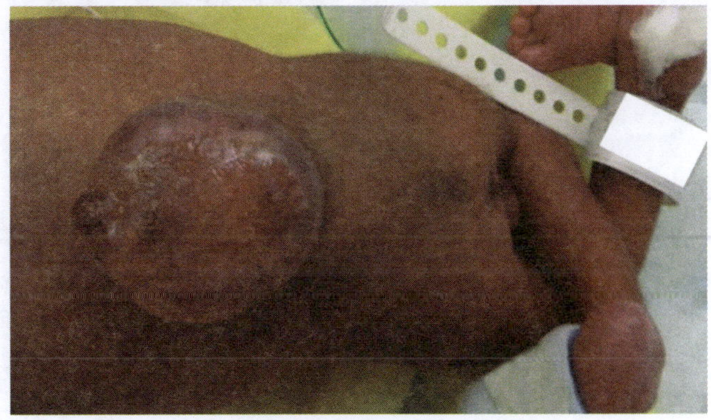

Meningomyelocele

Associated problems in meningomyelocele:

- Hydrocephalus is 80% (MC in thoracic defect)
- Chiari 2 malformation

Treatment:

- Repair in 24–48 hours (if delayed they develop CNS infection)
- Myofascial closure is advised.

ONCOSURGERY: SKIN CANCERS

- Basal cell Ca—most common
- Squamous cell Ca—2nd most common
- Melanoma

Basal Cell Cancer

- MC in men
- MC in age >40 years
- **MC site:** Face (inner canthus, nose and upper lip along tear flow area—tear cancer)
- MC in white-skinned individual
- **Spreads:**
    - **Direct spread (MC and only mode of spread):** Rolled out edge and Rodent ulcer is the other name.
    - **LN spread:** Not seen as the cells are large to enter lymphatics
    - **Hematogenous:** Rare (<0.01%)
- Wedge edge biopsy taken from the tumor
- Biopsy shows peripheral palisade pattern of cells**

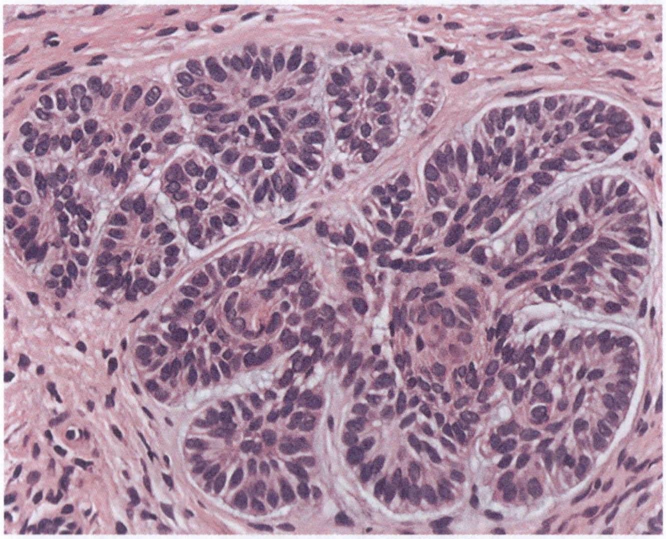

Peripheral palisading cells

- Predisposed by UV light (Strongest), arsenic, coal tar and aromatic hydrocarbon
- ***Clinical features:***
  - Nodular or ulcerated lesion in tear flow area

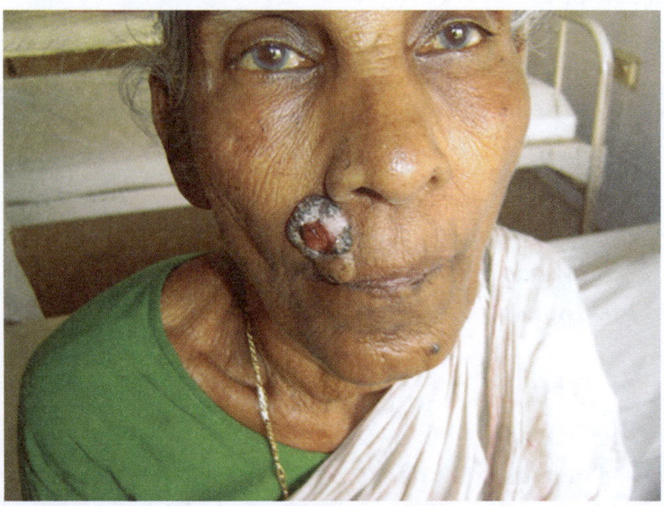

Basal cell cancer (BCC) in face

Squamous Cell Cancer

- 2nd MC
- Males > Females
- Arises from Malpighian/Prickle/Spinosum layer of skin
- ***Premalignant lesions:***
  - ***Bowen's disease:*** In situ squamous cell carcinoma (SCC) of skin/shaft of penis
  - ***Erythroplasia of Queyrat:*** In situ SCC of glans penis
  - Paget's disease
  - Leukoplakia
  - Erythroplakia
  - Senile keratosis

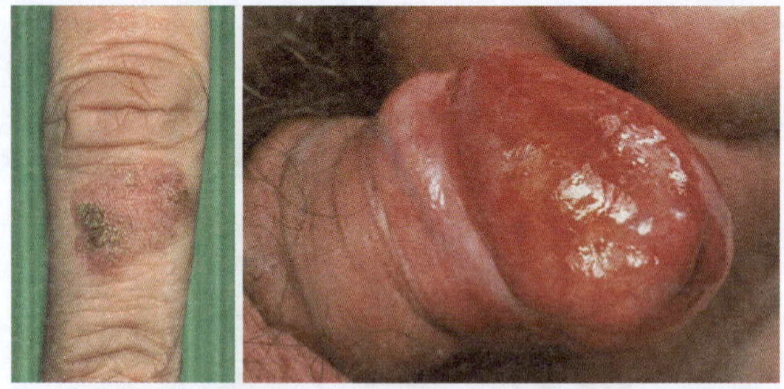

Bowen's disease and erythroplasia of Queyrat

- ***Risk factors:***
  - Radiotherapy
  - Longstanding scars or ulcers: Marjolin's ulcer
  - Sunlight
  - Xeroderma pigmentosa
  - Lupus vulgaris
  - HPV-5 and HPV-16
  - Prolonged exposure to ***irritants*****
- ***Irritants causing cancer:***
  - ***Kang cancer:*** Abdominal wall cancer in Kashmiris keeping hot pot on abdominal wall
  - ***Kangri cancer:*** Buttock cancer in Tibetans sitting on hot pot
  - ***Chimney sweeps cancer:*** Scrotal cancer
- On HPE, keratin pearls seen++ (onion skin appearance in epidermis)

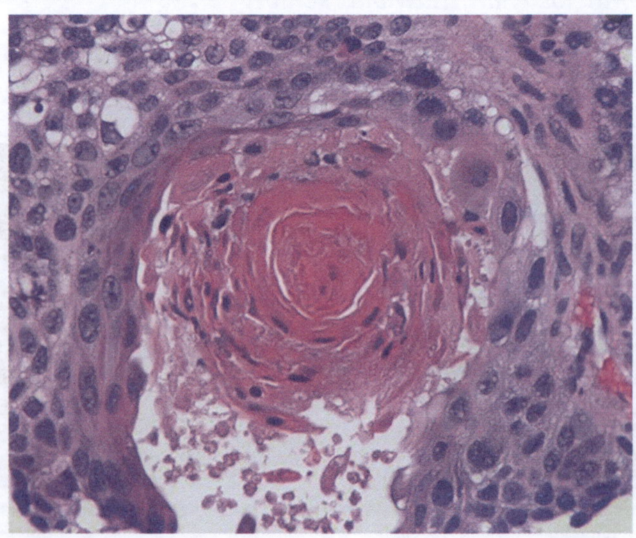

Keratin pearl (onion skin appearance in epidermis)

- Tumor marker for SCC: Cytokeratin 1 (CK1) and CK10

Treatment of BCC and SCC:

- Excision is the treatment of choice**
- Margin given 3 dimensionally is 4–6 mm margin for >2 cm size and 4 mm margin for <2 cm size.
- Larger tumors are given 1 cm margin.
- Cosmetic areas like face, penis, etc.—**Mohs micrographic surgery**—serial excision by shaving until the tissue becomes negative.

Malignant Melanoma

- Melanoma is the leading cause of death in women 20–40 years.
- MC cancer in age group from 20 to 39 years: Malignant melanoma.

Classical features of malignant melanoma: ABCDE

- **A:** Asymmetry
- **B:** Border irregularity
- **C:** Color variation
- **D:** Diameter >6 mm
- **E:** Evolution, Elevation, Enlargement

Types of melanoma:

- **Superficial spreading:** Most common
- **Acral lentiginous:** Most common in dark skin
- **Nodular:** Worst prognosis
- **Lentigo maligna:** Best prognosis
- Subungual melanoma

Superficial spreading melanoma:

- MC type occurring in white population
- Melanomas arising in preexisting dysplastic nevus are usually SSM.
- **MC sites:**
  Males: Trunk
  Females: Lower legs and back

Acral lentiginous melanoma:

- MC in black people
- MC in white areas—palms and soles
- Bad prognosis

Nodular melanoma:

- Second most common
- Can occur on any surface of the body
- MC site: Head, neck and trunk
- Only vertical growth, no radial spread
- High-risk group and **poor prognosis****

Lentigo maligna melanoma:

- Previously called as **Hutchinson's melanotic freckle**
- Common in face**
- Most commonly affects women than men
- In situ variant is called **lentigo maligna**
- Lowest metastatic potential
- Least common
- Least malignant
- Good prognosis

Subungual melanoma:

- MC below the nail bed
- Hutchinson's sign: Pigmentation extending to the nail lateral fold from the nail bed.

Tumor markers of melanoma:

- Melan-A
- HMB-45 (Hydroxymethyl bromide)
- S-100

Breslow thickness and Clark's level are the classification used for melanoma.

Treatment of malignant melanoma:

Excision biopsy with preferred margins 1–2 cm all directions.

TRANSPLANT SURGERY

Graft

- **Autograft:** Transplantation within same individual
- **Isograft:** Transplantation within identical twins
- **Allograft:** Transplantation within same species
- **Xenograft:** Transplantation between different species (Pigs are usually used for humans.)

Based on Placement of Graft

- **Orthotopic graft placement:** Graft is placed in same anatomical location, e.g.: liver, heart.
- **Heterotopic graft placement:** Graft is placed in a nonanatomical location, e.g.: kidney, pancreas.

Contraindications for organ donation—the following persons should not donate organ:

- HIV patient
- Creutzfeldt-Jakob disease
- Malignancy within 5 years (exclude SCC, BCC, cancer in situ uterus and brain tumors)
- HBV patients
- Death due to sepsis

Brain dead donor:

- Brain not working
- Heart is still beating.

In the United Kingdom, two doctors should certify to declare as brain dead.

- One should be a consultant.
- None of the two doctors must be a transplant surgeon.

Two doctors should separately examine the following in two separate occasions:

To condemn them as brain dead

- **Cranial reflexes:** CNS reflexes absent (pharyngeal, gag reflexes, etc.)
- **Motor response:** No response
- No spontaneous breathing on raising $PaCO_2$ >60 mm Hg

Donation after Cardiac Death (DCD) Donor

Maastricht classification of DCD donor:**

- **Category 1:** Dead on arrival at hospital
- **Category 2:** Dead even after attempt of resuscitation
- **Category 3:** Awaited cardiac arrest after withdrawal of supports (who is not brain dead)
- **Category 4:** Cardiac arrest while brain dead
- **Category 5:** Cardiac arrest in inpatient
- **Categories 3 and 4** are good donors because they have circulation in organs until death, they are controlled donors
- **Categories 1, 2 and 5:** Uncontrolled donors

Cold ischemic time: In surgery, the time between the chilling of a tissue, organ, or body part after its blood supply has been reduced or cut off and the time it is warmed by having its blood supply restored.

Cold ischemic solution: MC used is the University of Wisconsin Solution. Euro-Collins is another solution.

University of wisconsin solution components:

- **Lactobionate:** It prevents cell swelling.
- **AdENosine:** It provides energy.
- **Allopurinol:** It is a free radical scavenger.
- **Glutathione:** It is an antioxidant.

Organ	Optimum cold ischemic time (hours)	Maximum cold ischemic time (hours)
Kidney	<18	36
Liver	<12	18
Heart	<3	6
Lungs	<3	8
Pancreas	<10	18
Small intestine	<4	6

Must know points from various organ transplants:

- **MC indication of liver transplant in adults:** Cirrhosis (HCV >HBV)**
- **MC indication of liver transplant in children:** EHBA (Extrahepatic biliary atresia)**
- **MC indication for emergency transplantation:** Acute fulminant liver failure (PCM toxicity)
- **1st liver transplant was done by:** Starzl (1963)
- Domino liver transplant is a technique of using diseased amyloidosis liver to waiting list patient and using the donor liver to amyloidosis patients.
- **MC cause in adults:** Renal failure due to diabetic nephropathy.
- **MC cause in children:** Chronic glomerulonephritis
- It is always a heterotopic graft (Right iliac fossa > Left iliac fossa)
- **MC indication of small bowel transplant in adults/children:** Short bowel syndrome
- **MC cause of short bowel syndrome in adults:** Acute superior mesenteric artery ischemia
- **MC cause of short bowel syndrome in children:** Gastroschisis > Midgut volvulus
- **MC indication of pancreas transplant:** Type 1 DM with severe C peptide deficiency
- Pancreas is drained into either bladder or into intestine. Intestinal drainage is more physiological.
- **MC indication of heart transplant:** Dilated cardiomyopathy.

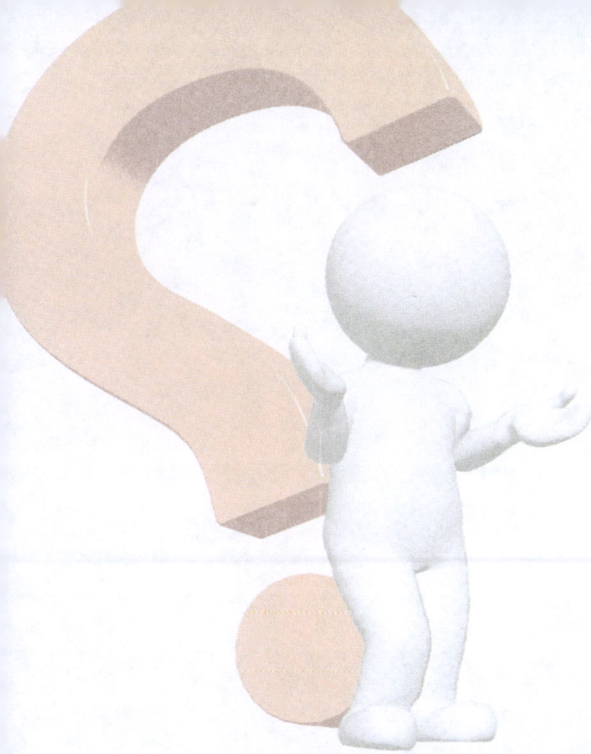

Latest Question Papers

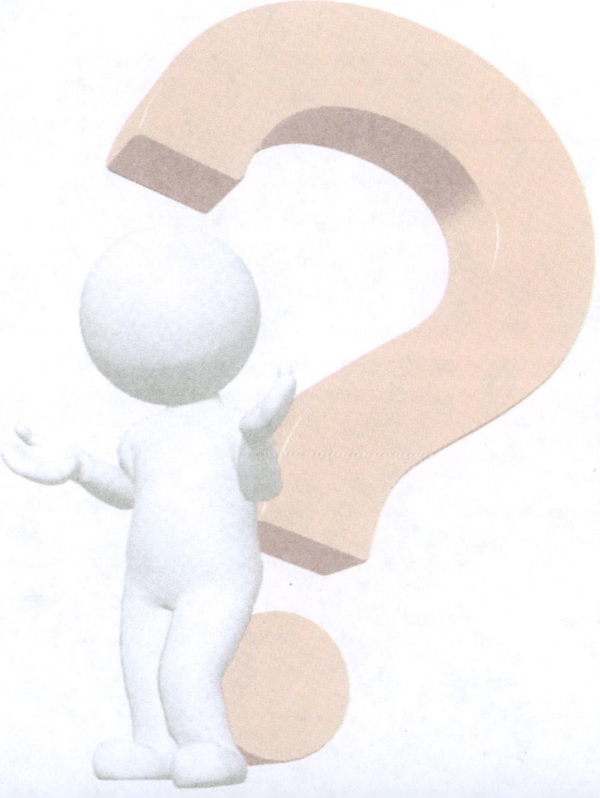

- → NEET PG 2023
- → NEET PG 2022
- → NEET PG 2021
- → INI-CET MAY 2022
- → INI-CET NOVEMBER 2021
- → INI-CET MAY 2021
- → INI-CET DECEMBER 2020
- → INI-CET NOVEMBER 2020
- → FMGE JANUARY 2023
- → FMGE JUNE 2022
- → FMGE DECEMBER 2021
- → FMGE JUNE 2021

NEET PG 2023

1. qSOFA score includes:

a. Respiratory rate >22/min, SBP <100 mm Hg, GCS <14
b. Temperature >100°C, SBP <100 mm Hg, GCS <14
c. Respiratory rate >22/minute, WBC count >12,000, GCS <14
d. Confused mental status, high temperature and low BP

Ans. a. Respiratory rate >22/min, SBP <100 mm Hg, GCS <14

(Ref. Surgery Sixer 6th Edition page 9)

Quick Sequential Organ Failure Assessment score includes:

- RR >22/min
- SBP <100 mm Hg
- Confused mental status (GCS measured)

2. Which is the true statement regarding the image shown:

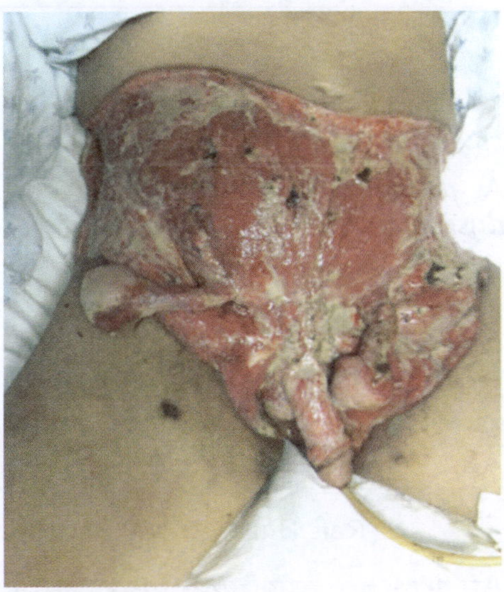

a. Bladder diversion done
b. Caused by mixed organisms
c. B/L orchidectomy done
d. Anti-gas gangrene serum used

Ans. b. Caused by mixed organisms

(Ref. Bailey 28th Edition page 58)

- This is a case of necrotizing fasciitis, in which there is a rapidly spreading gangrene via deep fascia.
- Multiple organisms are involved (MC being beta-hemolytic streptococci).
- Abdominal wall infection like this is known as Meleney gangrene.
- Fournier gangrene involves scrotum.
- This is usually spared testis and testis is not removed.

3. Calculate the GCS of a patient—opening eyes to pain, speaks inappropriate words and withdrawal seen on motor testing:

a. E2 V3 M4
b. E3 V3 M3
c. E4 V4 M2
d. E2 V4 M4

Ans. a. E2 V3 M4

(Ref. Bailey 28th Edition page 363)

- Eye opening to pain: 2
- Inappropriate words: 3
- Withdrawal response: 4

4. A patient developed acute chest pain radiating to back, widened mediastinum. Right and left arms—different BP. What is your diagnosis?

a. Aortic dissection
b. Acute coronary syndrome
c. Esophageal rupture
d. Myocardial contusion

Ans. a. Aortic dissection

(Ref. Bailey 28th Edition page 376)

Disproportionate BP between the limbs is a classical finding in Aortic dissection aneurysm.

5. Past H/o surgery, patient presents with scar in chest:

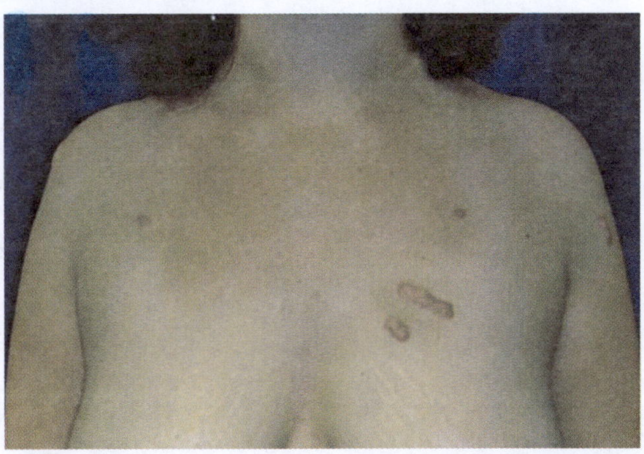

a. Keloid
b. Hemangioma
c. Thrombosis
d. Necrosis

Ans. a. Keloid

(Ref. Surgery Sixer 6th Edition page 37)

6. **An intern presented to you is shown here, he is agitated and tensed. What is elevated?**

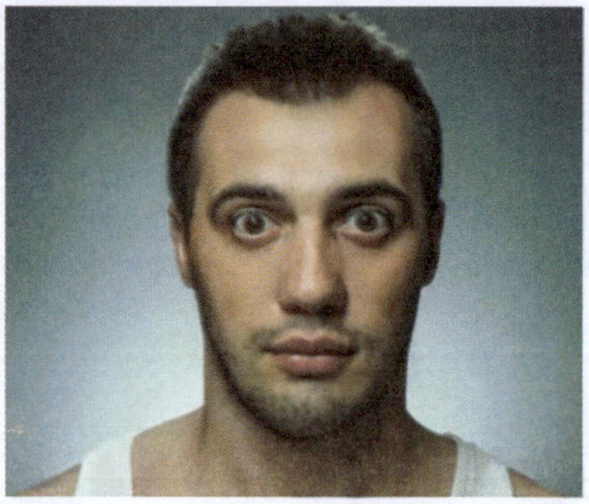

a. Anti-TPO
b. Anti-TSHR
c. Anti-TG
d. Thyrotropin

Ans. b. Anti-TSHR

(Ref. Bailey 28th Edition page 861)

Anti-TSHR also known as Long Acting Thyroid Stimulator (LATS) is seen in Graves disease cases.

7. **Which of the following is the good prognostic factor in BI-RADS 5 lesion?**

a. Ki-67 increase
b. Her2 positive
c. ER positive
d. Lymphovascular invasion

Ans. c. ER positive

(Ref. Bailey 28th Edition page 942)

The following are bad prognostic factors in cancer breast:

- Her2/neu positive
- Triple negative
- LVI+
- Extensive DCIS component
- High Ki-67 index

8. **Hernia seen medial to inferior epigastric artery is due to weakness of:**

a. Conjoint
b. Lacunar
c. Pectineal ligament
d. Inguinal ligament reflection

Ans. a. Conjoint

(Ref. Surgery Sixer 6th Edition page 179)

- Indirect hernia is seen lateral to IEA
- Direct hernia is seen medial to IEA via Hesselbach's triangle—the weakness in conjoint muscles.

9. **Post-laparoscopic hernia patient complains of pain. Which of the following nerve is injured?**

a. Lateral cutaneous nerve
b. Ilioinguinal nerve
c. Anterior cutaneous nerve
d. Femoral nerve

Ans. a. Lateral cutaneous nerve

(Ref. Surgery Sixer 6th page 182)

- MC nerve injured in open hernia repair—ilioinguinal nerve
- MC nerve injured in laparoscopic hernia repair—LCN**

10. **A swelling in neck moves with protrusion of tongue:**

a. Thyroid tumor
b. Thyroglossal cyst
c. Midline dermoid
d. Hyoid bursitis

Ans. b. Thyroglossal cyst

(Ref. Surgery Sixer 6th Edition page 143)

The only swelling moves with protrusion of tongue—thyroglossal (TG) cyst.

11. **A patient consumed alkali and has severe dysphagia. What is done next?**

a. Esophagojejunostomy
b. Gastrojejunostomy
c. Feeding jejunostomy
d. Esophagectomy

Ans. c. Feeding jejunostomy

(Ref. Bailey 28th Edition page 1130)

At present situation—for nutritional purpose, immediate feeding jejunostomy is done.

12. **Patient presented with hematemesis and melena, occasional alcohol intake+, H/o aspirin. What is the diagnosis?**

a. Peptic ulcer
b. Erosive gastritis
c. Variceal bleeding
d. Dieulafoy lesion

Ans. a. Peptic ulcer

(Ref. Bailey 28th Edition page 1165)

MC overall cause of UGI bleeding is peptic ulcer—duodenal ulcer*

13. Following APR surgery—a nerve is injured, which of the following complication is seen?

a. Sympathetic plexus—bladder dysfunction and impotence
b. Hypogastric nerve injury—retrograde ejaculation
c. Parasympathetic—impotence and atonic bladder
d. Pelvic plexus—erectile problems

Ans. b. Hypogastric nerve injury—retrograde ejaculation

(Ref. Sabiston 21st Edition page 1331, Image)

Superior hypogastric plexus (presacral plexus) contains only sympathetic fibers.

- Hypogastric nerves which descend from this plexus are purely sympathetic.
- A high IMA ligation damages superior hypogastric plexus resulting in sympathetic dysfunction characterized by retrograde ejaculation and bladder dysfunction.

Inferior hypogastric plexus (pelvic plexus)—lateral

- Present at the level of lateral stalks and contains both sympathetic and parasympathetic fibers.
- Injury to inferior hypogastric plexus (pelvic plexus) results in impotence and an atonic bladder.

14. Clonorchis sinensis causes the following cancer:

a. HCC
b. Bile duct cancer
c. GB cancer
d. Pancreas cancer

Ans. b. Bile duct cancer

(Ref. Bailey and Love 28th Edition page 1256)

The following infections are associated with bile duct cancer:

- Clonorchis sinensis
- Opisthorchis viverrini

15. In liver cirrhosis, the collaterals happen between the following veins; except:

a. Left gastric vein + Hemiazygos vein
b. Superior rectal vein with middle and inferior rectal veins
c. Left umbilical vein with superficial veins
d. Portal vein with IVC

Ans. d. Portal vein with IVC

(Ref. Surgery Sixer 6th Edition page 314)

- Portosystemic collaterals are formed in cirrhosis with portal hypertension in above areas.
- Most dangerous one is LGV with hemiazygos vein which results in esophageal varices*

16. Treatment of liver abscess—75 mL in a patient who had diarrhea:

a. Observe
b. Percutaneous aspiration
c. Percutaneous drainage
d. Injection metronidazole only

Ans. d. Injection metronidazole only

(Ref. Sabiston 21st Edition page 1459)

- From the history, this is an amebic abscess.
- Indications of aspiration of amebic abscess:
  - Size >5 cm (>125 mL is the capacity of 5 cm sphere)
  - Doubtful diagnosis
  - Not responding for 3–5 days
  - Left lobe abscess

17. A chronic pancreatitis patient with dilated PD >10 mm, and stones in PD. What is the treatment?

a. Gastrojejunostomy
b. Lateral pancreaticojejunostomy
c. Pancreaticoduodenectomy
d. Feeding jejunostomy

Ans. b. Lateral pancreaticojejunostomy

(Ref. Bailey 28th Edition page 1280, Image)

- For chronic pancreatitis, the dilated duct is laid open and anastomosis done with jejunum—procedure known as modified Puestow.
- The other procedures are: Frey, Beger (duodenum-preserving pancreatic head resection)

18. First-line treatment for the patient presenting with mass abdomen and CT image shown here:

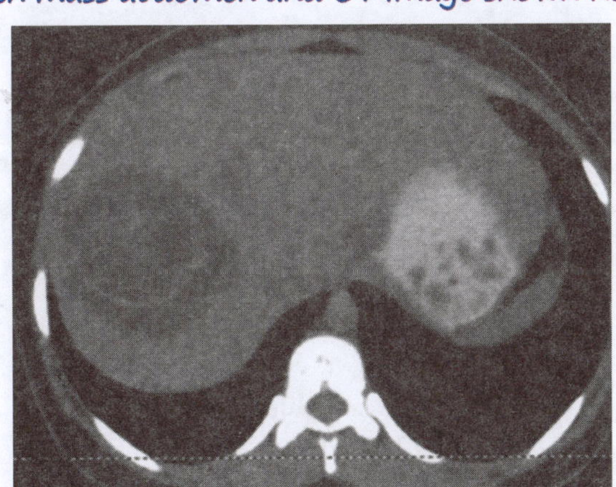

a. Medical treatment
b. PAIR
c. FNAC
d. Drainage

Ans. a. Medical treatment

(Ref. Bailey and Love 28th Edition page 75)

- PAIR is the ideal treatment for this hydatid cyst showing water-lily sign in CT scan.
- PAIR will be done only after the first line with albendazole.

19. A child presented with jaundice and IHBR and has collection in ducts. Liver biopsy shows bile ductular proliferation. What is your diagnosis?

a. EHBA
b. Choledochal cyst
c. Neonatal hepatitis
d. Primary sclerosing cholangitis

Ans. a. EHBA

(Ref. Bailey and Love 28th Edition page 268)

- This is a case of extrahepatic biliary atresia: Gold standard finding is ductal proliferation on liver biopsy.
- Emergency KASAI procedure is done and liver transplant is planned as early as possible.*

20. Alcoholic patient with increased AFP, AST and ALT normal:

a. HCC
b. Cholangiocarcinoma
c. Adenoma
d. Hemangioma

Ans. a. HCC

(Ref. Bailey and Love 28th Edition page 1215)

- Alpha-fetoprotein is the tumor marker for HCC, though only 70% sensitive.
- IOC for HCC is Triple phase CT scan.

21. CEAP classification of edema in limb:

a. C1 b. C3
c. C4 d. C5

Ans. b. C3

(Ref. Bailey and Love 28th Edition page 1030)

- C3 stands for edema of limb
- C4a: Pigmentation or eczema
- C4b: Lipodermatosclerosis or atrophie blanche
- C4c: Corona phlebectasia
- C5: Healed ulcer
- C6: Active ulcer

22. What is your diagnosis from this image?

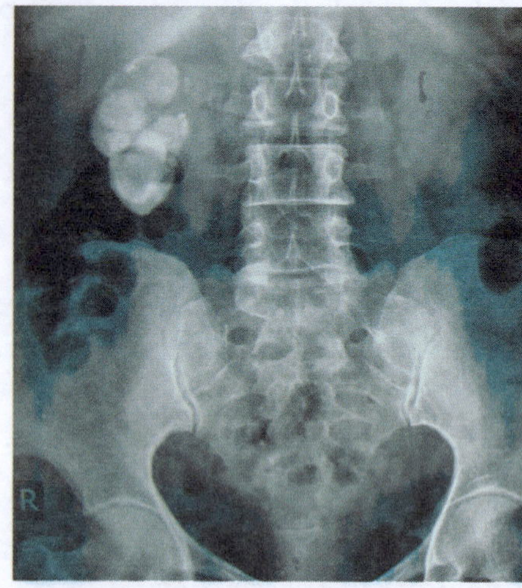

a. Putty kidney image
b. Staghorn stone
c. Congenital HUN
d. Xanthomatous glomerulonephritis

Ans. a. Putty kidney image

(Ref. Bailey 28th Edition page 399)

Chronic TB results in contracted calcified kidney known as Putty kidney.

23. What is the treatment of this lesion?

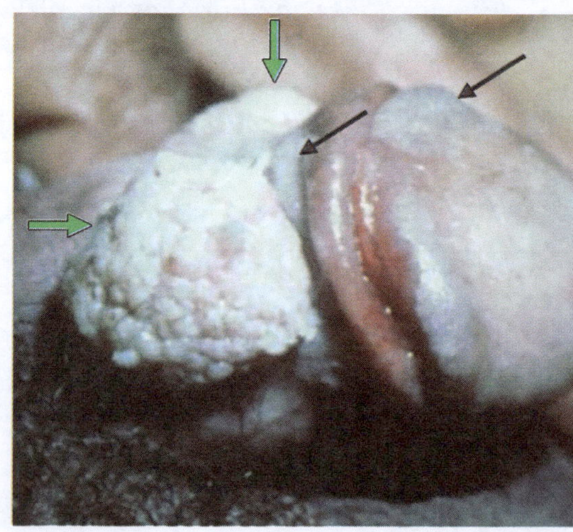

a. Excision b. Observation
c. Topical 5FU cream d. Antiviral drugs

Ans. a. Excision

(Ref. Bailey and Love 28th Edition page 1553)

- This is a case of Buschke-Lowenstein tumor: Locally invasive in nature.
- Histological pattern appears like verrucous carcinoma.
- Treatment is surgical excision.

24. **What type of ulcer is shown here?**

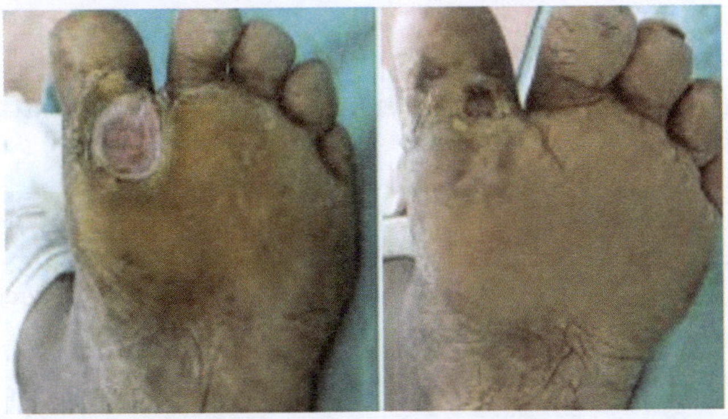

a. Venous ulcer
b. Arterial ulcer
c. Trophic ulcer
d. Infective ulcer

Ans. c. Trophic ulcer

(Ref. Short Cases in Surgery by Dr RRM)

Trophic ulcer is mainly due to loss of sensation and happens on bony prominences of sole of foot.

25. **A patient with hemoptysis presents with hypercalcemia and Horner syndrome. X-ray chest is shown here. What type of lung cancer is this?**

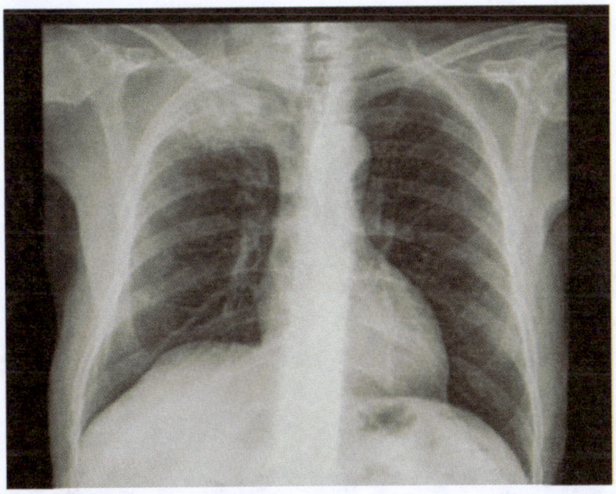

a. Squamous cell cancer
b. Adenocarcinoma
c. Small cell cancer
d. Large cell cancer

Ans. a. Squamous cell cancer

(Ref. Bailey and Love 28th Edition page 986, Image)

Pancoast tumor image is shown here—it is a finding in squamous cell carcinoma lung.

NEET PG 2022

26. **A patient with paraplegia is presenting with an ulcer in the gluteal region, identify the stage of this wound:**

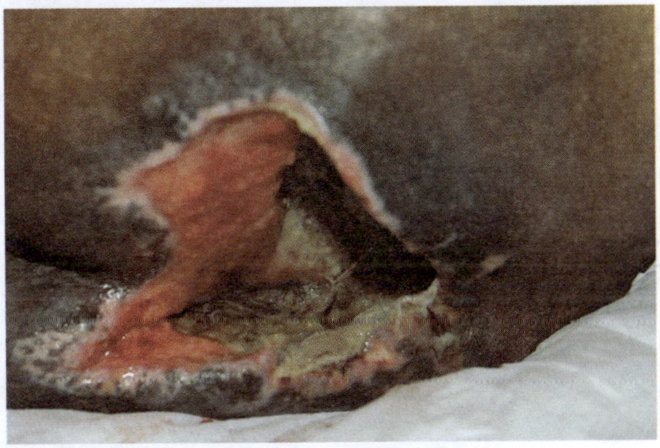

a. Stage 1
b. Stage 2
c. Stage 3
d. Stage 4

Ans. d. Stage 4

(Ref. Bailey and Love 27th Edition page 31, Table)

Classification of Pressure Sores:

- Stage 1: Nonblanchable erythema (no breech in epidermis)
- Stage 2: Partial thickness skin loss extending to epidermis and dermis**
- Stage 3: Full thickness skin loss extending to subcutaneous tissue (not to fascia)
- Stage 4: Skin loss extends to Fascia + Muscles + Bone or Tendon or Joint

27. **Identify the fluid based on the contents shown in image here.**

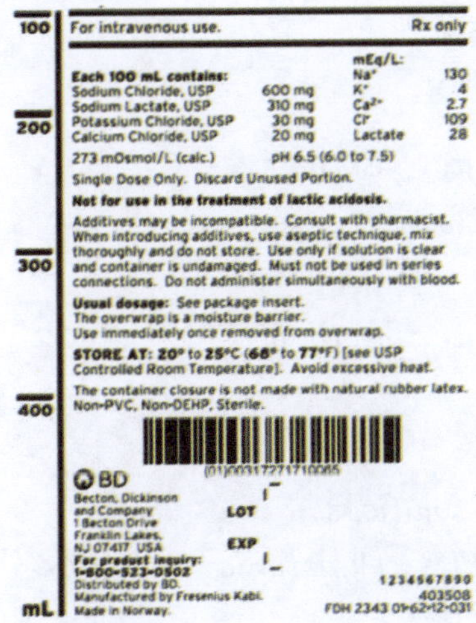

a. Ringer's lactate
b. Isolyte P
c. Isolyte M
d. Haemaccel

Ans. a. Ringer's lactate

(Ref. Bailey and Love 27th Edition page 281)

- Please remember the common fluids in ward—examiners will usually ask from basic fluids only. Especially here you can see the Ringer's lactate is asked—which contains—along with sodium, potassium, chloride—calcium and lactate.
- Please remember dextrose contains no electrolytes and provides water replacement and modest calories (1 L of 5% dextrose provides 400 kcal).
- A typical maintenance regimen must have combination 5% Dextrose+ Hartmann or NS to a volume of around 2 L**
- If hematocrit is below 21% blood transfusion is advised**

Fluids	Tonicity (ignores glucose)	Osmolarity (mOsmol/L)	Na+ (mmol/L)	K+ (mmol/L)	Cl− (mmol/L)	Dextrose (mmol/L)	Remarks
Plasma	Reference	288	140	4.5	103	–	Ca 2.5 mmol/L, Mg 1.25 mmol/L, buffer 24 mmol/L (bicarbonate)
0.9% NaCl							
0.9% NaCl	Isotonic	308	154	0	154	0	
0.9% NaCl + 5% dextrose	Isotonic	560	154	0	154	252	
0.9% NaCl + 20 mmol/L KCl	Isotonic	348	154	20	174	0	
Balanced solution							
Hartmann's solution	Isotonic	278	131	5	111	0	Ca 2 mmol/L, lactate 29 mmol/L
Ringer's lactate	Isotonic	273	130	4	109	0	Ca 1.35 mmol/L, lactate 28 mmol/L
Ringer's lactate + 5% dextrose	Isotonic	525	130	4	109	252	Ca 1.35 mmol/L, lactate 28 mmol/L
Plasma-Lyte 148 (pH 7.4)	Isotonic	294	140	5	98	0	Mg 1.5 mmol/L, acetate and gluconate
Plasma-Lyte 148 + 5% glucose	Isotonic	572	140	5	98	252	Mg 1.5 mmol/L, acetate and gluconate
Hypotonic solutions							
0.45% NaCl + 5% dextrose	Hypotonic	406	77	0	77	252	
0.45% NaCl + dextrose + 20 mmol/L KCl	Hypotonic	446	77	20	97	252	

28. **An old man presenting with tender scrotal swelling, H/o fever+. What is the diagnosis?**

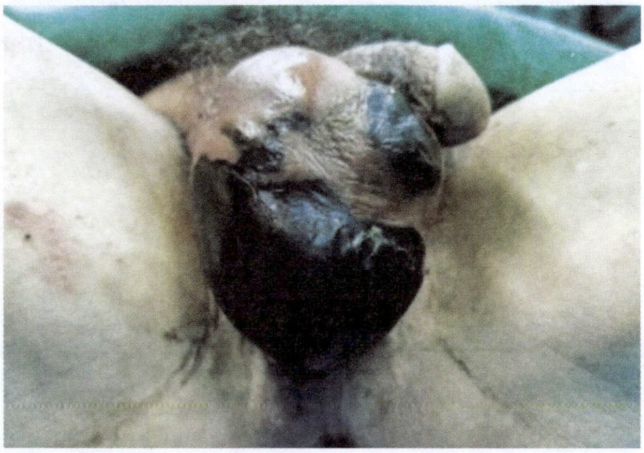

a. Fournier gangrene
b. Orchitis
c. Torsion of testis
d. Teratoma testis

Ans. a. Fournier gangrene

(Ref. Bailey and Love 27th Edition page 50)

29. **A young male shown in image sustained a stab injury on the anterolateral aspect of the abdomen and he is presenting with BP—120/80 mm Hg, PR—80/minute. Next step in the management is:**

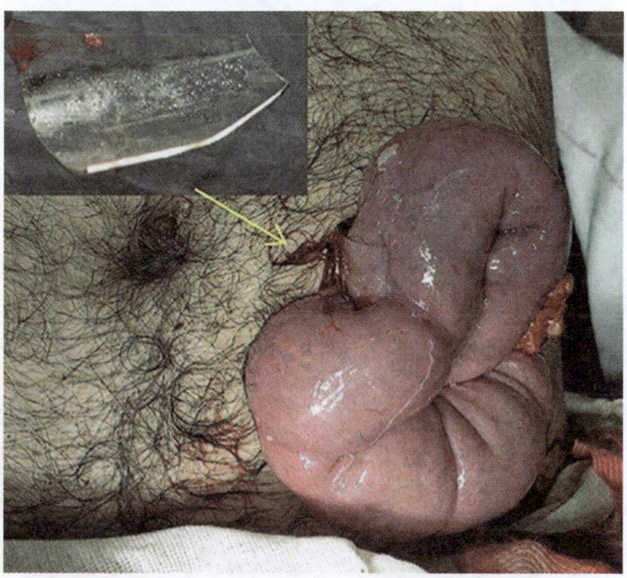

a. Wound cleaning and wait and watch
b. Immediate laparotomy
c. CT Abdomen
d. Need further investigations

Ans. b. Immediate laparotomy

(Ref. Sabiston 21st Edition page 414, Protocol)

When there is evisceration of contents in penetrating trauma, laparotomy is advised immediately.

30. **A 4-year-old child presented with burns as shown in image. What is the percentage of burns? (Burns were shown in right upper thorax, right half abdomen, thigh, arm up to axilla)**

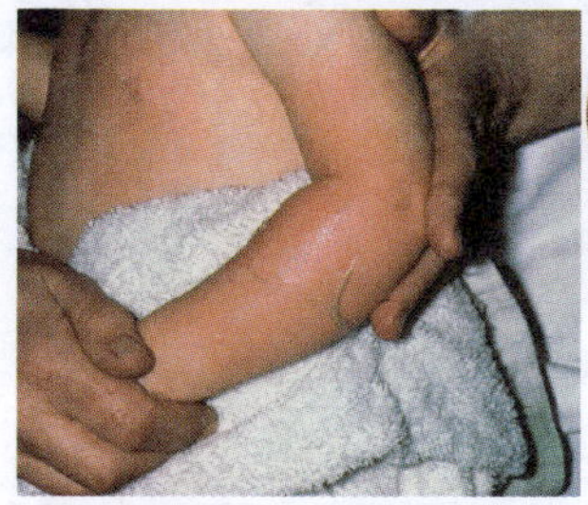

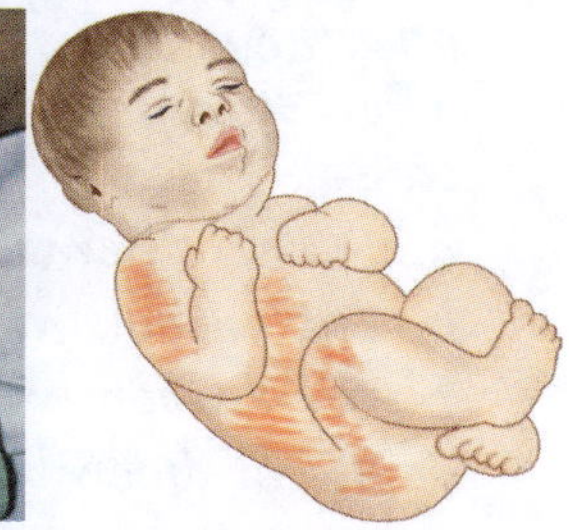

a. 25–30%
b. 35–40%
c. 10–15%
d. 15–25%

Ans. c. 10–15%

(Ref. Bailey and Love 27th Edition)

Accurate way of measuring the size of burns is to draw the burn on a Lund and Browder chart, which maps out the percentage TBSA of sections of our anatomy.

- This is the most accurate chart in children.
- Lund and Browder chart also takes into account different proportional body surface areas in children according to age.
- The "rule of nine" can be used as a rough guide to TBSA outside the hospital environment.
- As per the image: the percentage of burns is 10-15%.

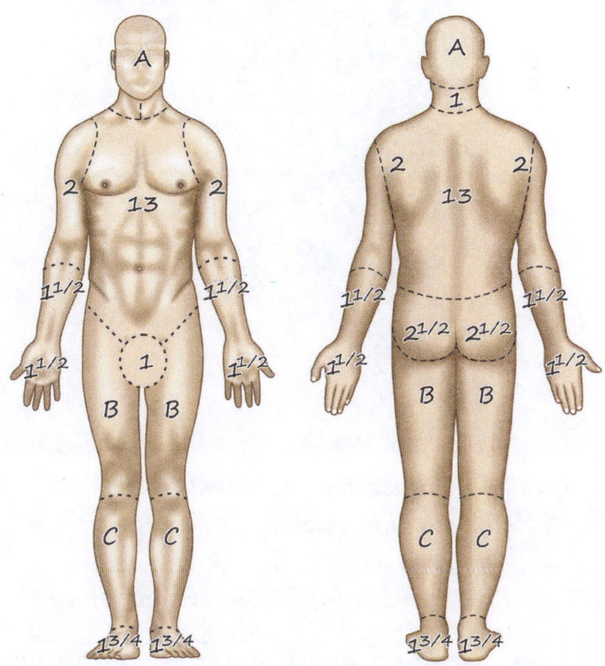

Relative percentage of area affected by growth

Age in years	0	1	5	10	15	Adult
A Head	9	8	6	5	4	3
B Thigh	2	3	4	4	4	4
C Leg	2	2	3	3	3	3

- Anterior half of trunk: 6.5%
- Right upper arm and axilla: 2%
- Anterior side of right thigh: 4%

31. A 25-year-old patient with history of massive RTA developed dyspnea and petechial rashes after 3 days of trauma. What is the most likely cause?

a. Massive hemorrhage
b. Fat embolism
c. Air embolism
d. Thromboembolism

Ans. b. Fat embolism

(Ref. Sabiston 21st Edition page 478)

Fat embolism syndrome (FES) is a condition characterized by respiratory distress, altered mental status, and skin petechiae. This is usually seen in fracture of long bones.

32. A 30-year-old patient presented to casualty following a motor bike accident. He has bruises over the chest. His pulse rate is 120 beats/min. BP is 90/60 mm Hg and respiratory rate is 40/min. A chest X-ray was performed which shown here. What is the next appropriate step in the management of this patient?

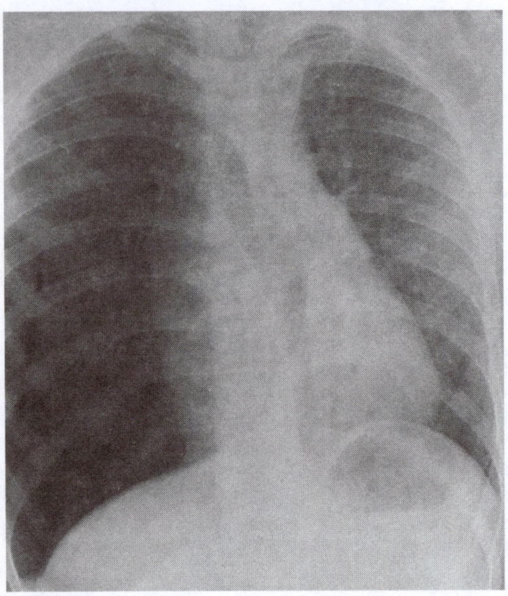

a. Immediate thoracotomy
b. Pericardiocentesis
c. Pleurodesis
d. Chest drain insertion and drainage

Ans. d. Chest drain insertion and drainage

(Ref. Bailey and Love 27th Edition page 367)

Explained in Question 34

33. In case of rupture of saccular aneurysm in brain, what type of hemorrhage occurs?

a. EDH
b. SDH
c. SAH
d. Hydrocephalus

Ans. c. SAH

(Ref. Bailey and Love 27th Edition page 335)

- MC cause of subarachnoid hemorrhage now is trauma.
- MC cause of spontaneous SAH is rupture of berry aneurysm (also known as saccular cerebral aneurysm).

34. A patient presented with road traffic accident, c/o breathlessness and decreased air entry into right lung and patient is hypotensive. What is the best step?

a. Wide bore needle insertion followed by ICD
b. Needle inserted in 5th ICS in MAL
c. Fluid resuscitation
d. Blood transfusion

Ans. a. Wide bore needle insertion followed by ICD

(Ref. Bailey and Love 27th Edition page 367)

For pneumothorax:

- Next treatment is needle thoracocentesis.
- Best treatment is intercostal tube drainage.
- Please remember ICD follows the needle insertion always.

35. A 60-year-old nondiabetic, chronic alcoholic patient has multiple oral lesions shown in image. The lesion is painful with burning sensation. What is the diagnosis?

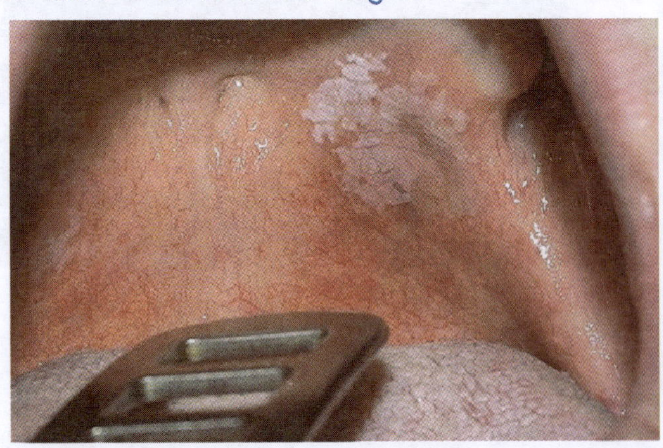

a. Erythroplakia
b. Leukoplakia
c. Submucous fibrosis
d. Melanoplakia

Ans. b. Leukoplakia

(Ref. Bailey and Love 27th Edition page 761)

36. **A 45-year-old female patient complains of recurrent swelling in one side of the neck. She is afraid of eating food as she immediately gets worse pain and swelling after eating. X-ray is shown here. What is the diagnosis?**

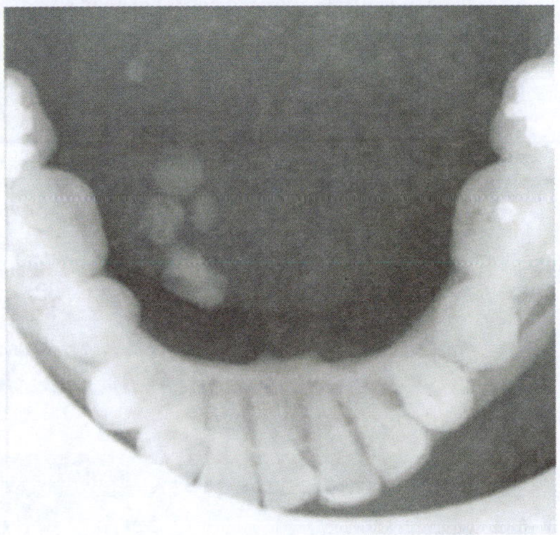

a. Sialolithiasis
b. Penetrated foreign body
c. Osteoma of floor of mouth
d. Cervical lymphadenopathy

Ans. a. Sialolithiasis

(Ref. Bailey and Love 27th Edition page 780)

37. **A young boy presented with painless swelling near angle of mandible as shown in the image. The swelling is nontender and firm. What is your diagnosis?**

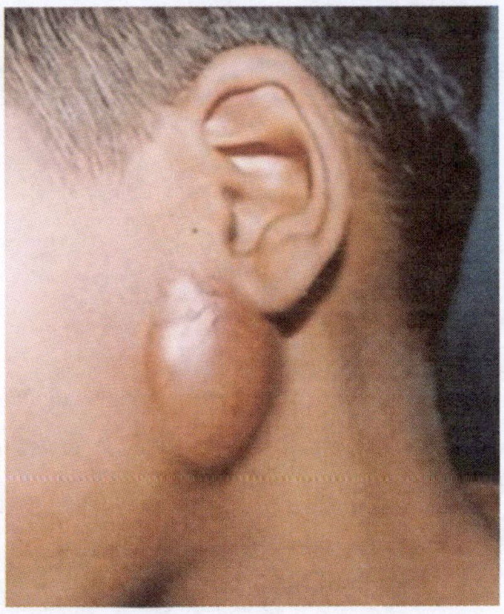

a. Bezold's abscess
b. Deep cervical node enlargement
c. Osteoma of mandible
d. Parotid swelling

Ans. d. Parotid swelling

(Ref. Bailey and Love 27th Edition page 787)

- Most tumors in parotid gland arise from superficial lobe and present as painless slow growing mass below the ear or in front of the ear or in the upper aspect of the neck.
- Bezold's abscess is a rare deep neck abscess and is an intratemporal complication of a coalescent mastoiditis, wherein the infection erodes through the lateral mastoid cortex medial to the attachment of the sternocleidomastoid (SCM) muscle.

38. **A patient is operated for thyroid nodule. Image of HPE is shown here. Which is the wrong statement?**

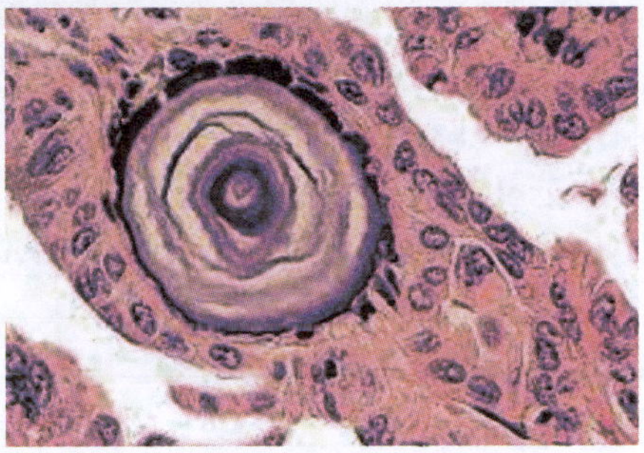

a. FNAC cannot diagnose
b. Nuclear features are diagnostic
c. Excellent prognosis
d. Metastasis to lymph node

Ans. a. FNAC cannot diagnose

(Ref. Bailey and Love 27th Edition page 818)

This is the image of psammoma bodies seen in papillary cancer.

39. **A 45-year-old female patient underwent thyroidectomy. On 3rd POD, she developed perioral numbness. Further investigation involves:**

a. Calcium, phosphate and PTH level
b. RAI scan
c. T3, T4 and TSH
d. Free T3 and T4

Ans. a. Calcium, phosphate and PTH level

(Ref. Bailey and Love 27th Edition page 815)

- Perioral numbness in a post-thyroidectomy case is suggestive of hypocalcemia due to hypoparathyroidism.
- MC cause is loss of blood supply to parathyroid glands.
- Immediately we must measure serum calcium level and PTH and phosphate can also be measured.

40. A female patient presented with a problem in breast. What is the reason for this presentation?

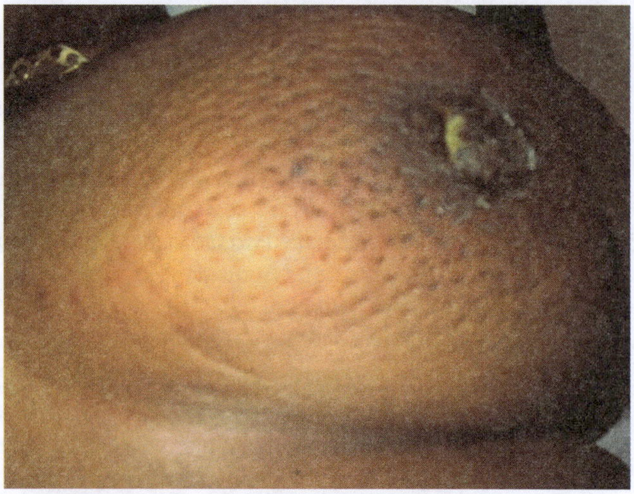

a. Blockage of subdermal lymphatics
b. Involvement of lactiferous ducts
c. Muscle involvement
d. Involvement of Cooper's ligament

Ans. a. Blockage of subdermal lymphatics

(Ref. Bailey and Love 27th Edition page 874)

Peau d'orange is a T4a lesion as per staging. It is due to blockage of subdermal lymphatics.

41. A 35-year-old patient presented with severe abdominal pain and vomiting. His vitals are stable. The radiograph is given here. What is the most effective way to treat this patient?

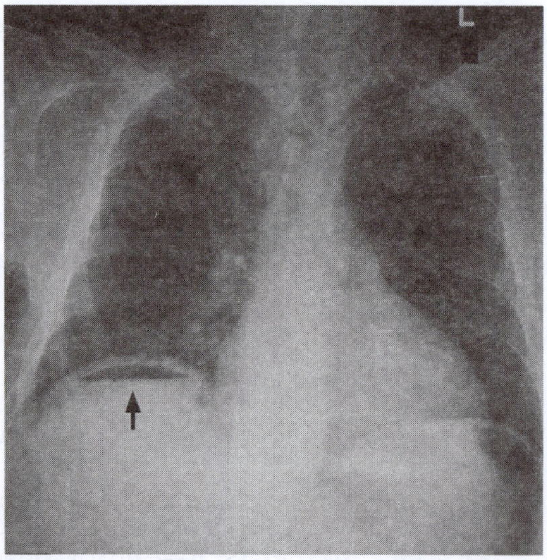

a. Gastric lavage with normal saline
b. Tracheostomy
c. Resuscitate and do laparotomy
d. Chest tube insertion

Ans. c. Resuscitate and do laparotomy

(Ref. Bailey and Love 27th Edition page 1125)

- X-ray showing air under diaphragm on the right side is a hundred times asked question and very important.
- All patients must undergo serum amylase test to differentiate from acute pancreatitis which will have very high values. (But please remember false high value can be seen in perforation also.)
- Initial priority—resuscitation and analgesics. There is no contraindication to give analgesics with fear of masking symptoms of peritonitis.
- Following resuscitation—principal treatment is surgical by upper midline laparotomy.

42. An infant presents with abdominal pain. Barium enema is done—image shown here. What is your diagnosis?

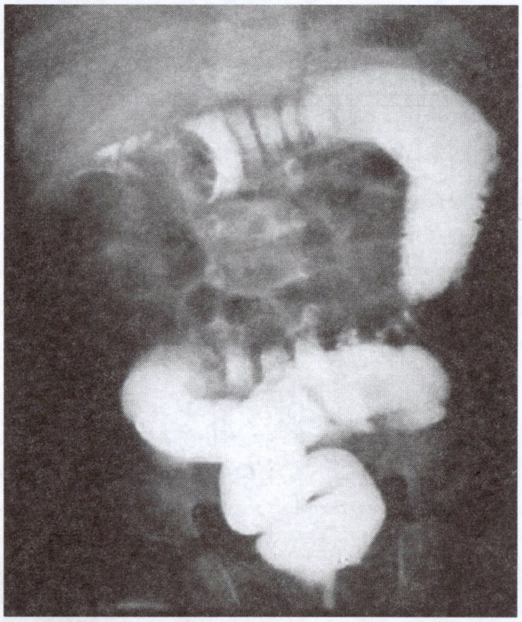

a. Volvulus
b. Malrotation of gut
c. Intussusception
d. Hirschsprung disease

Ans. c. Intussusception

(Ref. Bailey and Love 27th Edition page 1287)

- O/E, sausage-shaped lump with concavity toward umbilicus is seen.
- Le Dance empty right iliac fossa sign.
- Here barium enema shows claw/pincer sign.
- Treatment is hydrostatic air enema.

43. An Ola cab driver presented with a chronic discharging sinus with draining pus near the anal area as shown in the image. What is your diagnosis?

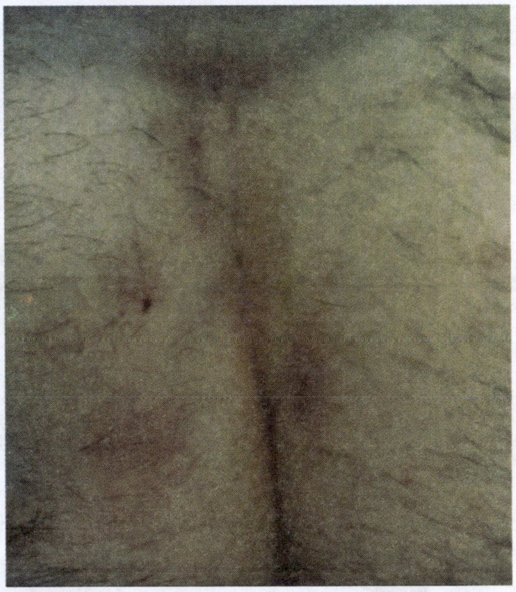

a. Anorectal fistula b. Pilonidal sinus
c. Furuncle d. Anal Fissures

Ans. b. Pilonidal sinus

(Ref. Bailey and Love 27th Edition page 1348)

If at all the image shows gluteal cleft area with too much of hair, think of pilonidal sinus especially if the history of cab driver is mentioned.

44. Which among the following areas is more prone for abscess formation?

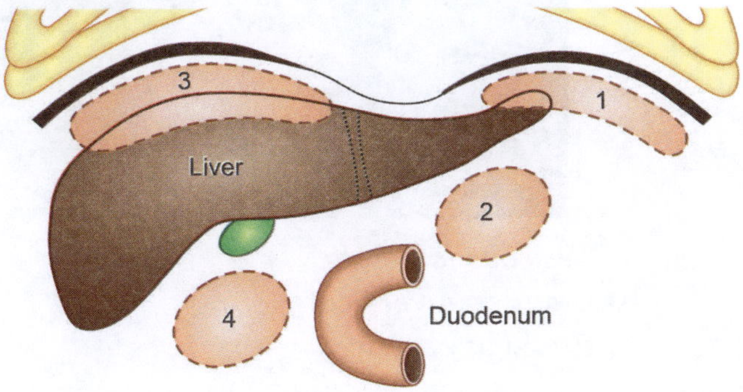

a. 1 b. 2
c. 3 d. 4

Ans. a. 1

(Ref. Bailey and Love 27th Edition page 1055)

This question is directly taken from Bailey.

The spaces in abdominal cavity are:

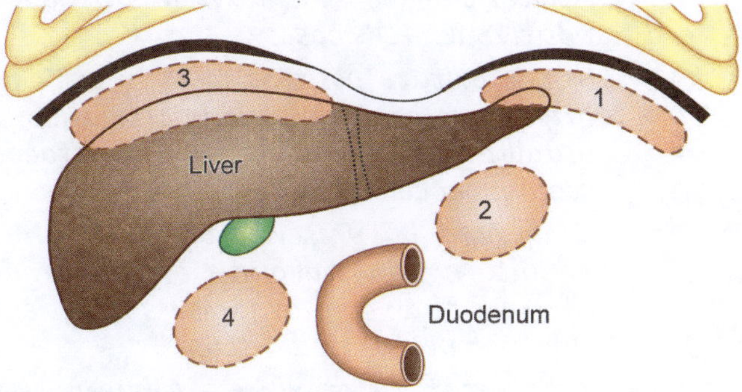

1. Left subphrenic space
2. Left subhepatic space (Lesser sac)
3. Right subphrenic space
4. Right subhepatic space (Rutherford Morison pouch)

45. A 35-year-old male presents with tender tense abdomen. Fluid analysis shows PMN >600 × 10^3 neutrophils. Paracentesis shows culture is negative. What is your diagnosis?

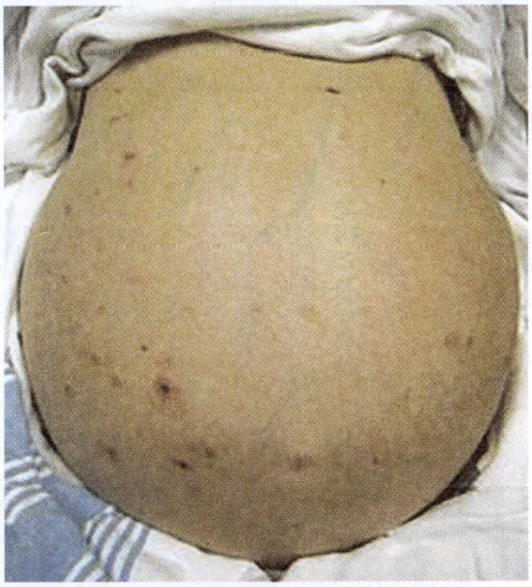

a. Malignant ascites
b. Intestinal perforation
c. Tuberculosis
d. Spontaneous bacterial peritonitis

Ans. d. Spontaneous bacterial peritonitis

(Ref. Bailey and Love 27th Edition page 1053)

Spontaneous Bacterial Peritonitis:
- Bacterial translocation from gut traversing the intestine into mesenteric lymph nodes lead to bacteremia and seeding of ascitic fluid*
- Predisposed by dehydration, bowel preparation and hypoproteinemia*

- MC in patients with GI hemorrhage
- Ascites culture is negative in 60% cases and positive in 40% cases
- In the culture positive cases, most common organisms are gram-ve bacteria like E. coli usually and gram+ve like streptococci or staphylococci usually*
- Diagnosed by presence of >250 PMN cells + Culture shows growth of one organism** (if more than two organisms are identified, think of perforated viscus)**
- Treatment: Cefotaxime + Albumin infusion
- Mortality: 20%

46. The IVP image of a female patient is shown here. What is your diagnosis?

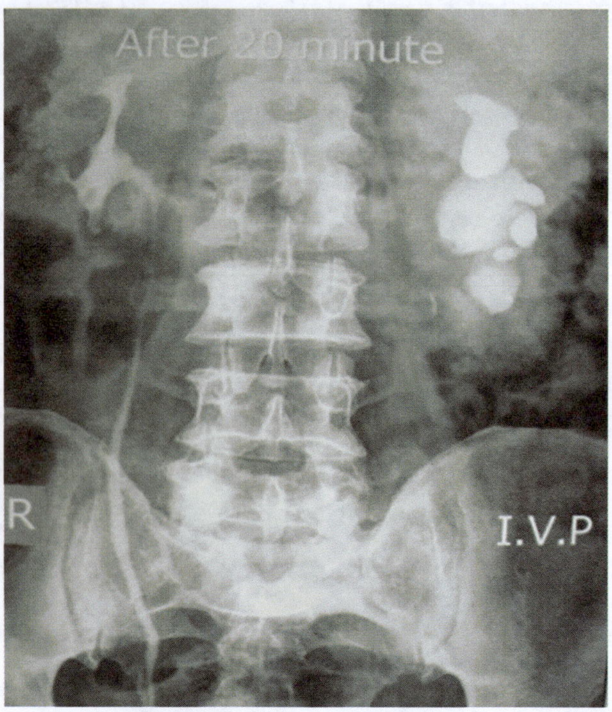

a. PUJ obstruction
b. Staghorn calculus
c. Putty kidney
d. Renal cyst

Ans. a. PUJ obstruction

(Ref. Bailey and Love 27th Edition page 1412)

- The IVP image shown here is classical image of right kidney showing normal contrast flow, but in left kidney there is contrast enhancement, but no flow in ureter.
- Hence the diagnosis is left PUJ obstruction.
- Staghorn calculi will take the shape of calyces.
- Putty kidney is a calcified contracted kidney as shown here.

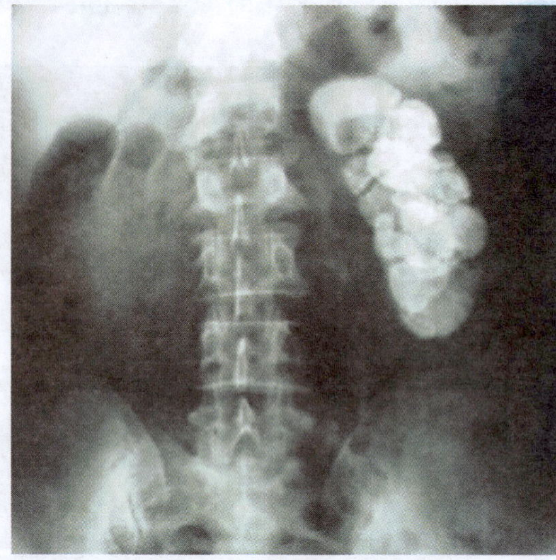

47. A child presented with recurrent UTI. Image is shown here. What is your diagnosis?

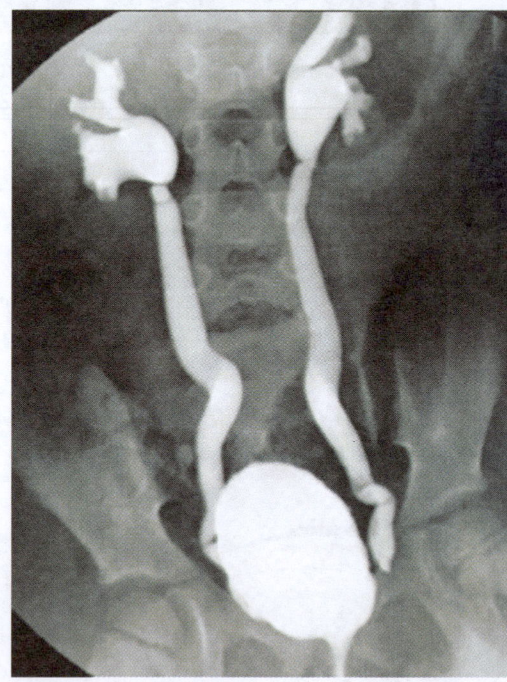

a. Vesicocolic fistula
b. Bladder diverticula
c. Bladder hernia
d. Vesicoureteric reflux

Ans. d. Vesicoureteric reflux

(Ref. Bailey and Love 27th Edition page 1400)

In VUR, there is reflux of urine into the ureter from the bladder which can be demonstrated by MCU as shown in the image.

48. A 40-year-old male patient presents with frequent micturition. On examination of his urine, there is sterile pyuria. X-ray is shown here. What is the diagnosis?

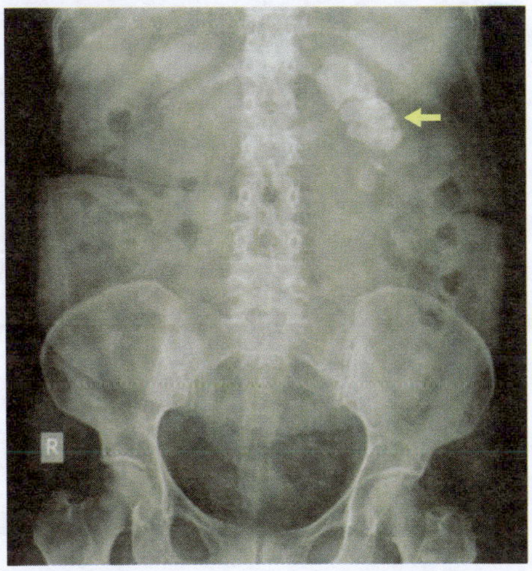

a. Nephrocalcinosis
b. Putty kidney
c. Staghorn calculi
d. Psoas calcification

Ans. b. Putty kidney

(Ref. Bailey and Love 27th Edition page 1411)

Putty kidney is a chronic calcified TB kidney. It is contracted and seen on CT scan as calcified kidney.

49. A young male patient had an RTA and presents with pelvic fracture and blood at urethral meatus. RGU is done—image shown here. What is the site of injury?

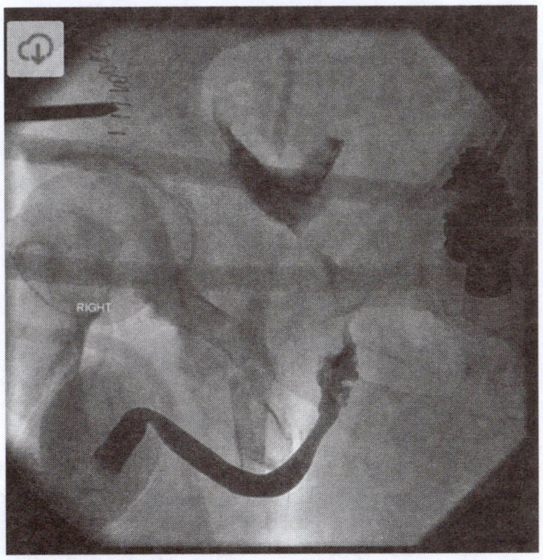

a. Bulbar urethral injury
b. Membranous urethral injury
c. Penile urethral injury
d. Spongy urethral injury

Ans. b. Membranous urethral injury

(Ref. Bailey and Love 27th Edition page 1480)

- Membranous urethral injury is due to pelvic fracture.
- The investigation shown is RGU—with narrowing at membranous urethra level.
- I am telling you a simple way, no need to even know the image—History is enough to come a conclusion of which part of urethra is injured.

50. A newborn baby after birth is presenting with the following finding as shown in image here. What is your diagnosis?

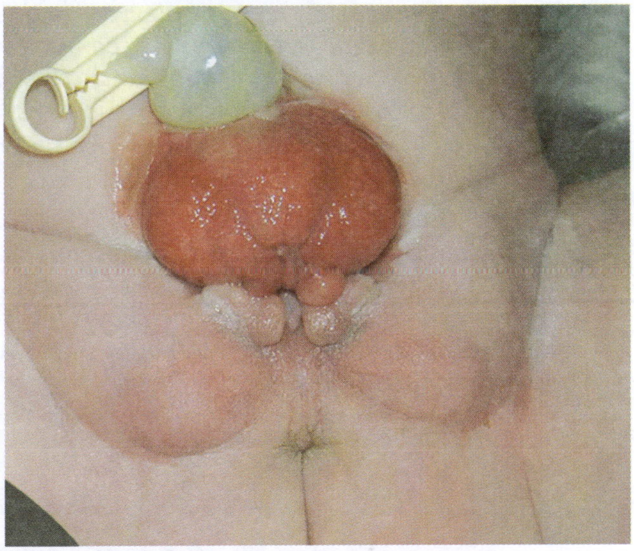

a. Exomphalos
b. Gastroschisis
c. Exstrophy of bladder
d. Omphalocele

Ans. c. Exstrophy of bladder

(Ref. Bailey and Love 27th Edition page 1424)

- 1,50,000 births (male: female ratio—4:1)
- In males, the penis is broad and short, and bilateral inguinal hernia may be present.
- There is separation of the pubic bones seen.
- In epispadias alone, the pubes are united and external genitalia are almost normal,
- In females, the clitoris is bifid.

51. Route of metastasis of prostate cancer to lumbar vertebra:

a. Transcoelomic
b. Lymphatics
c. Prostatic venous plexus
d. Inferior vesical vein

Ans. c. Prostatic venous plexus

(Ref. Internet Sources and Bailey 27th Edition page 1469)

- Spread by the bloodstream, it occurs particularly to bone; indeed, the prostate is the most common site of origin for skeletal metastases, followed in turn by the breast, the kidney, the bronchus and the thyroid gland.
- The bones involved most frequently by carcinoma of the prostate are the pelvic bones and the lower lumbar vertebrae.
- The femoral head, rib cage and skull are other common sites.
- The prostatic venous plexus drains into internal iliac vein which connects with vertebral venous plexus, and this is the route of bone mets of prostatic cancer.
- This venous plexus is known as Santorini's plexus—the prostatic venous plexus around the gland.

52. A patient who underwent cystoscopy showed multiple white plaques in the bladder. The histopathological examination shows infiltration of lamina propria layer as shown here. What is the diagnosis?

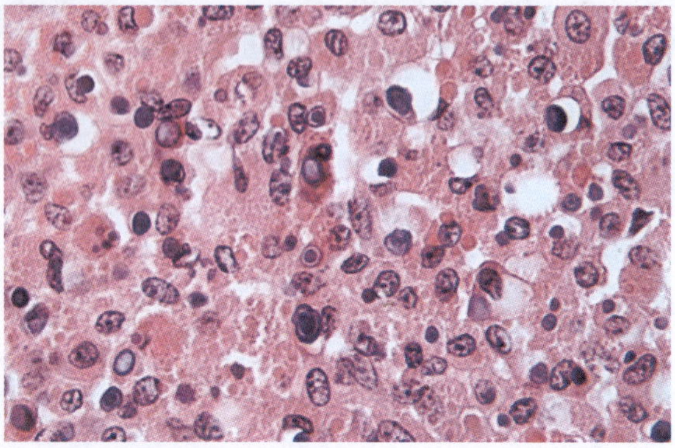

a. Malakoplakia
b. Interstitial cystitis
c. Acute cystitis
d. Chronic cystitis

Ans. a. Malakoplakia

(Ref. Internet Sources)

- Malakoplakia is characterized microscopically by the presence of foamy histiocytes (called von Hansemann cells) with basophilic inclusions called Michaelis-Gutmann bodies.
- These bodies are concentrically layered basophilic cytoplasm and are thought to represent the remnants of phagosomes mineralized by iron and calcium.

53. A male patient presented with bilateral toe gangrene with amputated digits and leg claudication. H/o impotence is seen. Where is the site of occlusion. See the image shown here.

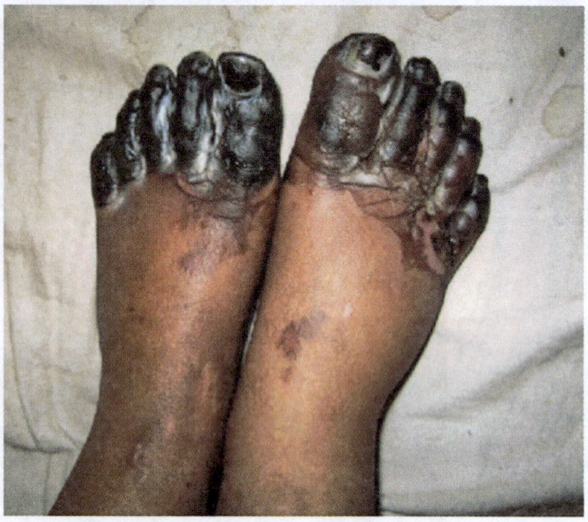

a. Aortoiliac
b. Bilateral internal iliac
c. Femoral
d. Popliteal

Ans. a. Aortoiliac

(Ref. Bailey and Love 27th Edition page 944, Table)

Aortoiliac occlusion is characterized by:

- Claudication in buttocks, thighs, calves
- Femoral and distal pulses absent in both limbs
- Bruit over aortoiliac region
- Impotence (Leriche syndrome)

54. Following surgery for varicose veins, patient started complaining of numbness along the medial aspect of leg. Which nerve is most commonly affected?

a. Superficial peroneal nerve
b. Deep peroneal nerve
c. Saphenous nerve
d. Sural nerve

Ans. c. Saphenous nerve

(Ref. Bailey and Love 27th Edition page 961)

- LSV stripping can injure—saphenous nerve
- SSV stripping can injure—sural nerve

55. Which of the following is not seen in MEN 2B syndrome?

a. Mucosal neuromas
b. Megacolon
c. Medullary cancer thyroid
d. Parathyroid adenoma

Ans. d. Parathyroid adenoma

(Ref. Sabiston 21st Edition page 1005)

56. A 65-year-old patient presented with a gradually increasing growth besides the nose near the medial canthus with ulceration. Histopathology image is shown here. What is the most likely diagnosis?

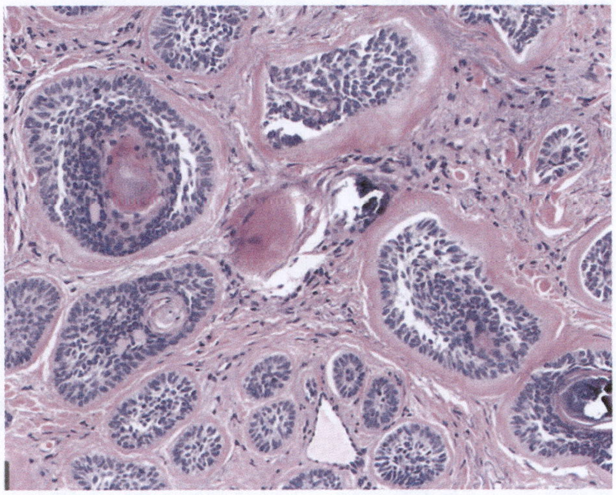

a. BCC
b. SCC
c. Melanoma
d. Nevus

Ans. a. BCC

(Ref. Bailey and Love 27th Edition page 604)

- Peripheral palisading of cells seen in basal cell cancer (BCC).
- It is only the outer layer of cells that actively divide, explaining why tumor growth rates are slower than their cycle speed and the reason behind why incompletely excised BCC will grow aggressively.
- Morphoeic BCC synthesizes type 4 collagenase and spreads rapidly.

NEET PG 2021

57. A male patient presents with below image. Which of the following is done?

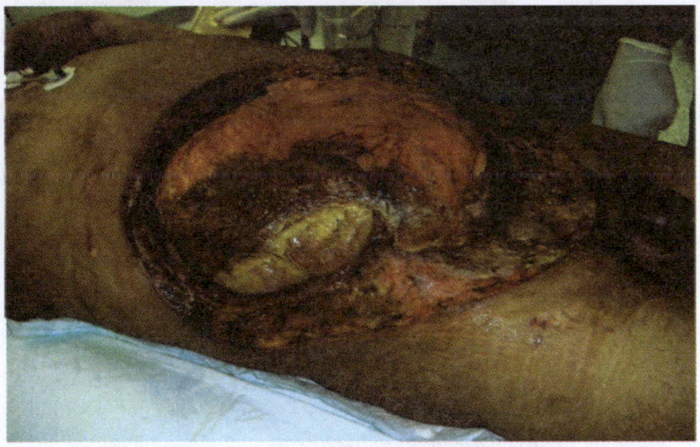

a. Orchidectomy done
b. Urinary diversion done
c. Mixed aerobic and anaerobic infection is seen
d. Anti-Gas gangrene serum given

Ans. c. Mixed aerobic and anaerobic infection is seen

(Ref: Bailey and Love 27th edition page 51)

- This is the image of Meleney's gangrene, synergestic infection of aerobic and anaerobic organisms.
- Not caused by clostridium.
- No need of Urinary diversion or Orchidectomy
- Usually testis is spared in Fournier gangrene and results in shameful exposure of testis

58. A patient presented with a road traffic accident after breathlessness and decreased air entry into right lung the patient is hypotensive. What is the best step?

a. Wide bore needle insertion followed by ICD
b. Needle inserted in 5th ICS in MAL
c. Fluid resuscitation
d. Blood transfusion

Ans. a. Wide bore needle insertion followed by ICD

(Ref: Bailey and Love 27th edition page 367)

For Pneumothorax:

- Next Treatment is Needle Thoracocentesis
- Best Treatment is Intercostal Tube drainage
- Please remember ICD follows the Needle insertion always

59. A patient presented in Emergency following a Blunt injury in a RTA, he had injuries in left hypochondrium. Patient is unstable. What will you do next?

a. CECT abdomen
b. E fast
c. Laparotomy and proceed
d. MRI

Ans. b. E fast

(Ref: Bailey and Love 27th edition page 373)

- E Fast is the first done investigation for Blunt injury abdomen. E fast is accurate in detecting >100 mL Blood.
- E Fast is not used in Penetrating injuries**

60. A patient with Blunt injury abdomen presents with Flank Ecchymosis. His vitals are stable. Which of the following investigation is best to localize the site of bleeding?

a. CECT abdomen
b. USG abdomen
c. RGU
d. X-ray

Ans. a. CECT abdomen

(Ref: Sabiston 21st edition page 413)

- CECT Abdomen is the IOC for stable patient
- FAST is done for unstable patient

Flowchart: Management of blunt trauma abdomen (BTA)

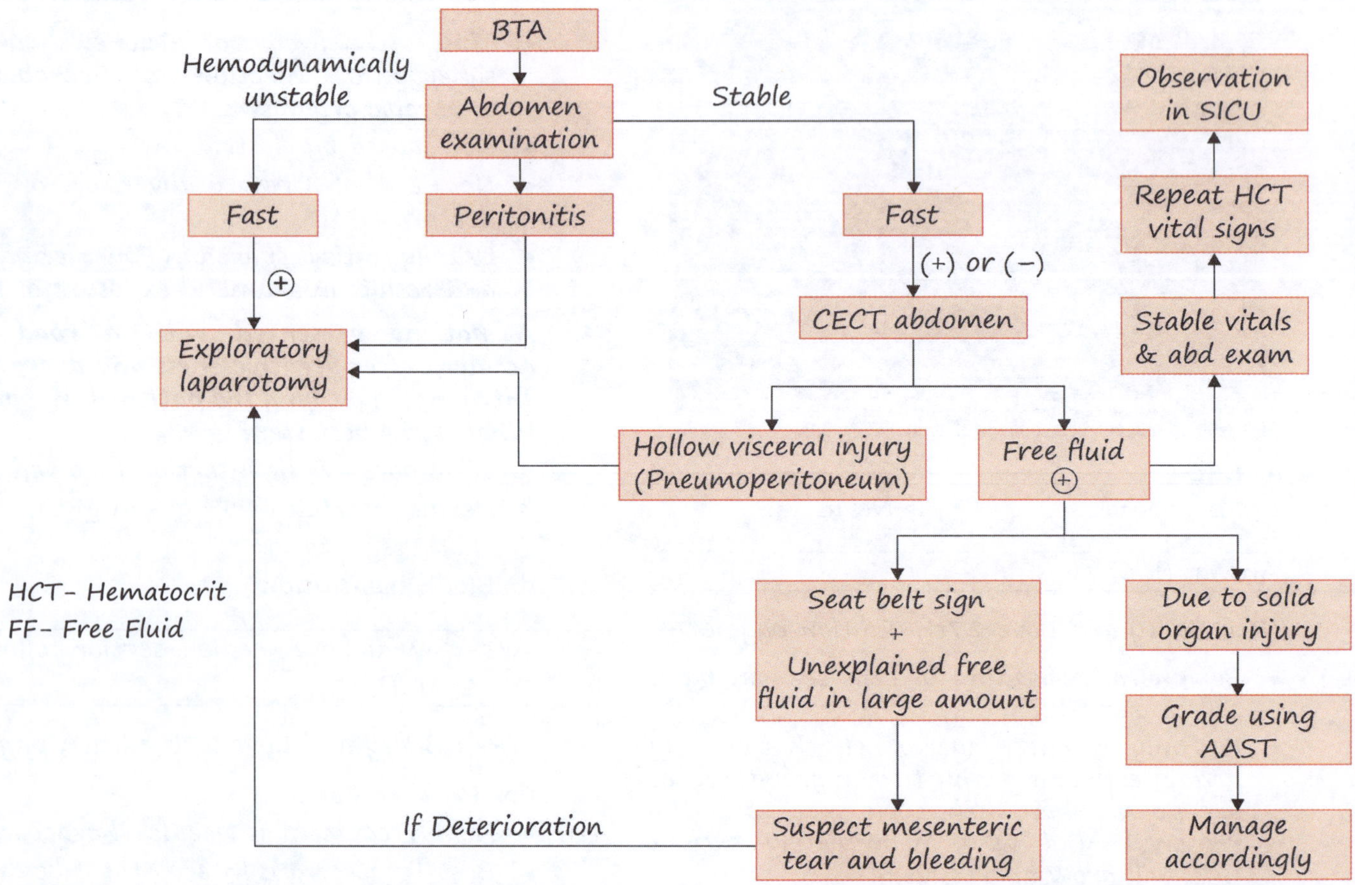

61. After total thyroidectomy, doctor is unable to extubate and patient shows cyanosis and respiratory distress. Cause of inability to extubate this:

a. BL recurrent laryngeal nerve palsy
b. UL recurrent laryngeal nerve palsy
c. Hemorrhage
d. Supralaryngeal nerve palsy

Ans. a. BL recurrent laryngeal nerve palsy

(Ref: Bailey and Love 27th edition page 815)

- UL RLN injury causes Hoarseness
- BL TLN injury causes Stridor

62. A patient underwent mastectomy for carcinoma breast and presents with upper limb swelling after 3 months. What is the diagnosis?

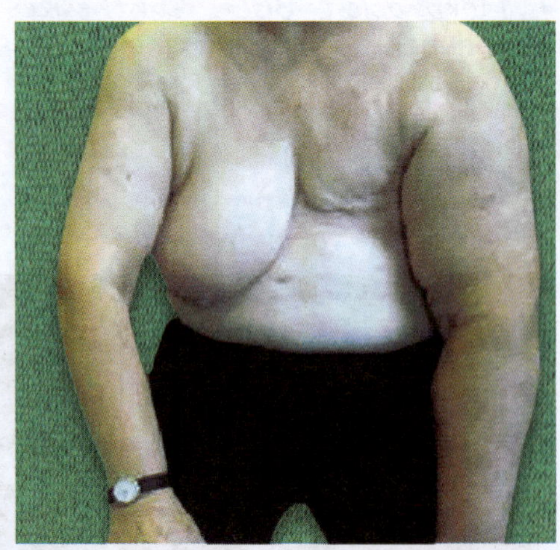

a. Upper limb Lymphangiosarcoma
b. Upper limb Lymphedema
c. Recurrence of Cancer
d. Cancer en cuirasse

Ans. b. Upper limb Lymphedema

(Ref: Bailey and Love 27th edition page 879)

- Lymphedema is rarely seen nowadays as RND and Radiotherapy are rarely combined now.
- It can occur any time, months to years after treatment.
- May also happen due to recurrence and neoplastic infiltration of axilla causing Lymphatic and venous blockage.
- Lymphangiosarcoma is a rare complication of lymphedema, onset many years after original treatment. It is characterized by multiple subcutaneous nodules. Forequarter amputation will be needed,
- Cancer en Cuirasse- Skin of chest infiltrated by tumor with appearance like a **coat.**

63. In operation theater, a hernia surgery is going on. The sac is found medial to inferior epigastric artery. Which type of hernia is this and what is the treatment for it?

a. Direct, Bassini repair

b. Indirect, Bassini repair

c. Direct, Lichtenstein repair

d. Indirect, Lichtenstein repair

Ans. c. Direct hernia and Lichtenstein repair

(Ref Bailey and Love 27th edition page 1033)

- Hernia medial to the Inferior Epigastric artery is Direct and hernia Lateral to the Inferior Epigastric artery is Indirect.
- Lichtenstein is the gold standard surgery for Direct hernia (and even for Indirect hernia)

64. A baby playing unsupervised complains of dysphagia for past few hours. What is the diagnosis as per the X-ray shown?

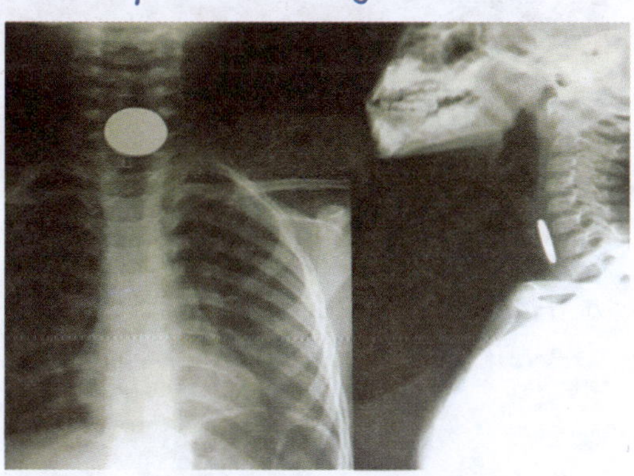

a. Tracheal foreign body

b. Esophagus having coin

c. Soft tissue calcification neck

d. Artifact

Ans. b. Esophagus having coin (Practical Radiology question)

- X-ray AP view cannot exactly find the location of FB in throat,
- X-ray Lateral view here shows the air shadow of trachea in front (anterior) and Esophagus having FB of coin posteriorly

65. A patient presented with vomiting and features of Gastric outlet obstruction. He has tumor infiltrating from Stomach to pancreas into duodenum and has multiple liver mets in right lobe liver. What is the ideal treatment for him?

a. Palliative Gastro jejunostomy

b. Right hepatectomy with radical gastrectomy

c. Whipple procedure

d. Palliative care

Ans. a. Palliative Gastro jejunostomy

(Ref: Bailey and Love 27th edition page 1138)

For inoperable and unresectable tumors in Stomach:

- Palliative procedure for distal stomach causing GOO- Palliative Anterior Gastro-jejunostomy or Roux loop GJ is done
- Palliative procedure for proximal stomach causing Dysphagia- SEMS or any other form of recanalization is acceptable

66. What is the metabolic finding seen in a baby with Congenital hypertrophic pyloric stenosis?

a. Hyperchloremic Hyper natremic metabolic alkalosis

b. Hypochloremic Hyponatremic metabolic acidosis

c. Hypochloremic Hyponatremic metabolic alkalosis

d. Hyperchloremic Hyponatremic metabolic alkalosis

Ans. c. Hypochloremic Hyponatremic metabolic alkalosis

(Ref: Bailey and Love 27th edition page 1130)

Electrolyte imbalances in GOO Cases:

- Vomiting of acid results in Hypochloremic alkalosis
- Initially as a compensation- Bicarbonate is excreted in urine, along with sodium and hence, Hyponatremia happens.
- Renin Angiotensin system comes into function when sodium decreases and tries to restore the sodium in the tubules. Instead

of sodium, potassium is lost and hence, Hypokalemia happens.

- The alkalosis leads to lowering of Ionized calcium and hence, Hypocalcemia and tetany occurs.
- At one stage from the tubules, instead of potassium, H+ ions get excreted and result in paradoxical renal aciduria, aggravating the alkalosis.

67. **Which part of the Bowel is shown in the specimen?**

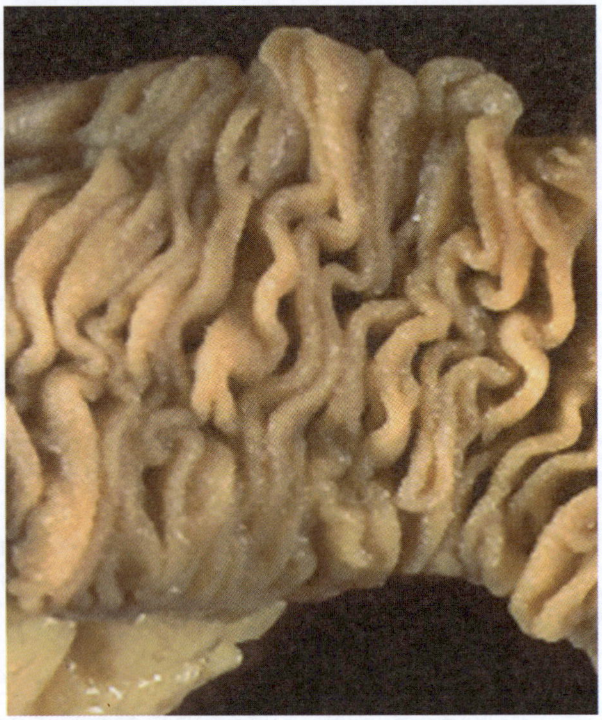

a. Jejunum
b. Ileum
c. Cecum
d. Ascending colon

Ans. a. Jejunum

(Ref: Bailey and Love 27th edition page 1241)

- Here jejunum is shown, which is identified by the Valvular conniventes/Valves of Kerckring.
- Ileum is featureless with no such valves
- These valves can be used to identify the jejunum in X-ray also.

68. **A patient presents with abdominal distension, features suggestive of intestinal obstruction. Which part of the bowel is distended here in image?**

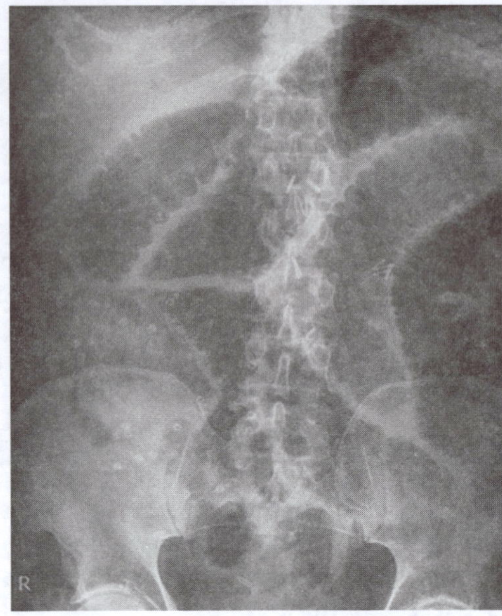

a. Jejunum b. Ileum
c. Colon d. Cecum

Ans. a. Jejunum

(Ref: Bailey and Love 27th edition page 1241)

- The distended bowel has prominent folds-which extend to full lumen diameter- these folds are Valvulae conniventes
- Similar appearing incomplete folds are Haustrations, which are seen in colon

69. **What surgery is shown here in the image?**

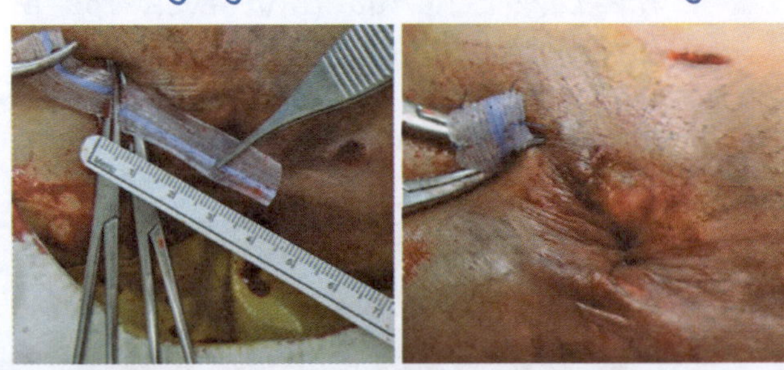

a. Thiersch wiring
b. Altemeier procedure
c. Hemorrhoidectomy
d. Well's operation

Ans. a. Thiersch wiring

(Ref: Sabiston 21st edition page 1395)

- Thiersch wiring is an anal encirclement operation that prevents rectum prolapsing down and is less commonly done now.
- It is done in extremes of age and has high recurrence rate

70. A 60-year-old female presents with increased bowel sounds. X-ray shows dilated bowel loops, with air in biliary tree. She gives History of Open hysterectomy done two years back. What is the diagnosis?
   a. Adhesions
   b. Gallstone ileus
   c. Mesenteric ischemia
   d. Large bowel obstruction

Ans. b. Gallstone ileus

(Ref: Sabiston 21st edition page 1502)

This is a case of Gallstone Ileus characterized by RIGLER triad:

- Cholecystoduodenal fistula
- Pneumobilia
- Tumbling Small bowel Obstruction

71. A patient underwent cholecystectomy and presented to hospital with Bile duct stones after two years. What is the name of such stones?
   a. Primary stone b. Secondary stone
   c. Retained stone d. Missed stone

Ans. a. Primary Stone

(Ref: Sabiston 21st edition page 1500)

- Primary stones are stones formed in Bile duct itself, they are usually Brown pigment stones.
- Primary stones are seen after two years of cholecystectomy in CBD and are also known as Recurrent stone and usually it's a brown stone
- Retained or missed stone is the name given for CBD stone in < 2 years after gallbladder removal.

72. A 40-year-old alcoholic male presents to emergency with acute abdominal pain and distention. A fluid-filled lesion is present in epigastric region. What is the abnormal investigation seen?
   a. Lipase b. GGT
   c. Bilirubin d. CEA

Ans. a. Lipase

(Ref: Sabiston 21st edition page 1541)

- Fluid-filled lesion in Epigastric swelling is more of a Pseudocyst pancreas.
- Serum amylase and lipase may be elevated in early stages of the pseudocyst formation.
- More diagnostic is EUS guided FNAC which shows elevated amylase and lipase levels with normal CEA levels. CEA is elevated in Cystic neoplasm of pancreas.

73. Mr Ramu faced an accident and had straddle injury, presented with Blood at urethral meatus. What will you do next?
   a. Do SPC and drain the urine
   b. Foley's catheter inserted
   c. Do retrograde urethrogram
   d. CECT pelvis is taken

Ans. a. Do SPC and drain the urine

(Ref: Bailey and Love 27th edition page 1480)

- Straddle injury causes rupture of the Bulbar urethra
- Foley catheter is contraindicated and immediate next step is to do SPC and drain the urine from Full bladder.

74. An 80-year-old male, with prostate lesion 2 × 2 cm. Serum PSA is 6. Gleason score is 6. What is the next management for him?
   a. Radical prostatectomy
   b. Active surveillance
   c. Brachytherapy
   d. Pelvic radiotherapy

Ans. b. Active surveillance

(Ref: Bailey and Love 27th edition page 1473)

- Low-risk prostate cancer (low PSA, small foci of Gleason 6 disease) can be managed by active surveillance.

- Here, with 3- to 6-monthly digital rectal examination (DRE) and PSA measurement and repeated prostate biopsy, a proportion can safely avoid the toxicity of radical treatment

75. A patient underwent CABG for which saphenous vein graft is taken and during the surgery GSV is removed. The complication that can occur is:

a. Saphenous nerve injury
b. Sural nerve injury
c. Common peroneal nerve injury
d. Deep peroneal nerve injury

Ans. a. Saphenous nerve injury

(Ref: Bailey and Love 27th edition page 890)

- On using the Long Saphenous vein for grafting, we will be dissecting the LSV and removing it fully as shown.
- During this procedure, Saphenous nerve can be injured.
- The patency of LSV is 60% at 10 years

76. A patient with no complaints presents with dilated veins. What is the CEAP staging for the image shown below?

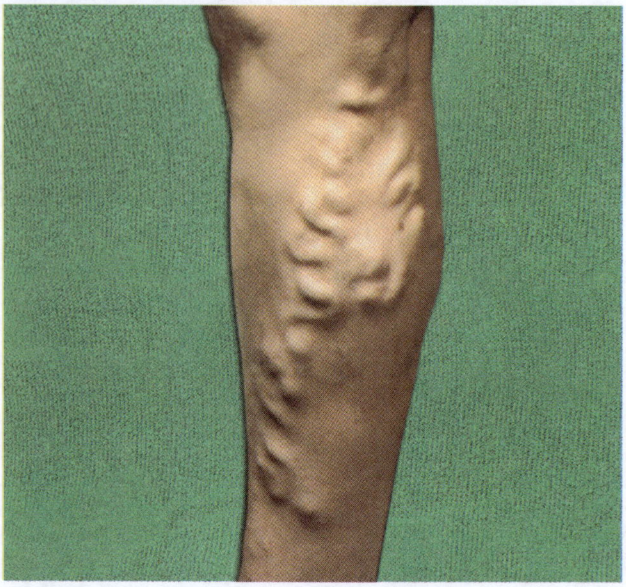

a. C2a b. C2b
c. C3a d. C3b

Ans. a. C2a

(Ref: Bailey and Love 27th edition, Page 974)

- Please remember "a" is asymptomatic case
- C2 is Varicose veins
- So, this image is C2a
- There is nothing like C2b** in classification of CEAP

77. A male smoker presents with claudication pain in right leg. Angiography is shown here. What will be the next treatment?

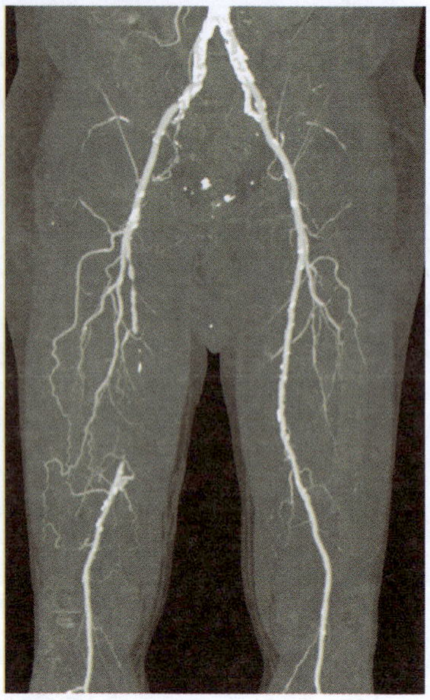

a. Aortofemoral graft
b. Iliofemoral graft
c. Endovascular stenting
d. No treatment needed

Ans. c. Endovascular stenting

(Ref: Bailey and Love 27th edition page 949)

- Please remember surgical treatment is reserved only patients in whom angioplasty is failed.

  Transluminal angioplasty and stenting:
- Following Seldinger needle puncture, the Balloon is passed via the catheter and is positioned at the lesion and inflated for 30 seconds and deflated.
- This Percutaneous Transluminal Angioplasty (PTA) is successful for Iliac, Femoropopliteal segments, the results below the knee are less satisfactory.
- Long occlusions are treated by Subintimal angioplasty.
- If vessel is not staying opened and getting coiled, we used to put a metallic self-expanding stent.

78. Which of the following is wrong statement regarding management of Pheochromocytoma?

a. 24 hours urinary metanephrine and normetanephrine
b. Urinary VMA is used in investigation
c. Beta blockers are used as initial treatment
d. Phenoxybenzamine is the DOC in preop preparation

Ans. c. Beta blockers are used as initial treatment

(Ref: Sabiston 21st edition Page 983, Bailey and Love 27th edition page 846)

Author's Note: If you are an INI-CET or NEET SS aspirant—you must know in-depth of this topic from (Sabiston page 983-986).

Biochemical diagnosis:

- Plasma metanephrine is the screening tool used to know whether patient is having Pheochromocytoma, but the problem is huge number of false positive.
- Hence, following plasma metanephrine, we have to test for 24 hours the urinary level of catecholamines and their metabolites (metanephrines, epinephrine, nor epinephrine, dopamine, Vanilly mandelic acid) are used.
- In case of equivocal elevation—Clonidine suppression test is used.

Please remember this flowchart from Sabiston 21st page 982

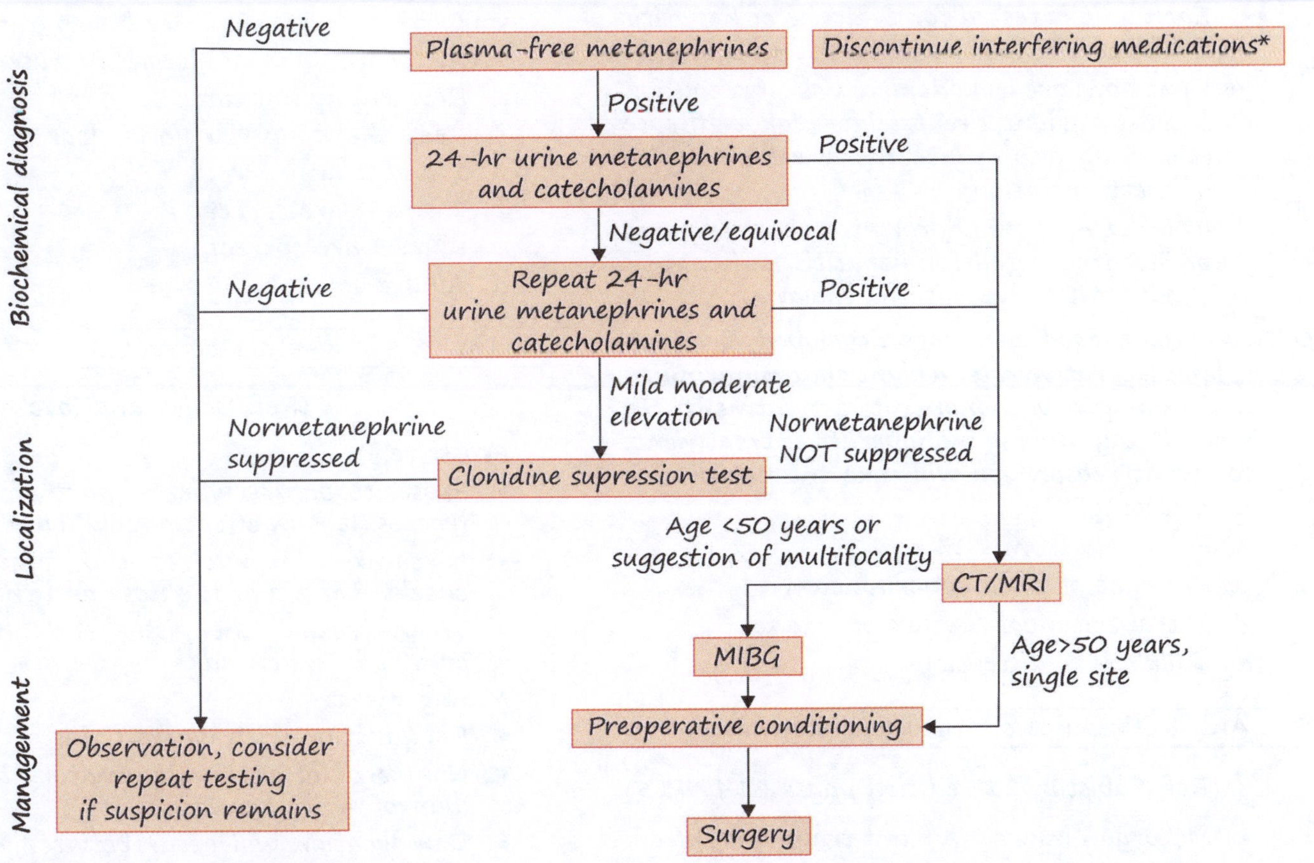

- In case of Localization of the lesion – Best is MRI
- Multifocal and malignant diseases suspected cases undergo-MIBG scan (I23 labeled-Meta Iodo Benzyl Guanidine scan)
- 68 Gallium Dotatate is the gold standard to diagnose the metastasis now.

Management:

Preop preparation:

- The drug should be started in Phenoxy benzamine (Alpha Blocker)- major complication is Postural hypotension
- After adequate alpha blockage is obtained, then only Beta blocker must be started for patients with persistent tachycardia and, for patients having epinephrine secreting tumors.
- If adequate alpha blockage is obtained—Nasal congestion occurs and it is an indicator.
- Laparoscopic adrenalectomy is the Gold standard treatment.

INI-CET MAY 2022

79. Blood from donor in Indian setup is usually screened for all; except:

a. Malaria
b. Hep B
c. HIV
d. Dengue

Ans. d. Dengue

(Ref: Bailey and Love 27th edition page 22)

- In the UK, up to 450 mL of blood is drawn, a maximum of three times each year.
- Each unit is tested for evidence of hepatitis B, hepatitis C, HIV-1, HIV-2 and syphilis.
- Donations are leukodepleted as a precaution against variant Creutzfeldt—Jakob disease (this may also reduce the immunogenicity of the transfusion).
- In India, it is mandatory to test every unit of blood collected for **hepatitis B, hepatitis C, HIV/AIDS, syphilis and malaria.**

80. A patient aged 30 years developed Grade 3 splenic laceration after a blunt abdominal injury and managed by nonoperative treatment. On second day during nonoperative treatment, for what reason you will take the patient for Laparotomy?

a. Fall in Hb from 12% to 10%.
b. Presence of pneumoperitoneum
c. Extraperitoneal rupture of bladder
d. Gallbladder distension

Ans. b. Presence of Pneumoperitoneum

(Ref: Sabiston 21st edition pages 414, 415)

- MC organ injured in blunt trauma is spleen.
- Isolated splenic injury is seen in 42%
- Patients who are nonresponders on fluid resuscitation with FAST will be operated immediately.
- Patients who respond to resuscitation are managed by nonoperative treatment. The rates of NOM for splenic injury is around 40-70% cases.

Nonoperative treatment of splenic injury:

- Overall success rate – 90%
- Due to increasing use of angiography and embolization- NOM can be done even for Grade 3 to 5.

Indications for Surgery in a patient in NOM:

- Patient becoming hemodynamically unstable
- Patient develops peritonitis (Pneumo-peritoneum in this question is a sign of perforation)

Other choices:

- Extraperitoneal rupture of bladder is not an indication for surgery
- Any patient in Nil oral will have GB distension and not an indication for surgery

81. Which of the following is true regarding FROSTBITE?

1. Extreme cases may need amputation
2. Antibiotics and analgesics not used
3. Rewarming not done
4. Keep the wound dry and clean

a. 1 and 2 are correct
b. 1 and 4 are correct
c. 1, 2, 3 are correct
d. All are correct

Ans. b. 1 and 4 are correct

(Ref: Bailey and love page 422)

Frostbite:

- Frostbite occurs when a part of the body freezes. It is in effect a 'cold' burn.
- It commonly involves the fingers, toes, cheeks, the tip of the nose and the ears.
- When frozen, the tissue feels hard and cannot be indented.

Management:

- Rehydration with warm fluids
- Nonsteroidal anti-inflammatory drugs like ibuprofen are beneficial.
- Demarcation will occur between dead and viable tissues and at this stage no surgery should be undertaken as there is often considerable deep recovery.
- **The injured area should be kept clean and dry; and efforts should be made to prevent further injury, as well as to prevent infection.**
- Definitive surgery to excise dead tissues can be left for many months.
- Recent developments, such as the use of tissue plasminogen activator (TPA) and nerve blocks, show promising results in reducing amputations, but have to be started within 24 hours and are seldom possible in the field.

82. Following blunt trauma, four chest X-ray are given. In which of them further investigation is required before inserting ICD?

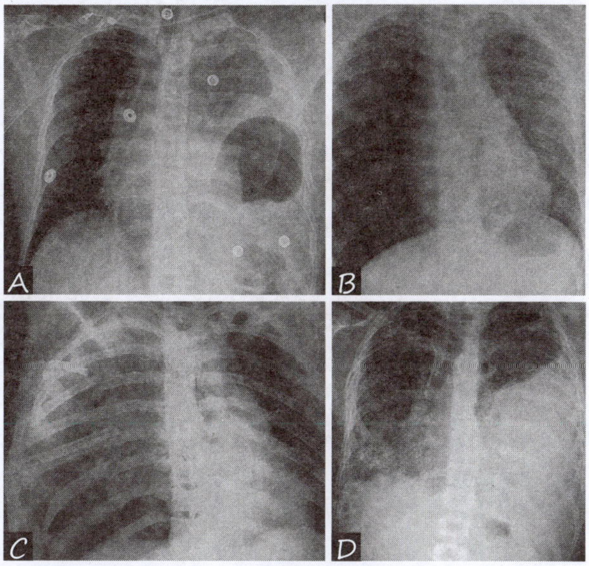

Ans. A

In this list;

Image A: Is a case of diaphragmatic hernia due to traumatic tear of left side of diaphragm and you can see the stomach has herniated into the chest. In such cases before putting ICD, we must rule out any other injury in abdomen by CECT abdomen. We cannot directly insert the ICD in these cases as we can injure the stomach.

Image B: Is a case of right side tension pneumothorax, here we must immediately insert an ICD, without any further investigation.

Image C: Is a case of flail chest, where more than three ribs are fractured at two or more places. The main treatment is to provide analgesics and oxygen support, They may need ICD, if there is associated Hemothorax. But if patient is stable, we will evaluate further with 3D CT Thorax to rule out pulmonary contusions. (Partially correct answer)

Image D: Is a case of hemothorax, which will need ICD tube.

83. A 37-year-old unmarried female, nulliparous is having regular intercourse, but on OCPs. Mother had cancer at 50 years of age. Sister had cancer at 40 years of age. What will you advise as next step?

a. Stop taking OCP
b. Do mammography
c. Genetic counseling for BRCA testing
d. Immediate mastectomy

Ans. c. Genetic counseling for BRCA testing

(Ref: Sabiston 21st edition page 823)

- The Couch model predicts risk for a mutation in the *BRCA1* gene.
- The BRCAPro model, developed by Myriad Genetics Laboratories, estimates the risk of *BRCA1* and *BRCA2* mutations.

Indications for consideration of genetic testing

- Include breast cancer diagnosed before age 50,
- Bilateral breast cancer,
- Breast and ovarian cancer in the same individual,
- Breast cancer in men.

Other factors that may be indications for testing:

- A family history (maternal or paternal) of two or more individuals with breast and ovarian cancer,
- A close male relative with breast cancer,
- A close relative with early-onset (<50 years) breast or ovarian cancer,
- *BRCA1* or *BRCA2* mutation in the family.

84. A patient is on Tamoxifen after a breast cancer surgery. For around 5 years, she was on Tamoxifen. When will she stop Tamoxifen if she wants to conceive?

a. One month before.
b. No need to stop.
c. Stop 2 months before conceiving
d. Must continue even in pregnancy

Ans. c. Stop 2 months before conceiving

(Ref: JournalPublished online 2011 Oct 21. doi: 10.1634/theoncologist.2011-0121)

- The relatively high frequency of severe congenital abnormalities indicates that a reliable birth control method is mandatory during tamoxifen treatment.
- The half-life of tamoxifen and its metabolites is rather long.
- The patient should be informed about a washout period of 2 months before conceiving.
- If an inadvertent pregnancy occurs, the potential risks for the fetus and new born should be discussed with the patient, along with the possible options.

85. **A patient developed loss of sensation in root of penis after a laparoscopic hernia surgery. Which of the following nerves would have been damaged?**

a. Ilio-inguinal nerve
b. Ilio-hypogastric nerve
c. Genitofemoral nerve
d. Lateral cutaneous nerve

Ans. a. Ilio-inguinal nerve

(Ref: Internet sources, applied anatomy Question)

- From the following image, you can note the root of penis is supplied by Ilio-inguinal nerve.
- But please remember, the most common nerve injured in laparoscopic hernia surgery is lateral cutaneous nerve.

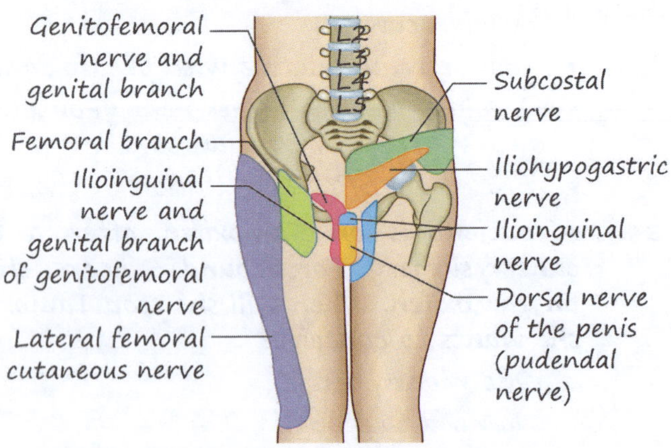

86. **A patient presented with dysphagia. Barium swallow is done. What investigation is not needed and not done in this case?**

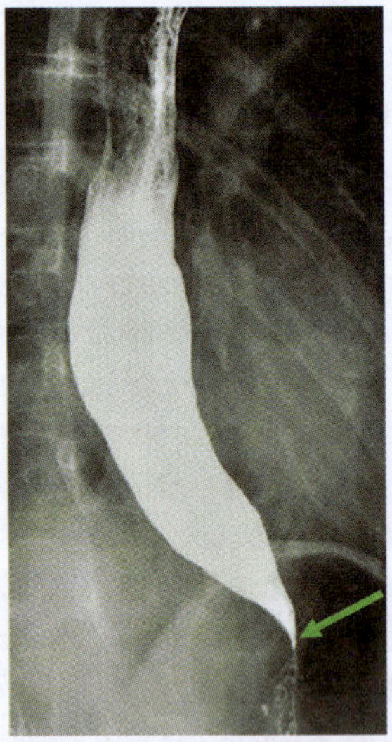

a. Manometry
b. 24 hours pH
c. Endoscopy
d. CECT chest

Ans. b. 24 hours pH

(Ref: Bailey and Love 27th edition page 1097)

(For achalasia cardia, Bird Beak sign in Barium swallow)

- IOC is High resolution manometry
- Barium swallow will give a clue of achalasia by Bird beak Abrupt cut off.
- Endoscopy is always done to rule out pseudo achalasia due to malignancy* in Cardia of stomach.
- CECT Chest can also be done to look for any causes of pseudo achalasia.
- 24 Hours pH monitoring is not needed in achalasia.

87. **Nutritional complications are more with which fistula?**

a. Pancreatic fistula
b. Duodenal
c. Colonic
d. Distal ileal

Ans. b. Duodenal

(Ref: Schwartz 11th edition page 1241)

The loss of enteric luminal contents, particularly from high-output fistulas originating from the proximal small intestine, results in dehydration, electrolyte abnormalities and malnutrition.

88. **Most common ectopic tissues found in Meckel's diverticulum is/are?**

1. Gastric
2. Thyroid
3. Pancreatic
4. Adrenals

a. 1 and 3
b. 1 and 2
c. 1 and 4
d. 2 and 3

Ans. a. 1 and 3

(Ref: Sabiston 21st edition page 1289)

- The cells in vitellointestinal duct are pluripotent and hence, ectopic mucosa is common.
- MC is Gastric (seen in 50% of Meckel's) and pancreatic mucosa (seen in 5%). Rarely colonic mucosa may also be seen.

89. **Mark the correct statements about IBD:**

1. Crohn's disease has skip lesions
2. Childhood IBD is genetic
3. Crohn's is mucosal and UC is transmural
4. Crohn's is fully curable

a. 2,3 are correct
b. 1 and 2 are correct
c. 1,2,3 are correct
d. All are correct

Ans. b. 1 and 2 are correct

(Ref: Sabiston 21st edition page 1265)

- Please remember Crohn's is incurable as it involves from mouth to anus and recurrence is very common.
- Crohn's is a transmural disease and Ulcerative colitis is mucosa*

90. **The following are the perineal procedures; except:**
   a. Thiersch
   b. Altemeier operation
   c. Delorme
   d. Ripstein

Ans. d. Ripstein

(Ref: Sabiston 21st edition page 1395)

Perineal approach	Abdominal approach
• Delorme's mucosectomy operation of removal of rectal mucosa and plicating the muscle layer* • Thiersch anal encirclement operation • Altemeier's perineal recto-sigmoidectomy procedure with Coloanal anastomosis*- Resection procedure**	• Ripstein's anterior rectopexy • Well's posterior rectopexy • Resection rectopexy (Frykman and Goldberg) for redundant sigmoid colon • Anterior resection

91. **Psoas abscess presents as:**
   1. Fluctuant mass in thigh
   2. Pott's spine can present as psoas abscess
   3. Pain during passive extension of hip
   4. Hematogenous spread of TB in immunocompromised
   a. 1, 2 and 3 are correct
   b. 1 and 2 are correct
   c. 1, 2, 3, 4 are correct
   d. 1 and 4 are correct

Ans. c. 1, 2, 3, 4 are correct

(Ref: Sabiston 21st edition page 1100)

Applied Anatomy

- Psoas muscles attached from vertebra to lesser trochanter is involved in flexion of hip.
- Psoas muscle are supplied by venous blood from Lumbar spine and lymphatics from nearby intra-abdominal organ.

Etiology

- Secondary psoas abscess is due to spread of infection from vertebra or from intra-abdominal organ infections from Crohn's disease, Appendicitis, Diverticulitis, etc.
- Less common infection also can develop in Perinephric abscess, LSCS, Retroperitoneal hematoma or from Genitourinary infections.
- It can spread in TB by hematogenous or direct spread from Pott's spine

Clinical Features of retroperitoneal abscess:

- The most common symptoms of retroperitoneal abscesses include abdominal or flank pain (60%–75%), fever and chills (30%–90%), malaise (10%–22%), and weight loss (12%).
- Patients with psoas abscesses may have referred pain to the hip, groin, or knee. The duration of symptoms is usually longer than one week.
- Patients with retroperitoneal abscesses often have concurrent, chronic illnesses such as renal lithiasis, diabetes mellitus, HIV infection, or malignancies.
- There is severe pain on passive extension and internal rotation of hip in psoas abscess

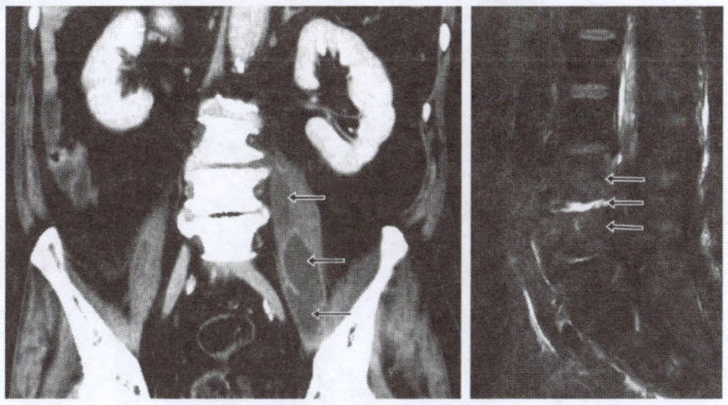

Iliopsoas abscess

Management

- IOC to diagnose the abscess is CECT Abdomen.
- Treatment is by CT guided drainage by Percutaneous approach.

92. **Identify the specimen shown below:**

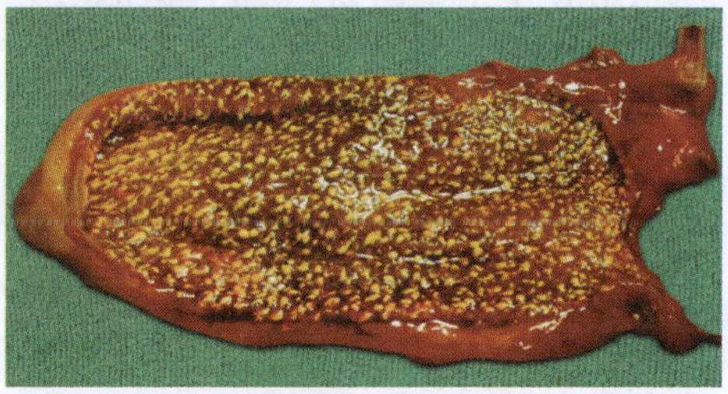

   a. Strawberry gallbladder
   b. CA gallbladder
   c. Cholelithiasis
   d. Multiple polyps

Ans. a. Strawberry gallbladder

(Ref: Bailey and Love 27th edition page 1201)

- Chronic inflammatory changes in Gallbladder are known as Cholesterosis in which hyperplasia of tissue elements is seen.
- In fresh state, the interior looks like a strawberry in some patients as shown in image, the yellow specks are submucous aggregations of Cholesterol Crystals and cholesterol esters.
- It may be associated with cholesterol stones.

93. A 60-year-old male presented with a cancer and the illustration of the surgery is shown here. Which cancer is operated here?

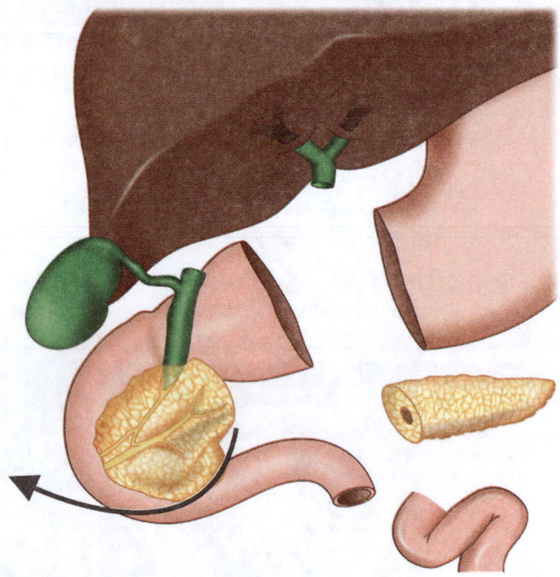

a. Cancer gallbladder
b. Carcinoma periampullary cancer
c. Cholangiocarcinoma
d. Chronic pancreatitis

Ans. b. Carcinoma periampullary cancer

(Ref: Sabiston 21st edition page 1557)

Whipple procedure (Pancreaticoduodenectomy): Indications:

- Distal CBD cancer
- Pancreatic Head cancer
- Periampullary cancer
- Cancer in second part duodenum

After the specimen is removed: three anastomoses are done

- Pancreaticojejunostomy
- Hepaticojejunostomy
- Gastrojejunostomy

94. A patient's Hydatid cyst of kidney is shown in image. State the wrong one:

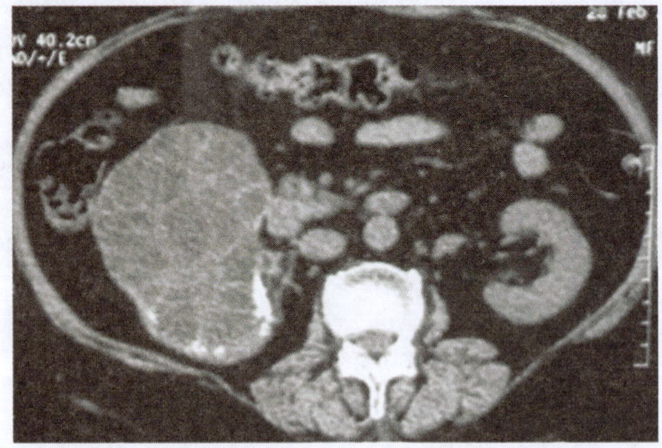

a. FNAC or Biopsy required before surgery
b. Albendazole is given preop
c. Caused by Dog tapeworm
d. Leakage of the cyst can cause anaphylaxis

Ans a. FNAC or Biopsy required before surgery

(Ref: Bailey and Love 27th edition page 66)

- Hydatid cyst is caused by Dog tapeworm-Echinococcus granulosus.
- Leakage of cyst fluid can cause anaphylaxis.
- FNAC or Biopsy is contraindicated due to the risk of leakage or rupture.
- CT scan is the IOC
- Surgical Treatment or PAIR is done under cover of T. Albendazole**

95. A 30-year-old male had a blunt injury to abdomen. No blood at tip of meatus. Foley's catheter was put but urine was almost nil. Retrograde Cystogram image is shown below. How will you manage the patient?

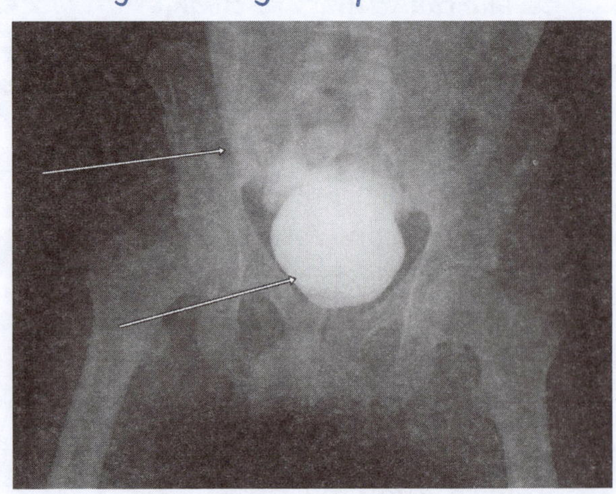

a. Suprapubic catheterization
b. Per urethral catheterization
c. Laparotomy
d. Pelvic packing with B/L nephrostomy.

Ans. c. Laparotomy

(Ref: Bailey and Love 27th edition page 1425)

- Intraperitoneal rupture is usually secondary to a blow or fall on a distended bladder, and more rarely to surgical damage.
- Extraperitoneal rupture is caused by blunt trauma or surgical damage.
- Gross hematuria can be absent.
- **Intraperitoneal rupture patients may present with Shock; and abdomen distends due to urinary peritonitis.**
- Peritonitis does not follow immediately if the urine is sterile; varying degrees of rigidity are present on examination
- A lower midline laparotomy should be performed; the edges of the rent are trimmed and sutured with a single-layer 2/0 absorbable suture.

96. **Volume of prostate:**

a. 20 mL
b. 50 mL
c. 70 mL
d. 100 mL

Ans. a. 20 mL

(Ref: Anatomy Chaurasia)

- The normal prostate gland has measurement of 3 × 3 × 5 cm approximately or a volume of **25 mL.**

97. **A deep ulcer in the heel of a patient given:**

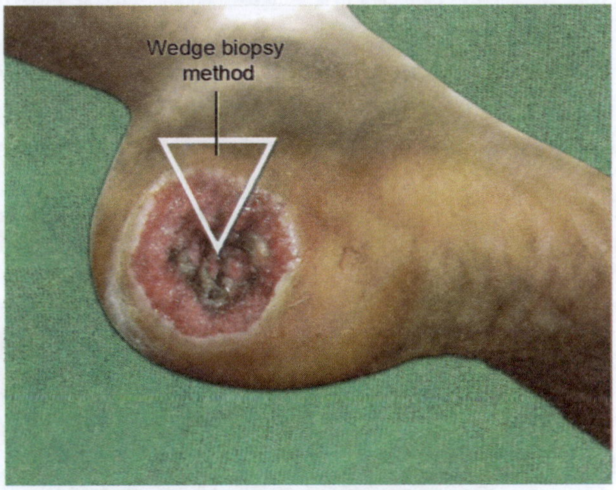

a. Positive Trendelenburg test
b. Absent distal pulses
c. Decreased sensation
d. Pain on passive movement of calf muscles

Ans. c. Decreased sensation

(Ref: Short Cases in Surgery By Dr Rajamahendran)

Trophic Ulcer

- It is due to impaired nutrition, blood supply and added neurological deficit.
- Important causes: diabetes, tabes dorsalis, leprosy, peripheral neuritis, etc.
- Also called neurotrophic/ neuropathic ulcer.
- Painless ulcer
- MC location- pressure points like foot, back (bedsores), etc.
- Punched out
- Base formed by underlying bone
- Immobile

Venous ulcer will be seen over the medial malleolus.

Arterial ulcer will be seen on the dorsal aspect of foot.

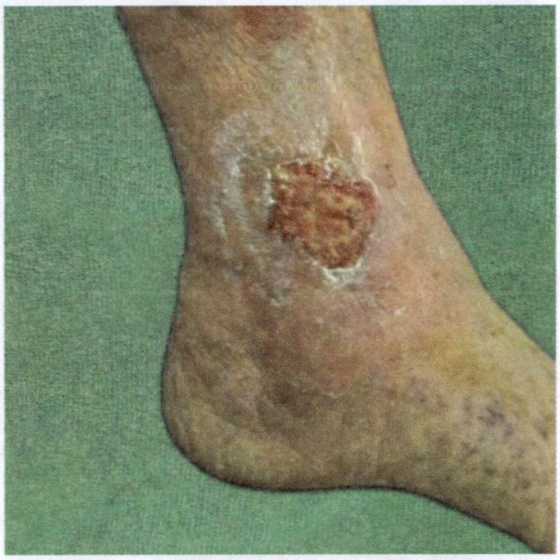

Venous ulcer

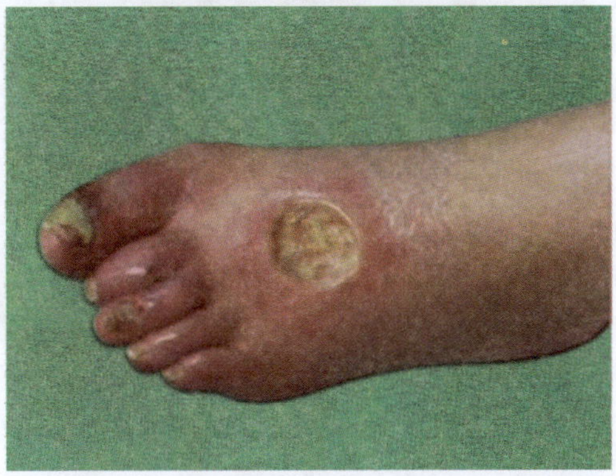

Arterial ulcer

98. **Reagarding difference between partial thickness and full thickness graft, correct statements are:**

1. Primary contraction more with SSG
2. Secondary contraction more with SSG
3. Primary contraction more with full thickness graft.

4. Secondary contraction more with full thickness graft
   a. 1 and 2 are correct
   b. 1 and 3 are correct
   c. 2 and 3 are correct
   d. 3 and 4 are correct

Ans. c. 2 and 3 are correct

(Ref: Schwartz 11th edition page 1976)

This is based on the table in Schwartz, please remember this table:

	STSG (thin)	STSG (thick)	FTSG
Dermal content	+	++	+++
1° contraction	+	++	+++
2° contraction	+++	++	+
Engraftment	+++	++	+
Durability	+	++	+++
Pigmentation	+++	++	+
Resist desiccation	+	++	+++
Recipient bed	+	++	+++
Appearance	+	++	+++

INI-CET NOVEMBER 2021

99. A patient underwent mastectomy and a drain is kept. What type of drain is this?

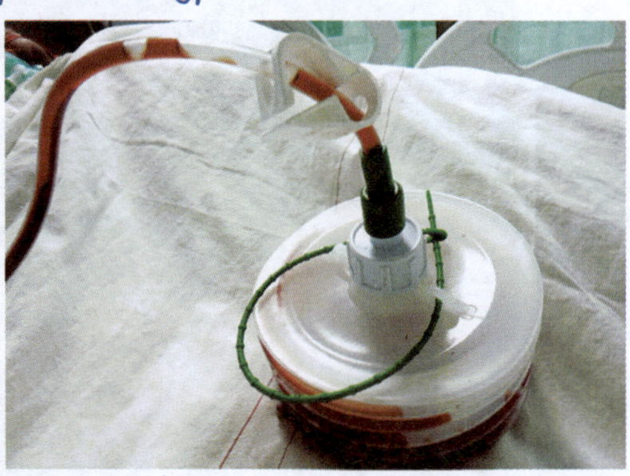

a. Semi open b. Semi closed
c. Open d. Closed

Ans. d. Closed

(Ref: Bailey and Love 27th edition page 99-101)

- Drains are inserted to allow the fluid or air that might collect at operation site or in a wound to drain freely to the surface.
- They are used as Prophylactic in elective surgery and as therapeutic in emergency surgery.
- Three types of drains are used:

1. Open drains that utilize the principles of gravity
2. Semi open drains that work on principle of capillary effect
3. Closed drains that utilize the Suction

- There are huge controversies in usage of the drains by the surgeons in various places- the only area in alimentary tract where it is still routinely advocated is ESOPHAGEAL Surgery**

100. Nasogastric tube length is measured by:
   a. Nose to ear and Xiphoid process
   b. Nose to Xiphoid and umbilicus
   c. Nose to mouth and Pubic symphysis
   d. Nose to Xiphisternum

Ans. a. Nose to ear and Xiphoid process

(Ref: Bailey and Love 27th edition page 285)

- NEX rule- Nose to Ear and Ear to Xiphoid process is used to calculate the length of Nasogastric tube.
- MC complication of the Nasal tubes is blockage. All tubes must be washed with water at least twice daily.
- Chymotrypsin may salvage a partially obstructed tube
- Guidewires must not be used as they may perforate the tube and cause contiguous damage.
- Fine bore tubes <3 mm diameter are used if feeding is used for >1 week.

101. For cannula shown below, what is the flow rate/minute?

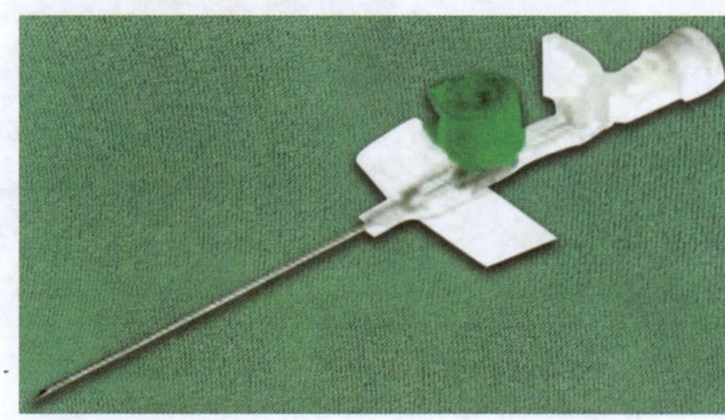

a. 66 mL b. 86 mL
c. 106 mL d. 56 mL

Ans. b. 86 mL

(Ref: Internet Sources)

Gauge	Color Code	Ext. Dia. mm	Length mm	Flow Rate mL/mm	Indications
14G	Orange	2.1	45	240	Trauma, surgical procedures
16G	Gray	1.8	45	180	Trauma, surgical procedures
18G	Green	1.3	32 / 45	90	Trauma, quick blood transfusion
20G	Pink	1.1	32	60	Normal IV or blood transfusion
22G	Blue	0.9	25	36	Children, older adults
24G	Yellow	0.7	19	20	Neonates, children, old elderly
26G	Violet	0.6	19	13	Neonates

102. A patient had chest trauma, which of the following must not be done?

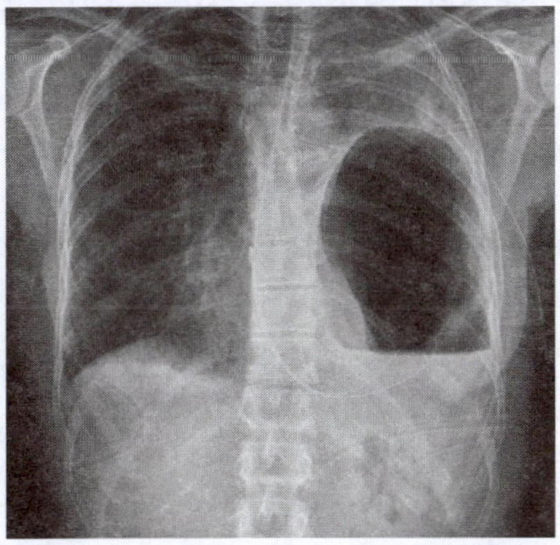

a. Log roll
b. ICD Tube
c. NG Tube
d. Epidural anesthesia

Ans. b. ICD tube

(Ref: Bailey and Love 27th edition page 370)

- Nasogastric tube insertion and taking an X-ray chest will give a clue that stomach has herniated to the chest. Added contrast via NG tube will give added conclusive evidence.
- Most accurate investigation is VATS or Diagnostic laparoscopy
- Bag and mask is contraindicated, if oxygen deprivation occurs. Always provide oxygen by intubation.
- ICD tube if inserted without operating for diaphragmatic hernia, can cause gastric injury or other bowel injury which has herniated into the thorax.
- Repair is done via abdomen and not via chest. After surgery, ICD will be put for drainage.

103. What will be the most common complication that will happen when we put an incision along the line shown in the X-ray below?

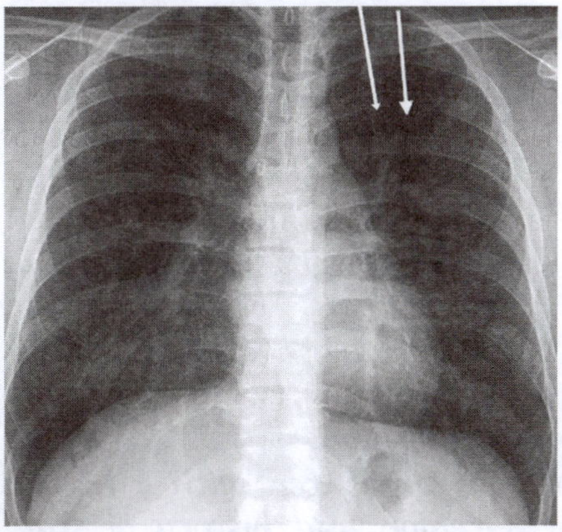

a. Chylothorax
b. Thrombophlebitis
c. Arterial Bleeding
d. Empyema of thorax

Ans. c. Arterial Bleeding

(Ref: IJCIIS Journal, Craik Kombau)

Complications of Central Venous Catheter insertion:

- Failure to place catheter- 22%
- Arterial puncture- 5%
- Malposition- 4%

- Pneumothorax—1%
- Subcutaneous hematoma—1%
- Hemothorax—1%
- Cardiac arrest—<1%

Arterial Puncture: Management:

- If inadvertent injury happens: Two options are there:
    1. Immediate removal of catheter with pressure can result in uncontrolled hemorrhage or AV fistula
    2. Prolonged arterial catheterization without removing can result in Thrombosis and Neurological deficits and Stroke
- Recent studies say—leaving the catheter in place and prompt repair carry less morbidity and mortality compared to giving pressure

Chylothorax:

Left sided IJV or SCV carries a high risk of lymphatic injury due to anatomic location of the thoracic duct, but lymphatics injury can happen at right side also.

Catheter related sepsis:

New concepts from Bailey and Love 27th Edition:

- Previously if we suspected catheter related sepsis, we removed the catheter and sent the Tip for C/S and did Blood C/S and if both were same organisms, we confirmed whether it was a sepsis due to catheter.
- Now- no need to remove the catheter: we can do swab from central vein catheter or Take blood sample from Central vein catheter and do C/S and compare with peripheral blood aspirated C/S. If they are same organisms, we will remove the catheter and insert a new catheter in opposite side.

104. A man presented with a hematoma over the arm region and history of stab injury in the arm. On examination, radial and ulnar pulse are not felt. Brachial artery has a 3.5 cm longitudinal cut. Ideal repair is:

a. Primary repair
b. Repair with prosthetic graft
c. Repair with reverse saphenous graft
d. Repair with saphenous vein patch

Ans. c. Repair with reverse saphenous graft

(Ref: Sabiston 21st edition page 1806)

Brachial artery injury:

- Brachial artery is exposed by a Longitudinal incision along the medial aspect of the upper arm over the groove between the Triceps and Biceps muscles.
- Primary repair of undamaged ends of vessel by End- to End Anastomosis should be performed if repair is tension free.
- Saphenous vein interposition should be chosen whenever vessel injury is extensive or if primary repair is not feasible.
- PTFE is a second choice to autologous veins in Brachial and forearm vessel injuries.

Combined Ulnar and Radial artery:

- It requires repair of only one vessel.
- Ulnar artery is usually larger in proximal arm and is better target for repair.
- Either saphenous vein or direct repair is done

Isolated Ulnar or Radial artery:

- Simple ligation is enough, no need to repair if adequate circulation is seen *via* the other vessel

Please remember venous injuries do not need to be repaired and they can be simply ligated in Upper limb**

105. A midline neck swelling moves with deglutition-patient has tachycardia and exophthalmos. What are the investigations to be done?

1. Thyroid scan
2. FNAC
3. Thyroid function test
4. USG neck

a. 1 and 2
b. 1, 3 and 4
c. 1, 2, 3 and 4
d. 2, 3 and 4

Ans. b. 1, 3 and 4

(Ref: Bailey and Love 27th edition page 807)

- This is a case of Graves disease from history
- The investigations that are not done for Graves are:
    - FNAC
    - Biopsy

106. A 40-year-old female had carcinoma breast and surgery is done. During surgery, the surgeon ordered Frozen section study. This procedure will be useful for all; except:

a. For Margins positivity
b. For Sentinel Node study
c. For confirming the diagnosis of malignancy
d. For confirming the malignancy in Node showing high activity in Gamma camera for preop evaluation of axillary nodes.

Ans. c. For confirming the diagnosis of malignancy

(Ref: Bailey and Love 27th edition page 877)

- Frozen section is usually done for Confirming the margin positive or negative in Breast conservative surgery cases.
- Frozen section is a part of SNB protocols, whether it is done by Blue dye injection or by radiolabeled colloid.
- Please know statement "d" is also sentinel node biopsy
- If frozen section of nodes is negative, we avoid further axillary dissection.
- Other methods to confirm the tumor in SNB study are by Touch imprint cytology and by molecular methods of detecting the Cytokeratin 19 or mammoglobin**

107. A patient who has McBurney's incision is converted to Rutherford Morrison incision. What are the structures cut?

1. External oblique
2. Internal oblique
3. Transversus abdominis
4. Rectus abdominis

a. 1, 2, 3 b. 1 and 2
c. 2 and 3 d. 1, 2, 3, 4

Ans. a. 1, 2, 3

(Ref: Bailey and Love 27th edition page 1309)

- In cases of Paracecal and retrocecal and fixed appendix we need to extend the Grid iron incision to Rutherford muscle cutting incision of cutting the muscles-Internal Oblique and Transversus abdominis in the line of incision.
- (In the same page in last line 1309- Bailey mentions—all layers are divided in the line of incision—which is actually the correct answer- all layers EO, IO and TA are all cut in muscle cutting Rutherford Morrison Incision)

108. Which of the following are correct regarding HCC and treatment?

1. Increasing incidence
2. TACE is done
3. Ipilimumab is used for advanced cases
4. NASH and NAFLD are risk factors

a. 1, 2, 3 are correct
b. 1, 2, 3, 4 are correct
c. 2 and 3 correct
d. 1 and 2 correct

Ans. b. 1, 2, 3 ,4 are correct

(Ref: NCCN Guidelines for HCC Version 1.2022- March 29, 2022)

- The incidence of HCC is increasing in the United States, particularly in the population infected with HCV. The annual incidence rate of HCC among patients with HCV-related cirrhosis has been estimated to be between 2 and 8%
- Globally, HBV is the leading cause of HCC incidence and mortality. Approximately 1.5 million people in the United States are chronically infected with HBV
- Prospective studies have demonstrated that downstaging (prior to transplant) with percutaneous ethanol injection (PEI), RFA, TACE, TARE with Y-90 microspheres, and transarterial chemoinfusion are associated with improved outcomes
- Based on results of the REFLECT trial, the FDA approved lenvatinib in 2018 as first-line treatment of patients with unresectable HCC.
- Lenvatinib is an inhibitor of VEGFR, fibroblast growth factor receptor, platelet-derived growth factor receptor (PDGFR), and other growth signaling kinases
- The NCCN Guidelines include combined nivolumab and ipilimumab as well as pembrolizumab as "other recommended regimens."
- Ipilimumab is a human IgG1 that binds CTLA-4, preventing T-cell inhibition signal pathway.

109. A patient after undergoing cholecystectomy presents with Intrahepatic biliary radicle dilatation and Jaundice. What is the investigation of choice?

a. MRI b. CECT
c. PTC d. USG

Ans. a. MRI

(Ref: Bailey and Love 27th edition page 1192)

- MRI of biliary system is known as MRCP. It is the best investigation for studying Biliary pathology.
- This case is due to some obstruction in Bile duct, which is best picked by MRCP.
- ERCP is the gold standard only for CBD stones as the management of stone can be done simultaneously.

110. A 60-year-old male patient presented with hematuria, urine microscopic examination reveals- Transitional cell cancer. CT scan shows 2x2 cm mass in bladder invading the muscle with no regional nodal metastasis. What is the management?

a. TUR bladder tumor
b. Radical cystectomy
c. Hemicystectomy with bladder cancer reconstruction
d. Neoadjuvant chemotherapy

Ans. b. Radical cystectomy

(Ref: Bailey and Love 27th edition page 1448)

- Muscle-invasive disease (pT2) accounts for 25% of new cases.
- Such tumors carry a much worse prognosis because they are subject to local invasion and distant metastasis.
- Radical primary treatment options include radical cystectomy, urinary diversion and thorough lymph node dissection, which tends to be offered as first line, or radical external beam radiotherapy
- Neoadjuvant chemotherapy improves survival rates as well as adjuvant chemo-therapy in some cases, particularly in the presence of nodal and distant diseases

111. Which of the following is not a LUTS ?

a. Urgency b. Hesitancy
c. Frequency d. Pyuria

Ans. d. Pyuria

(Ref: Bailey and Love 27th edition page 1459)

Lower urinary tract symptoms (LUTS) can be described as:

Voiding symptoms

- Hesitancy (worsened if the bladder is very full)
- Very Poor flow (unimproved by straining)
- Intermittent stream – Urine stops and starts
- Dribbling (including after micturition)
- Sensation of poor bladder emptying
- Episodes of near retention

Storage Symptoms

- Increased frequency
- Nocturia
- Urgency
- Urge incontinence
- Nocturnal incontinence (enuresis)

112. Which is most common cause of urinary obstruction in Male neonate?

a. PUV b. Hypospadias
c. Epispadias d. Phimosis

Ans. a. PUV

(Ref: Bailey and Love 27th edition page 1475)

- Incidence 1 in 5000 males
- The valves are distal to verumontanum and cause obstruction to urethra of boys.
- This is the most common cause of urinary obstruction in males.

INI-CET MAY 2021

113. Angle between skin and needle when performing intermittent sutures:

a. 70° b. 90°
c. 45° d. 60°

Ans. b. 90°

(Ref: Bailey and Love 27th edition page 91)

Interrupted skin sutures:

- The needle needs to be inserted at right angles to the incision and then pass out at right angles to the incision.
- The distance (X) from the entry point of the needle to the edge of the wound should be equal to the same depth (X) of the tissue being sutured.
- The distance between the successive sutures must be twice this distance (2X)

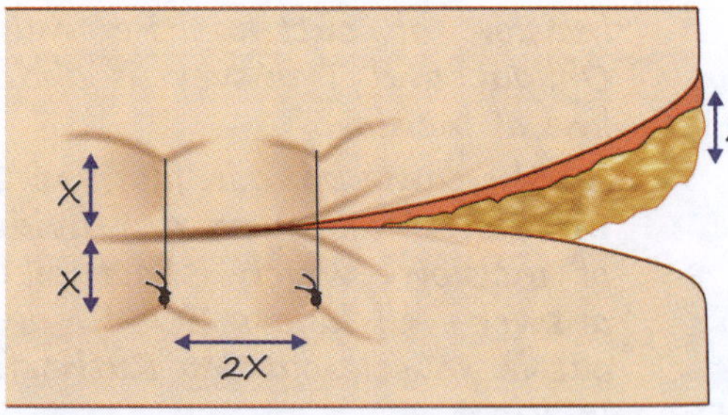

114. Inflation during laparoscopy is done with help of which instrument?

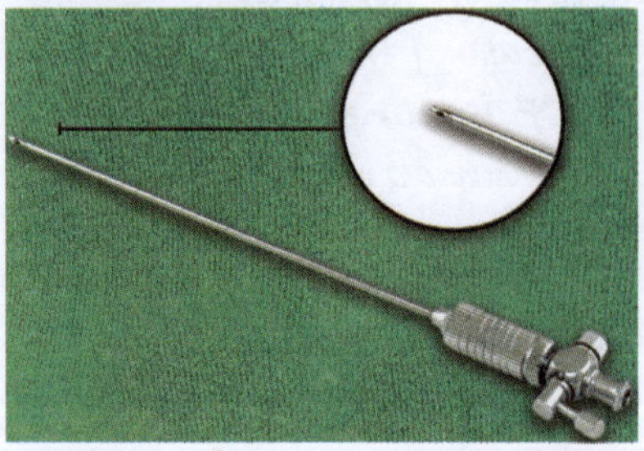

a. Jacob b. Mathew
c. Veress needle d. Alex

Ans. c. Veress needle

(Ref: Bailey and Love 27th edition page 112)

- Closed method involves blind puncture using a Veress needle into abdominal cavity for creating pneumoperitoneum.
- This method is fast and relatively safe.
- There is small but significant potential for intestinal and vascular injury on introduction of needle or Trocar.

115. Match the following:

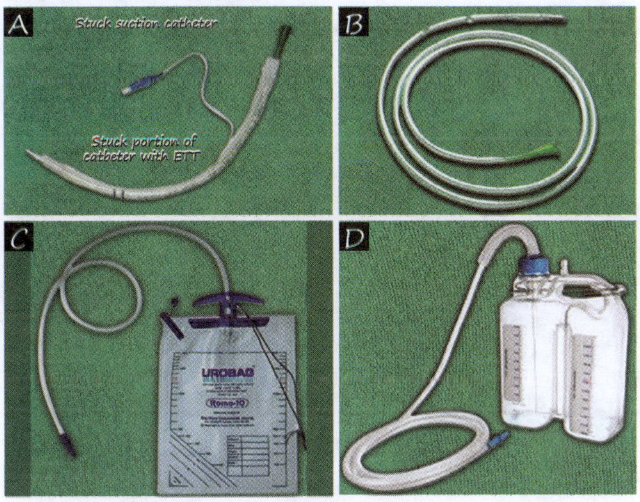

1. ET and oral suction tube
2. Ryle's tube
3. Urobag
4. Underwater seal

a. A-1, B-2, C-3, D-4
b. A-2, B-3, C-4, D-1
c. A-2, B-4, C-3, D-1
d. A-3, B-4, C-2, D-1

Ans. a. A-1, B-2, C-3, D-4 (Practical Question)

- These are very basic practical questions which you must have learnt in CRRI period..
- **Author's note:** If you are a Final year/ CRRI student reading this book- please remember whatever you ignore casually in ward during internship is being focused by the examiners more than book contents nowadays in exams.

116. Which is the most common cause for readmission after day care surgery?

a. Hypotension
b. Nausea and vomiting
c. Bleeding
d. Apnea

(c) Bleeding

(Ref: Bailey and Love 27th edition page 305)

- The risk of postoperative hemorrhage occurring once the patient has returned home is often stated as a major reason to keep the patient in hospital overnight (Straight line from Bailey and Love 27th Edition)

Surgical Hemorrhage:

- Reactionary hemorrhage—Occurs in 4-6 hours after surgery and is caused by Slipping of ligature, clot displacement or cessation of vasospasm after mobilization or even after cough.
- Secondary Hemorrhage—occurs >24 hours after surgery and is due to infection eroding vessel.

117. An asymptomatic patient recovered from Covid infection. You are planning for an elective surgery. When will you do?

a. 4 weeks
b. 6 weeks
c. 8–10 weeks
d. 12 weeks

Ans. a. 4 weeks

(Ref: ASA- APSF Joint Statement on Elective Surgery and Anesthesia for Covid 19 patients)

After how many weeks an elective surgery is done:

- **4 weeks for an asymptomatic** patient or recovery from only mild nonrespiratory symptoms
- **6 weeks for a symptomatic patient** (Cough and Dyspnea) Who does not require hospitalization
- **8-10 weeks for a symptomatic patient** who is diabetic, immunocompromised or hospitalized
- **12 weeks for a patient** who is admitted to an intensive care unit due to Covid infection.

118. Triage is defined as:

a. To classify according to severity
b. To classify according to site
c. To classify according to depth
d. To categorize the number of injuries

Ans. a. To classify according to severity

(Ref: Bailey and Love 27th edition page 413)

- Triage has been derived from French word- to sort out

- It aims to identify and treat the patients who will benefit from early treatment
- By sorting out minor injuries-triage lessens the immediate burden on the medical facilities.
- Triage must be done by a senior person with experience and it must be undertaken in the field, before evacuation and at Hospital.
- A system of color coded tags attached to the patient's wrist or neck is done.
- The color denotes the degree of urgency which a patient requires treatment

Priority - Color	Medical need	Clinical status	Examples
1st - Red	Immediate	Critical – but likely to survive if treated early	Severe facial trauma Tension pneumothorax Profuse external bleeding Hemothorax Flail chest Major intra-abdominal bleed EDH
2nd - Yellow	Urgent	Critical – likely to survive if treated in hours	Compound fractures Degloving injuries Ruptured abdominal viscus Pelvic fractures Spinal injuries
3rd - Green	Non- Urgent	Stable, Treatment can be delayed from hours to days also Walking wounded	Simple fractures Sprain Minor lacerations
4th - Black	Unsalvageable	Not breathing Pulseless Severely injured and unable to save the patient	Severe Brain damage Extensive burns Major disruption of chest wall or abdominal wall structures

119. A female patient with lump present in right breast upper outer quadrant 4cm*3cm, axillary lymph node is negative, mammography reveals BIRADS 4; Patient underwent BCS, final HPE report reveals DCIS with high grade, what will be done next?

a. Follow up after 6 months and thereafter 2 years
b. Adjuvant RT
c. Adjuvant CT
d. Trastuzumab

Ans. b. Adjuvant RT

(Ref: Bailey and Love 27th edition page 872)

From the history and data given in the question, we can come to a conclusion that this is a case of DCIS and further management after surgery depends on:

- **Van Nuys System:**
  - Patient age
  - Type of DCIS
  - Presence of microcalcification
  - Extent of resection margin
  - Size of lesion
- Patients with high grade have benefit from Radiotherapy after complete excision.
- Patients with low grade whose tumor is completely excised will need no further treatment.

120. A 45-year-old female patient comes for examination of her breast. A 4.5 cmx 3cm size irregular mass is felt in the Left upper quadrant of the Right breast which is not fixed to the pectoralis major muscle and no skin changes, a 2cmx1.5cm lymph node is also palpated in the Right axilla. No mass is felt in the opposite breast. Which investigations will you do to this patient?

a. Mammography
b. PET scan
c. Biopsy of the Breast mass
d. USG guided biopsy of the enlarged axillary LN

1. a, b, c and d 2. a and c
3. a, b and c 4. a, c and d

Ans. 2 (a and c)

(Ref: AJCC, 8th edition)

The TNM stage of the Breast cancer is

- Size: 4.5 cm = T2 (2–5 cm)- no skin and Chest wall involvement seen
- Node: Ipsilateral 2*1.5 cm size node seen = N1
- T2 N1: Stage II (Early Breast Cancer)
- For Early Breast Cancer, PET CT is not a part of Investigation protocol. For LABC, PET CT is must.
- Axillary nodes if present it's malignant unless proved otherwise and we don't need to take Biopsy to confirm that.

121. A patient underwent Cholecystectomy and had abdominal pain in postoperative period. Patient had tachycardia. WBC count 11000 cells/mm^3 USG done shows a collection 5x 5 cm in right hypochondrium. What is the next step?

a. Pig tail drainage USG guided
b. ERCP
c. Reopen the abdomen
d. Observation

Ans. a. Pig tail drainage USG guided

(Ref: Bailey and Love 27th edition page 1204)

- This is a case of Bile duct injury and leak causing a collection in subhepatic space and fever.
- Immediate treatment is to call the interventional radiologist and to bring out the percutaneous drainage (Pig tail catheter) via the USG guidance

122. A patient has multiple Cholelithiasis with CBD diameter of 12 mm. Serum Bilirubin 0.8. Alkaline phosphatase is around 380. GGT is normal. What will be next step of management?

a. ERCP b. MRCP
c. Lap cholecystectomy d. CECT abdomen

Ans. b. MRCP

(Ref: Bailey and Love 27th edition page 1192)

- Elevation of Alkaline phosphatase is an important finding to say there is obstructive jaundice.
- CBD diameter of 12 mm is a sign of Distal obstruction.
- So to find out the cause of the obstruction- the next best investigation is MRCP

123. Identify the Urinary Crystal shown below.

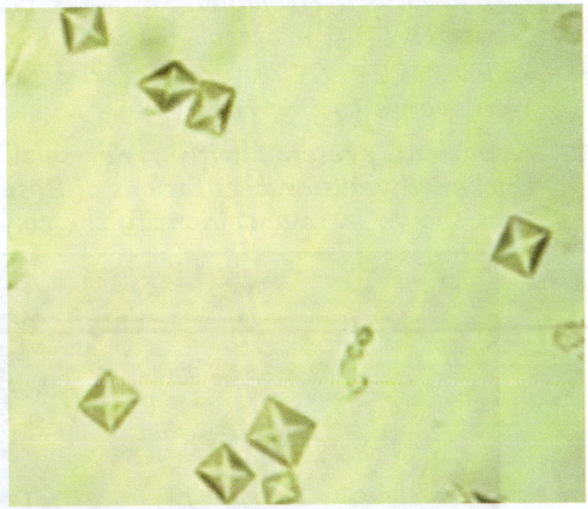

a. Calcium phosphate
b. Calcium oxalate
c. Uric acid
d. Cysteine

Ans. b. Calcium oxalate

(Ref: Pathology sources)

Pyramidal or envelope shaped—Calcium oxalate

124. A 3-year-old child was brought by her mother noticing an abdominal swelling with Ballottable nature. The mother says H/O Hematuria which resolved 2 days before. O/E ballottable abdominal swelling is the only significant finding. Which of the following investigations you will do?

1. CECT 2. PET CT
3. Urine VMA 4. FNAC

a. 1, 2, 3 are correct
b. 1, 2, 3, 4 are correct
c. 3, 4 are correct
d. 1, 2, 4 are correct

Ans. d. 1, 2, 4 are correct

(Ref: Sabiston 21st edition page 1873)

- From the History, this is a case of Wilms Tumor.
- Urine VMA is not needed for Wilms Tumor, it is elevated in Catecholamine secreting tumors—neuroblastoma, pheochromocytoma, and other neural crest tumors
- USG is the first done investigation and CECT abdomen is the IOC.

- MC site of metastasis is Chest—hence, CT Chest and X-ray chest are done.
- We have to do FNAC of the lesion, if we are planning a Neoadjuvant Chemotherapy as per NWTSG protocol.
- FDG PET CT is useful for assessing the response to Chemotherapy.

125. A patient presents with renal swelling with thickened walls and septations of Bosniak Type 3 as shown in image. Identify the condition.

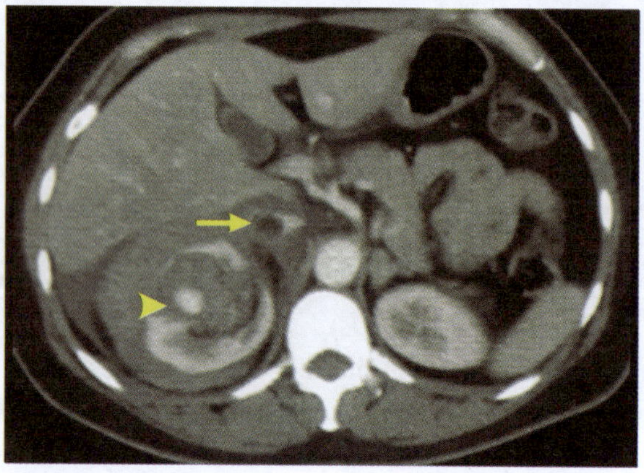

a. Angiomyolipoma b. Renal cyst
c. RCC d. Oncocytoma

Ans. a. Angiomyolipoma

(Ref: Bailey and Love 27th edition page 1416 and 1389)

- Type 3 Bosniak is Indeterminate mass with cystic lesions having thickened wall and septations showing enhancement
- Angiomyolipoma comes under Type 3 Bosniak Cyst classification
- It has high fat content and has a typical appearance on CT scan.
- Malignant elements are present in 1/4th cases.

126. A boy with perineal injury came to emergency department. On examination, blood is present at meatus and he has not passed urine. Bladder is not full. Next step of management is:

a. Suprapubic catheterization
b. Wait and send home
c. Foley's catheter insertion
d. Wait for bladder to fill and urge to urinate

Ans. d. Wait for bladder to fill and urge to urinate

(Ref: Bailey and Love 27th edition, Page 1479)

- Perineal injury usually results from a straddle injury which can cause bulbar urethral rupture.
- This case is a Bulbar urethral injury and hence Foley's must not be inserted. We must wait for the Bladder to fill and do a Suprapubic catheterization after the bladder is full.
- Please understand the basics- SPC is a blind procedure which is done when Bladder is full and palpable in lower abdomen, if you put it without inflated- you will do bowel injury.

127. A young patient presented with painless enlargement of testis. LDH values are increased. Next step is:

a. FNAC
b. Biopsy
c. High orchidectomy
d. Tumor markers

Ans. d. Tumor markers

(Ref: Bailey and Love 27th edition page 1508)

- Painless enlargement of testis with elevation of LDH is suggestive of Seminoma
- USG is the first step to be done.
- Tumor markers used are- AFP, hCG. These markers are used to assess the response to treatment.
- Tumor markers should be measured prior to orchidectomy.
- Staging work up is done with CT Chest, Abdomen and Pelvis.

128. Best investigation to localize Parathyroid tissue:

a. Sestamibi scan
b. CECT
c. USG abdomen
d. MRI

Ans. a. Sestamibi scan

(Ref: Bailey and Love 27th edition page 827)

- Sestamibi (2 methoxy 2 methyl propyl iso nitrile) is the most accurate and reliable method to image the parathyroid gland.
- It can find out ectopic position better than USG
- Parathyroid adenomas are picked up based on Oxyphilic cells with high mitochondria content.
- Hurthle cell nodules all exhibit oxyphil cells and can give false positive, which can be reduced by adding Tc99m Pertechneate subtraction Sestamibi scans.

129. Identify the Hernia shown below:

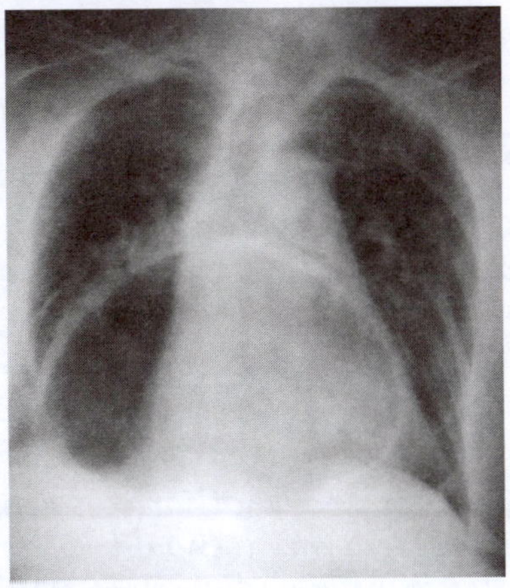

a. Bochdalek hernia
b. Morgagni hernia
c. Gastric volvulus
d. Eventration of diaphragm

Ans. b. Morgagni Hernia

- Anterior to heart and defect is in Larrey's space
- Ideally we need the lateral X-ray to make the diagnosis perfectly or a CECT chest and abdomen

INI-CET DECEMBER 2020

130. Which of the following are components of q-SOFA scoring?

A. Respiratory rate B. Blood pressure
C. CNS features D. Leukocyte count
1. A, B, C and D 2. A, B and C
3. B, D and C 4. A, C and D

Ans. 2. A, B and C

(Ref: Sabiston 21st edition page 62)

q-SOFA is a quick sequential organ failure assessment score, is calculated by Tachypnea, Altered mental status and Hypotension.

131. What is the size of cannula shown below?

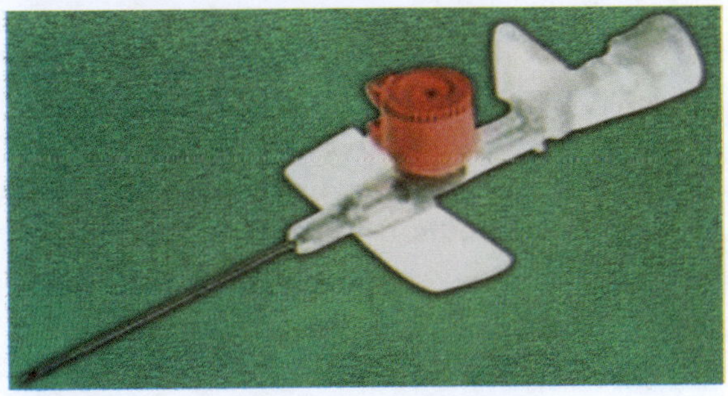

a. 14G b. 16G
c. 18G d. 20G

Ans. d. 20G (Multiple repeat question)

Pink Cannula—20 G size is used in adults for elective fluid transfusions.

132. Name this position of the patient in Operation theater.

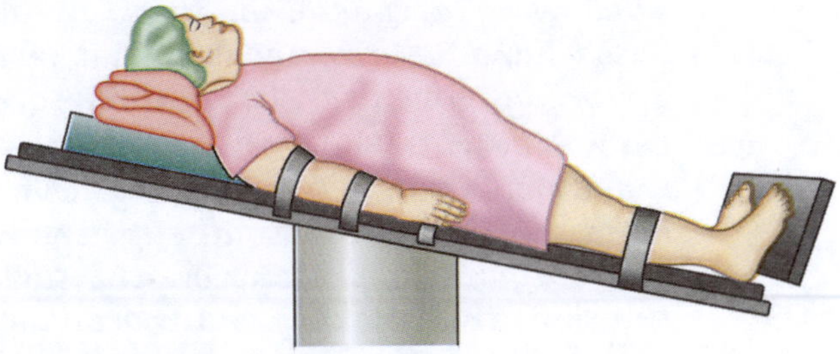

a. Trendelenburg
b. Lloyd-Davies position
c. Reverse Trendelenburg
d. Jack knife position

Ans. c. Reverse Trendelenburg

- In Trendelenburg position, the foot end is elevated; and in reverse Trendelenburg, the head end is elevated.
- Trendelenburg position – Varicose vein surgery done
- Reverse Trendelenburg position– Thyroid and neck surgery

133. In which of the following conditions sanitizer can be used:

a. Before examining the patient
b. After examining the patient
c. After touching patient's surroundings
d. When hands are soiled.
1. a, b, c and d 2. a, b and c
3. a and b 4. a, b and d

Ans. 2. a, b and c

(Ref: Internet Sources)

Don'ts of using hand sanitizers

1. Do not use a hand sanitizer if your hands are **dirty or greasy** as it does not work well on dirty hands. Wash your hands with soap and warm water instead to thoroughly clean them.
2. Don't rush while using hand sanitizer as it would not be effective if you rinse or wipe your hands before it dries on its own. You must rub your hands with the sanitizer for at least 20 seconds.
3. If your hands are contaminated with **chemicals such as pesticides and heavy metals**, sanitizers would not be able to clear

them off your hands. You need to wash your hands with soap and warm water if you've come in contact with these chemicals.

4. Rather than using hand sanitizer, **children** should be encouraged to wash their hands as they can ingest the sanitizer. A child swallowing a tiny amount of an alcohol-based hand sanitizer could result in alcohol poisoning, which can be fatal for some.
5. Do not overuse hand sanitizers as they can make your skin extremely dry. **Overuse** of hand sanitizers can also disrupt the healthy microorganisms present on the surface of the skin, thus making one more vulnerable to infections. Overuse can also break down the skin, leaving it cracked and chapped, thus allowing the germs to enter through these crevices easily.
6. You must wash your hands after using hand sanitizer and before eating or cooking food. **Consumption of 1-propanol**, one of the ingredients found in some hand sanitizers, can lead to central nervous system depression. A person exposed to 1-propanol would present with symptoms such as confusion, decreased consciousness, and slower heart rate and breathing.
7. Do not use hand sanitizers to clean your **food such as vegetables and fruits.**

134. A 25-year-old male patient came to ER with history of trauma, his RR is 35/min and BP is 100/60 mm Hg, on percussion hyper resonance is heard over entire Right side of the chest. FAST was performed by the doctor in ER room and is normal. After looking at the chest X-ray, what is the next step in management of this patient?

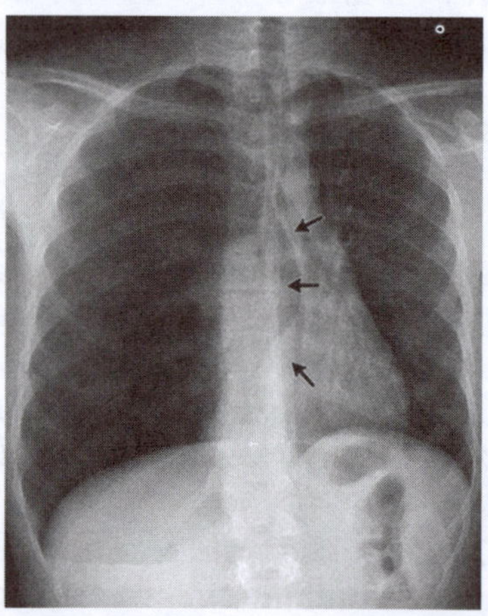

a. Wide bore needle insertion in the 5th ICS
b. Wide bore needle insertion followed by intercostals drain in the 5th ICS
c. Aspirate the collection
d. No intervention needed

Ans. b. Wide bore needle insertion followed by intercostals drain in the 5th ICS

(Ref: Bailey 27th edition page 367)

- This is a case of Pneumothorax.
- Clinical examination may reveal tracheal deviation this is a late finding and is not necessary to clinically confirm diagnosis.
- There will also be hyper-resonance and decreased or absent breath sounds over the affected hemithorax.
- Tension pneumothorax is a **clinical** diagnosis; and treatment should never be delayed by waiting for radiological confirmation
- Treatment consists of immediate decompression, initially by rapid insertion of a large-bore cannula into the second intercostal space in the mid-clavicular line of the affected side, then followed by insertion of a chest tube through the fifth intercostal space in the anterior axillary line.
- The only line which doesn't suit in this paragraph- FAST can diagnose Pneumothorax- which will show Stratosphere sign**

135. What is the additional benefit of doing e-FAST?

a. Pelvic trauma can be identified
b. Chest trauma can be identified
c. Sub dural and dural trauma can be identified
d. Retroperitoneal trauma can be identified

Ans. b. Chest trauma can be identified

(Ref: Bailey 27th edition page 372)

- Efast is extended to two more regions apart from FAST focused four regions.
- They are both side chest to rule out chest injury.
- Pneumothorax appears as Stratosphere sign/Bar Code sign.

136. A young male with head injury was brought to the emergency in unconscious state. The patient was not able to breathe properly, put on ventilatory support. On examination, GCS was 8 with findings of raised ICT. NCCT brain and spinal imaging were normal. What is the most probable diagnosis?

a. Diffuse axonal injury
b. Posterior circulation stroke
c. Post concussion syndrome
d. Posterior reversible encephalopathy syndrome (PRES)

Ans. a. Diffuse axonal injury

(Ref: Bailey 27th edition page 336)

Diffuse axonal Injury:

- This is a form of primary brain injury, seen in high-energy accidents, and which usually renders the patient comatose.
- It is strictly a pathological diagnosis made at postmortem, but hemorrhagic foci in the corpus callosum and dorsolateral rostral brainstem on CT may be suggestive, although the CT often appears normal.
- MRI is IOC for DAI

137. A 25-year-old female presents with rapid weight gain and loss of appetite. Patient has very low T4 and high TSH. What is your diagnosis?

a. Graves disease
b. Hashimoto's thyroiditis
c. De Quervain's thyroiditis
d. Papillary cancer

Ans. b. Hashimoto's thyroiditis

(Ref: Sabiston 21st edition page 884)

- Hashimoto's thyroiditis is the most common cause of hypothyroidism in the world
- It is characterized by Hypothyroidism after a brief episode of hyperthyroidism initially.
- Weight gain and loss of appetite and low T4 and high TSH all suggest hypothyroidism
- De Quervain's presents with pain and swelling along with transient hyperthyroidism.

138. A 40-year-old female has a massive enlargement of her left breast over 30 days, it is mobile over chest wall and local rise of temperature is seen, what is your likely diagnosis?

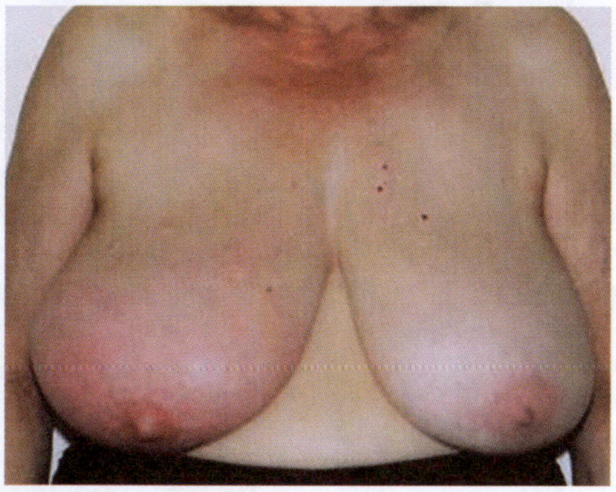

a. Galactorrhea
b. Inflammatory breast cancer
c. Lymphatics obstruction
d. Phyllodes tumor

Ans. b. Inflammatory Breast Cancer

(Ref: Bailey 27th edition page 872, Sabiston 21st edition page 851)

- 1% to 5% of all breast tumors
- Most aggressive subtype of breast cancer.
- The hallmark of inflammatory breast cancer is diffuse tumor involvement of the dermal lymphatic channels within the breast and overlying skin, often without a discrete underlying tumor mass.
- Inflammatory breast cancer manifests clinically as **erythema, edema, and warmth of the breast** as a result of lymphatic obstruction.
- There may be no abnormality on mammography beyond skin thickening, and a palpable mass is not required for the diagnosis. The term *peau d'orange* is used to describe the orange-peel appearance of the skin resulting from edema and dimpling at sites of hair.
- The history should reveal a rapid onset of the disease, with progression over weeks to 3 months.
- Inflammatory cancer is a clinical diagnosis and can occur with tumors of ductal or lobular histology.
- The pathologic hallmark of inflammatory cancer is the presence of tumor cells within dermal lymphatics.
- Axillary nodal metastases are common, and there is a significant risk for distant metastases.

139. Identify the size of this instrument used in taking Biopsy from breast.

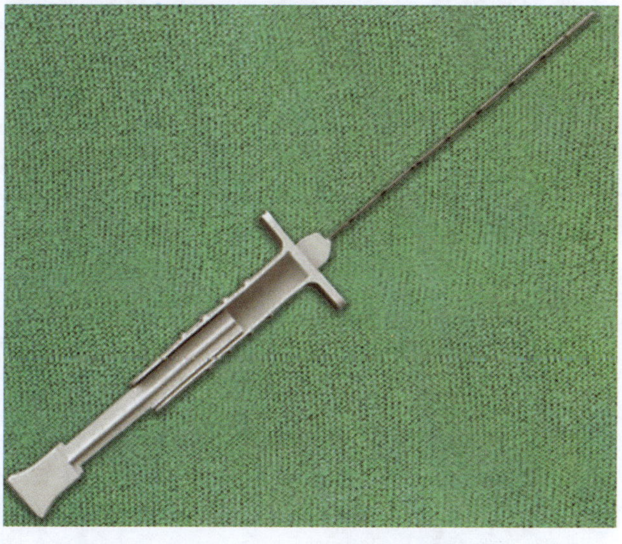

a. 24 G
b. 22 G
c. 20 G
d. 18 G

Ans. d. 18 G

(Ref: Internet Sources)

- This is Trucut biopsy needle used to take biopsy from breast.
- Sizes are 18 G and bigger.
- Gauge size number increases the sample taken, diameter decreases.
- 22 G is smaller than 18 G size.
- 22 G is FNAC, 18 G is Trucut.
- Trucut is more confirmatory than FNAC and yields more material for study.

Author's note: Don't get confused with Fr (French) units.

- As the French size increases the diameter increases—14 Fr < 16 Fr < 18 Fr
- As the gauge size increases the diameter decreases—18 G > 22 G > 24 G
- 1 French unit = 3 mm size**

140. As per European Hernia Society Classification-Incisional hernia at level of Umbilicus is given the term

a. M1 b. M2
c. M3 d. M4

Ans. c. M3

(Ref: Internet sources)

European Hernia Society classification for incisional abdominal wall hernias

EHS Incisional Hernia Classification			
Midline	subxiphoidal	M1	
	epigastric	M2	
	umbilical	M3	
	infraumbilical	M4	
	suprapubic	M5	
Lateral	subcostal	L1	
	flank	L2	
	iliac	L3	
	lumbar	L4	
Recurrent incisional hernia?		Yes ○	No ○
length:	cm	width:	cm
	W1	W2	W3
Width	<4 cm	≥4–10 cm	≥10 cm
cm	○	○	○

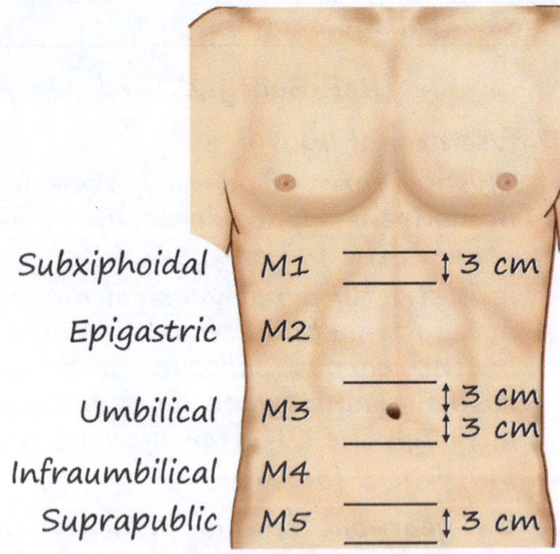

141. Regarding the Boundaries of laparoscopic anatomy of Inguinal hernia, false statement is:

a. Medial boundary of Triangle of Doom is Vas deferens
b. Lateral boundary of Triangle of pain is Iliopubic tract
c. Myopectineal orifice is bounded by Internal oblique and Transversus abdominis superiorly
d. Myopectineal orifice bounded by Iliopubic tract inferiorly

Ans. d. Myopectineal orifice bounded by Iliopubic tract inferiorly

(Ref: Long cases of Surgery by Rajamahendran)

Myopectineal Orifice of Fruchaud

- Medial—Rectus sheath
- Lateral—Iliopsoas
- Superior—Conjoint Tendon
- Inferior—Pecten Pubis

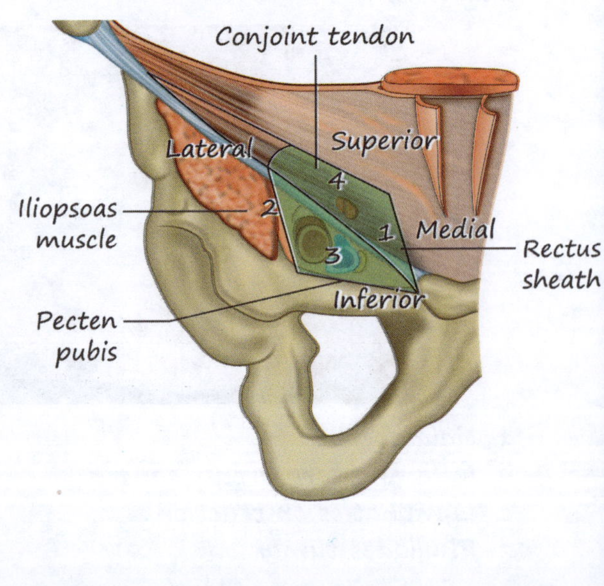

142. Match the following (nerves injured in surgery):

Nerve Injured	Surgery
1. External laryngeal nerve	A. Laparoscopic hernia surgery
2. Long thoracic nerve	B. Video assisted thymectomy
3. Phrenic nerve	C. Modified radical mastectomy
4. Hypoglossal nerve	D. Thyroidectomy
5. Lateral Cutaneous nerve	E. Submandibular gland surgery

Ans. 1-D, 2-C, 3-B, 4-E, 5-A

- Long Thoracic nerve of Bell can be injured in MRM which results in Winging of Scapula.
- External laryngeal nerve is the most common nerve injured in Thyroidectomy
- Phrenic nerve is injured in VATS thymectomy.
- Lingual and Hypoglossal nerves are injured in submandibular gland excision.
- LCN of thigh is the MC nerve injured in TAPP for Hernia

143. A 25-year-old female patient presents with progressive dysphagia to solids and liquids, barium swallow was done. What are the investigations needed to confirm your diagnosis?

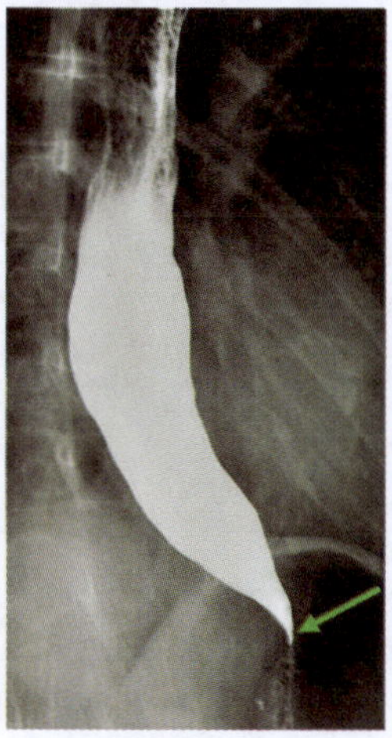

a. Endoscopy + 24 hours pH monitoring
b. Endoscopy + Esophageal manometry
c. Endoscopy + CT chest
d. Endoscopy + biopsy

Ans. b. Endoscopy+ Esophageal manometry

(Ref: Sabiston 21st edition page 1026)

- The Barium swallow shows Bird's Beak appearance here
- Manometry is the Gold standard to diagnose this case of Achalasia cardia.
- Endoscopy must also be performed in all suspected cases of Achalasia to rule out narrowing due to pseudoachalasia (GEJ tumors, Strictures, Neuropathy)

144. Which of the symptoms given below are seen in the child with the following X-ray?

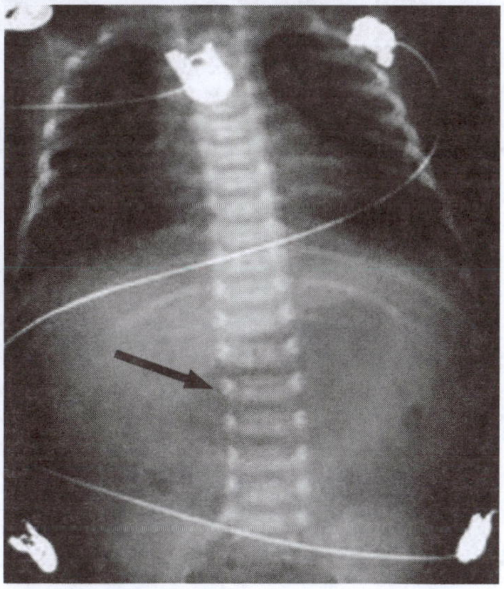

a. Bilious vomiting
b. Palpable mass
c. Hypochloremia and Hypokalemia
d. Metabolic alkalosis

1. a, b, c and d
2. a, b and d
3. b, c and d
4. a, b and c

Ans. 3. b, c and d

(Ref: Bailey 27th edition page 128)

- Infantile CHPS is common between 2-8 weeks and never happens after 13 weeks
- We can easily differentiate from other causes of vomiting like infections because CHPS babies have severe Hunger**
- In the UK, it affects 1:300 infants, with a male:female ratio of 4:1.
- CHPS is readily treated by surgery but the infant must be adequately rehydrated and the hypochloremic hypokalemic alkalosis corrected; this may take 48 hours if the chloride is 85 mmol/L or lower.
- In most babies, the dehydration and alkalosis can be corrected by giving 150–180 mL/kg/day of 0.9% saline with 0.15% KCl in 5% glucose.
- Oral feeding is discontinued and the stomach emptied with an 8–10 Fr nasogastric tube; ongoing gastric losses should be replaced intravenously.

145. A 35-year-old male patient of peptic ulcer disease came with pain in abdomen of two days duration and obstipation for 2 days, X-ray erect abdomen was done. What is the next line of management of this patient?

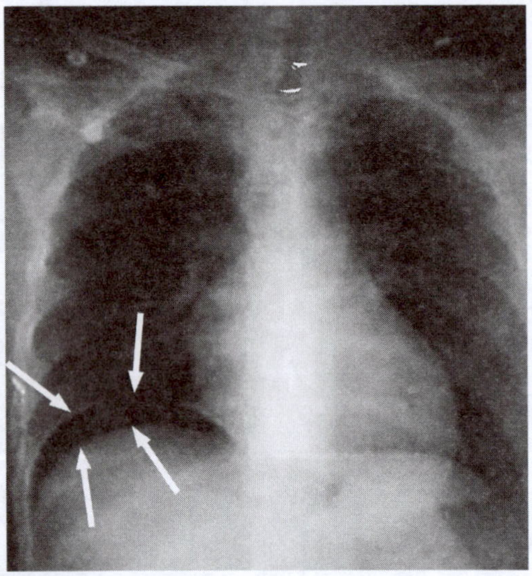

a. USG abdomen
b. IV fluids
c. Exploratory laparotomy
d. Keep the patient in observation

1. b and c 2. b and d
3. a and b 4. b, a and c

Ans. 1. b and c

(Ref: Sabiston 21st edition page 1213

- Perforation of duodenal ulcer is the common cause of this pneumoperitoneum.
- Urgent Laparotomy is advised with resuscitation.
- <1 cm perforation: Closed primarily and Buttress with vascularized omentum
- 1-3 cm perforation: Graham's omental patch closure
- > 3cm: Pyloric Exclusion with Roux En Y limb Jejunal serosal patch (If omental is unhealthy) + GJ performed

146. A 40-year-old patient, with previous history of MI, presented to the emergency with history of multiple episodes of vomiting, pain abdomen and blood in stool. On examination, BP-90/60 mm Hg, PR 112/min and pulse were irregularly irregular. Abdomen was soft, non-distended and bowel sounds were absent. What is the most probable diagnosis?

a. Ruptured aortic aneurysm
b. Peptic ulcer perforation
c. Acute mesenteric ischemia
d. Severe acute pancreatitis

Ans. c. Acute mesenteric ischemia

(Ref: Sabiston 21st edition page 1255)

- The History of MI and irregularly irregular Pulse point to Atrial fibrillation, which can result in Embolus from heart to mesenteric vessels resulting in Acute mesenteric Ischemia.
- In Acute mesenteric ischemia, there will be gangrene of bowel with absent bowel sounds and soft abdomen.
- The signs will be out of proportion to symptoms.

147. Which of the following is correct about Peutz-Jeghers syndrome?

1. Congenital hypertrophy of retinal pigment epithelium is most common extra-intestinal manifestation
2. Arborizing pattern
3. STK11 mutation
4. Autosomal recessive
5. Multiple GI polyps seen

a. 1, 3 and 5 b. 2, 3 and 5
c. 1, 2 and 4 d. 1, 2, 3 and 5

Ans. b. 2, 3, 5

(Ref: Sabiston 21st edition)

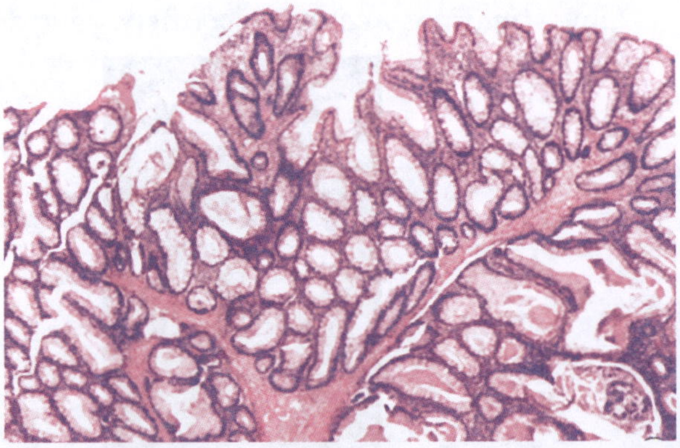

- The histologic hallmark of Peutz-Jeghers polyps is the presence of smooth muscle fibers in an arborizing pattern, and it is often assumed that this is a reliable indicator of Peutz-Jeghers polyps and Peutz-Jeghers syndrome throughout the gastrointestinal tract.

Peutz-Jeghers Syndrome:

- Autosomal Dominant
- 39% life time risk of CRC
- Mucocutaneous pigmentation seen (CHRPE is a feature of FAP**)
- MC site of Polyps is Small bowel at jejunum, also seen in colon

- PJS caused by STK 11 mutation in Chr 19p
- PJS differs from juvenile polyps histologically as PJS polyps are due to overgrowth of muscularis mucosa rather than lamina propria.

148. Match the following:

1. ET tube
2. Ryles tube
3. Underwater drain
4. Urine drain bag

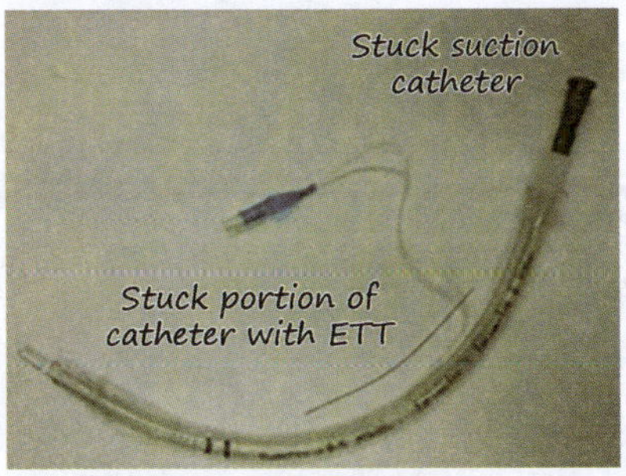

A

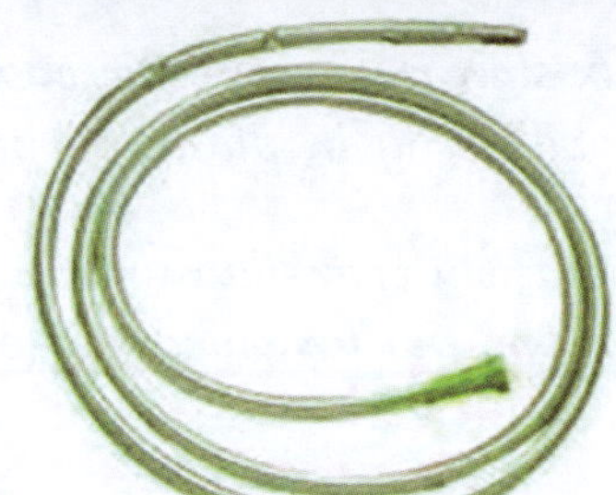
B

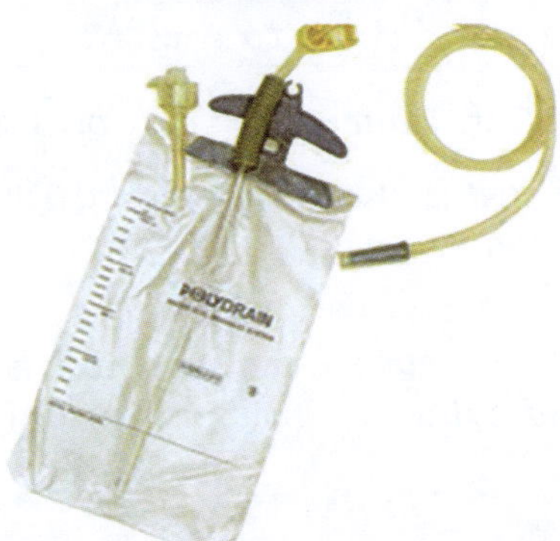

C

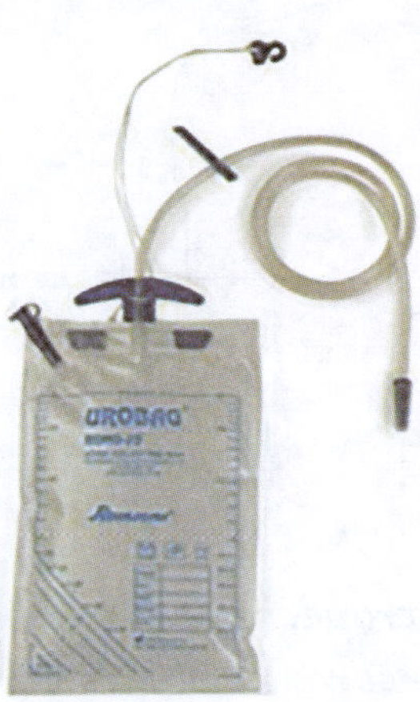

D

a. 1-A, 2-B, 3-C, 4-D
b. 1-B, 2-A, 3-D, 4-C
c. 1-D, 2-C, 3-A, 4-B
d. 1-D, 2-B, 3-A, 4-C

Ans. a. 1-A, 2-B, 3-C, 4-D

- From the pictures, you might get confused only with underwater drain and Urobag.
- Please observe closely in Underwater bag- the external tube goes deep inside, so that we can pour water above the level to prevent air entering inside.

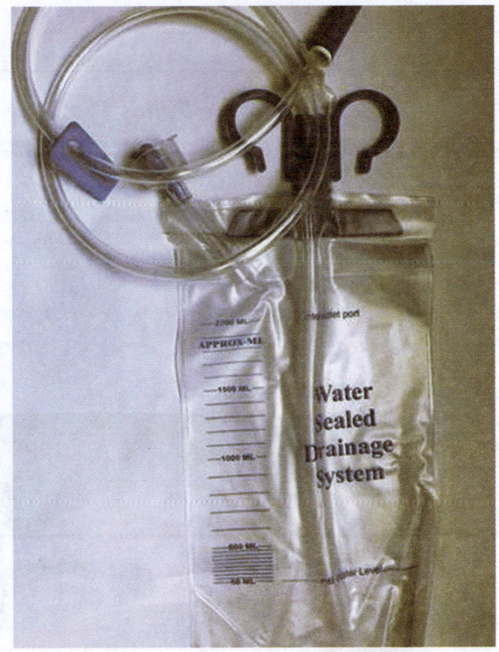

Note the external tube entering up to lower part of the bag. In Urobag, it will be ending at the top of the bag.

INI-CET NOVEMBER 2020

149. While doing Parotid Surgery, the following Landmarks are used to identify the Facial nerve Trunk; except:

a. Tragal Cartilage Pointer
b. Posterior Belly of Digastric insertion
c. Inferior Belly of Omohyoid
d. Mastoid Process

Ans. c. Inferior Belly of Omohyoid

(Ref: Bailey and Love 27th edition page 791)

Methods to identify the facial nerve while doing parotidectomy:

- Identify the Conley's pointer (Inferior portion of cartilaginous canal)
- Upper border of posterior belly of digastric
- Squamo tympanic fissure
- Styloid process (nerve is superficial to it)
- Mastoid process can be drilled and nerve identified more proximally
- Retrograde technique

150. A patient after parotid surgery on awakening noticed lower lip paralysis. Otherwise she is able to close his eyes normally. Which of the following nerve is most likely injured?

a. Cervical Branch of facial nerve
b. Facial Nerve main trunk
c. Parotid duct
d. Temporal branch of facial nerve

Ans. a. Cervical branch of facial nerve

- Cervical branch supplies Platysma muscle.
- The majority of muscles responsible for depression of the lip are supplied via the **marginal mandibular branch of the facial nerve.**
- The platysma, which is also involved in depression of the lower lip, receives its innervation via the cervical branch of the facial nerve

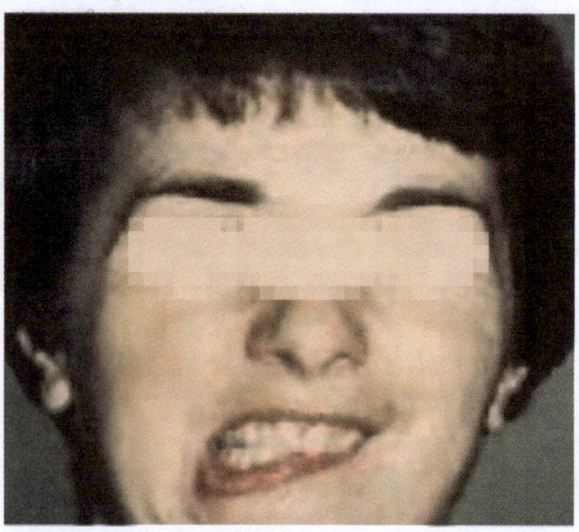

Lower lip movement by Marginal branch of Facial nerve and Cervical branch of facial nerve

Below is the illustrated image of all muscles supplied by various branches

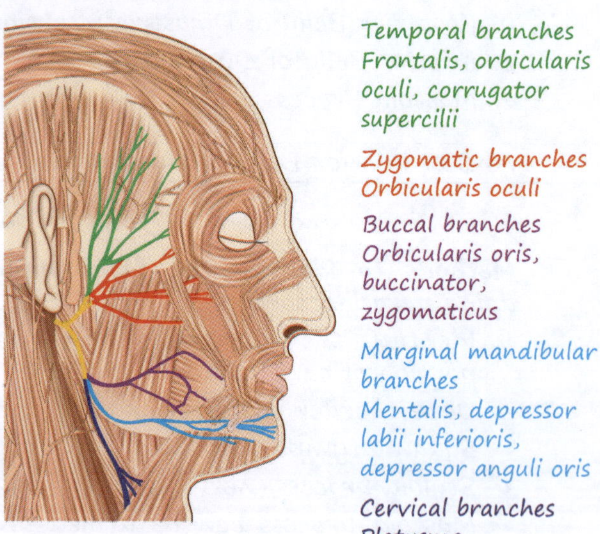

151. A male patient is diagnosed with carcinoma Colon. Which of the following gene mutations is likely to be present?

a. Kras, APC, DCC
b. APC, K-ras, P53
c. BRCA1, K ras, APC
d. APC, Kras and loss of 10 on myc

Ans. b. APC, K-ras, P53

(Ref: Sabiston 21st edition page 1364)

This is FEARON VOGELSTEIN SEQUENCE based order of mutation.

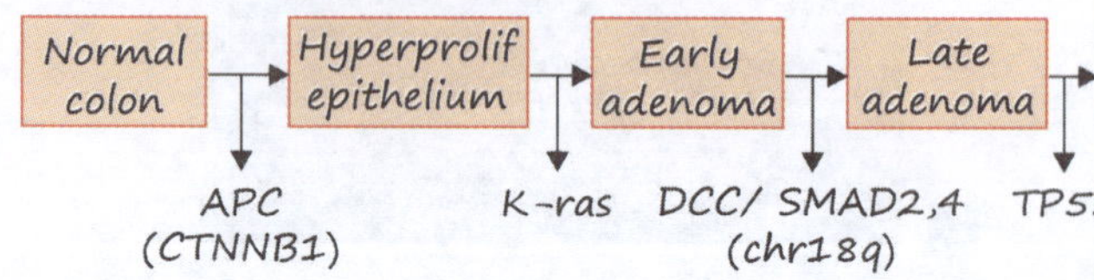

152. What is Tillaux sign in mesenteric cyst?

a. Mass is mobile only in plane perpendicular to mesentry
b. Mass is brilliantly transilluminating
c. Mass felt in the periumbilical region
d. Fluctuation positive

Ans. a. Mass is mobile only in plane perpendicular to mesentry

(Ref: Bailey 27th edition page 1063)

Mesentric cyst is characterized by Tillaux Triad:

- Central dullness due to mass
- Zone of resonance around the mass
- Mesentric cyst movement is possible perpendicular to mesentry only (Tillaux sign)

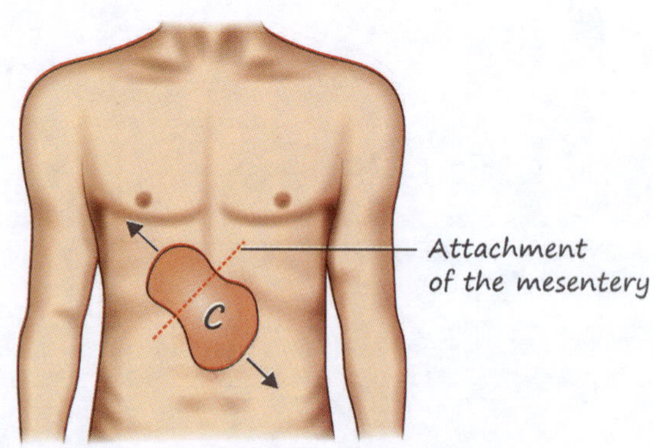

153. Most common retroperitoneal tumor:

a. Rhabdomyosarcoma
b. Liposarcoma
c. Leiomyosarcoma
d. Neuroblastoma

- PJS caused by STK 11 mutation in Chr 19p
- PJS differs from juvenile polyps histologically as PJS polyps are due to overgrowth of muscularis mucosa rather than lamina propria.

148. Match the following:

1. ET tube 2. Ryles tube
3. Underwater drain 4. Urine drain bag

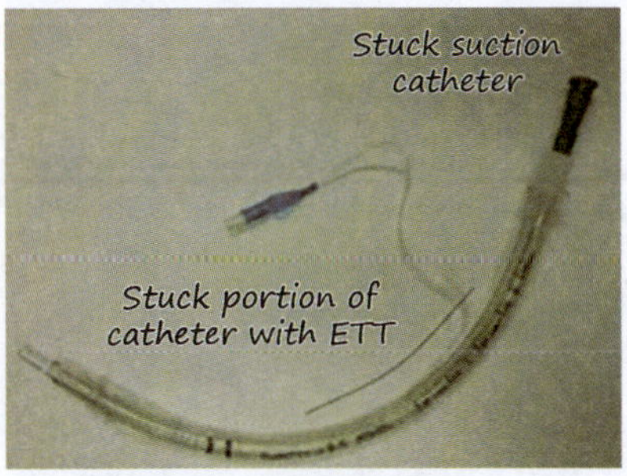

A

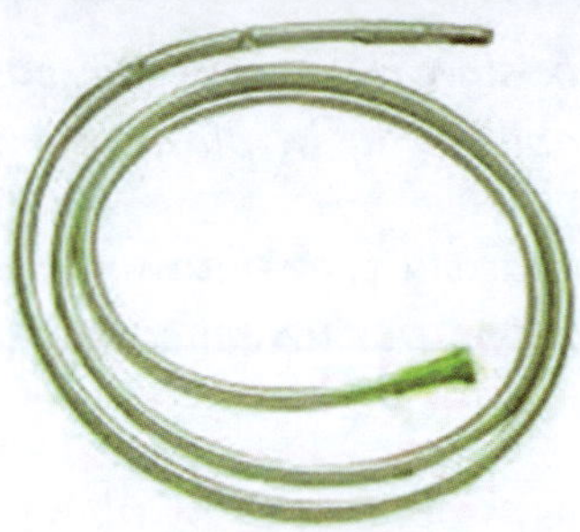

B

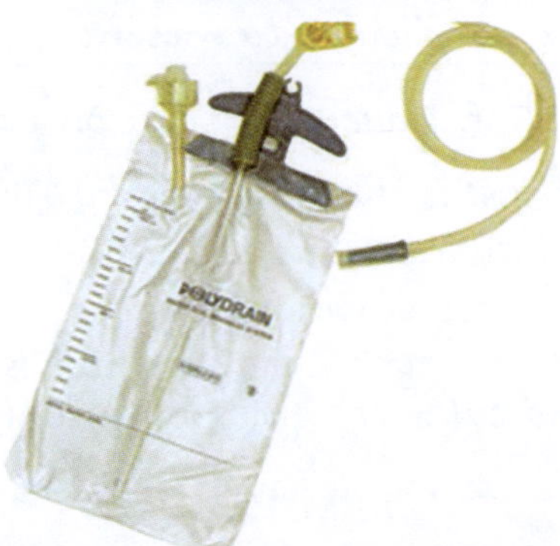

C

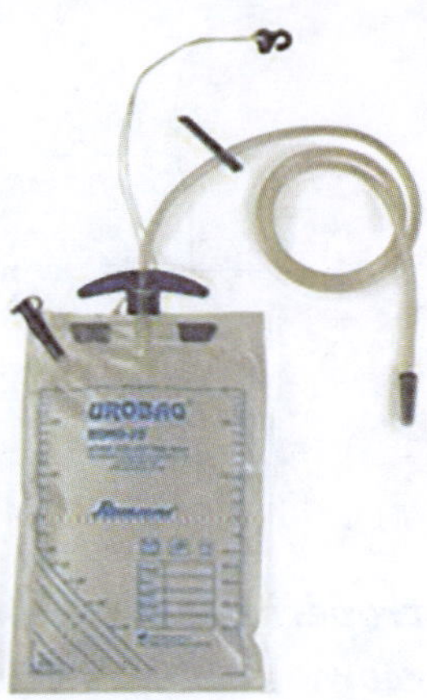

D

a. 1-A, 2-B, 3-C, 4-D
b. 1-B, 2-A, 3-D, 4-C
c. 1-D, 2-C, 3-A, 4-B
d. 1-D, 2-B, 3-A, 4-C

Ans. a. 1-A, 2-B, 3-C, 4-D

- From the pictures, you might get confused only with underwater drain and Urobag.
- Please observe closely in Underwater bag- the external tube goes deep inside, so that we can pour water above the level to prevent air entering inside.

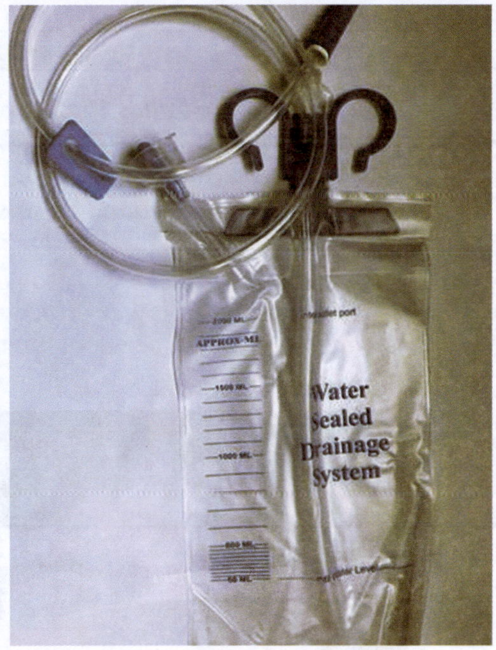

Note the external tube entering up to lower part of the bag. In Urobag, it will be ending at the top of the bag.

INI-CET NOVEMBER 2020

149. While doing Parotid Surgery, the following Landmarks are used to identify the Facial nerve Trunk; except:

a. Tragal Cartilage Pointer
b. Posterior Belly of Digastric insertion
c. Inferior Belly of Omohyoid
d. Mastoid Process

Ans. c. Inferior Belly of Omohyoid

(Ref: Bailey and Love 27th edition page 791)

Methods to identify the facial nerve while doing parotidectomy:

- Identify the Conley's pointer (Inferior portion of cartilaginous canal)
- Upper border of posterior belly of digastric
- Squamo tympanic fissure
- Styloid process (nerve is superficial to it)
- Mastoid process can be drilled and nerve identified more proximally
- Retrograde technique

150. A patient after parotid surgery on awakening noticed lower lip paralysis. Otherwise she is able to close his eyes normally. Which of the following nerve is most likely injured?

a. Cervical Branch of facial nerve
b. Facial Nerve main trunk
c. Parotid duct
d. Temporal branch of facial nerve

Ans. a. Cervical branch of facial nerve

- Cervical branch supplies Platysma muscle.
- The majority of muscles responsible for depression of the lip are supplied via the **marginal mandibular branch of the facial nerve.**
- The platysma, which is also involved in depression of the lower lip, receives its innervation via the cervical branch of the facial nerve

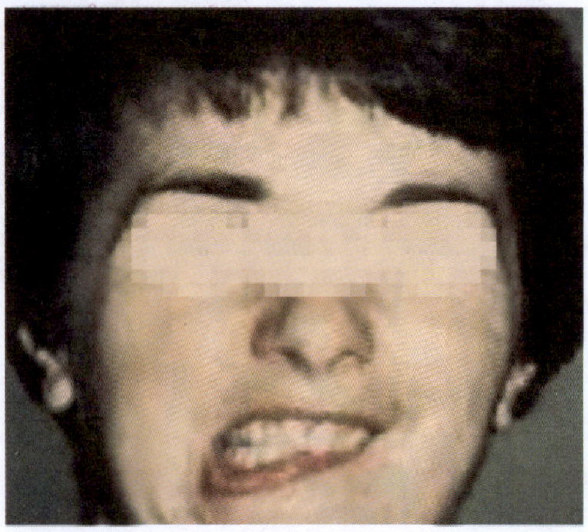

Lower lip movement by Marginal branch of Facial nerve and Cervical branch of facial nerve

Below is the illustrated image of all muscles supplied by various branches

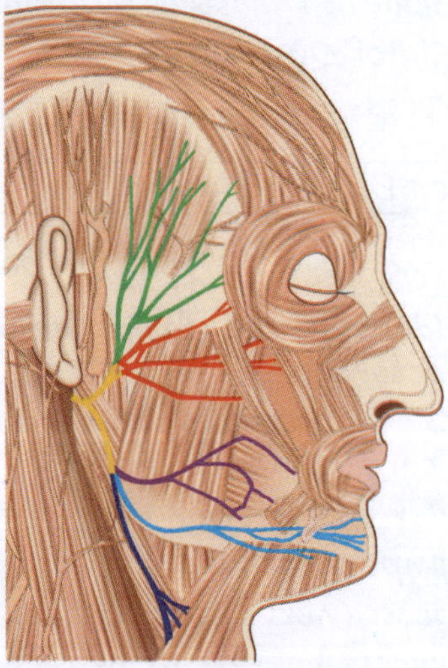

151. A male patient is diagnosed with carcinoma Colon. Which of the following gene mutations is likely to be present?

a. Kras, APC, DCC
b. APC, K-ras, P53
c. BRCA1, K ras, APC
d. APC, Kras and loss of 10 on myc

Ans. b. APC, K-ras, P53

(Ref: Sabiston 21st edition page 1364)

This is FEARON VOGELSTEIN SEQUENCE based order of mutation.

Normal colon → Hyperprolif epithelium → Early adenoma → Late adenoma →

APC (CTNNB1) | K-ras | DCC/ SMAD2,4 (chr18q) | TP53

152. What is Tillaux sign in mesenteric cyst?

a. Mass is mobile only in plane perpendicular to mesentry
b. Mass is brilliantly transilluminating
c. Mass felt in the periumbilical region
d. Fluctuation positive

Ans. a. Mass is mobile only in plane perpendicular to mesentry

(Ref: Bailey 27th edition page 1063)

Mesentric cyst is characterized by Tillaux Triad:

- Central dullness due to mass
- Zone of resonance around the mass
- Mesentric cyst movement is possible perpendicular to mesentry only (Tillaux sign)

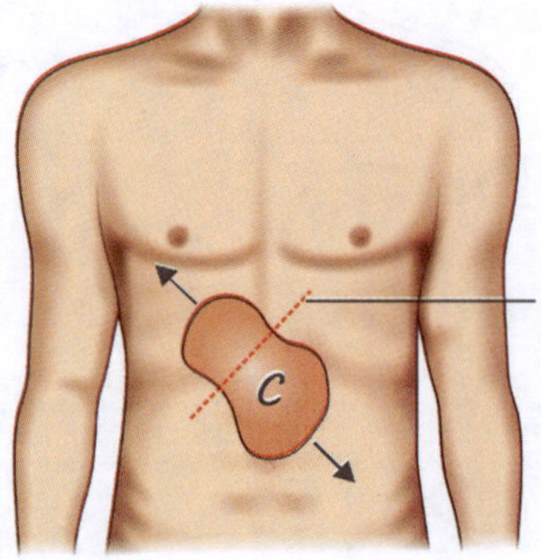

153. Most common retroperitoneal tumor:

a. Rhabdomyosarcoma
b. Liposarcoma
c. Leiomyosarcoma
d. Neuroblastoma

Ans. b. Liposarcoma

(Ref: Sabiston 21st edition page 1101)

- Approximately 15% of soft tissue sarcomas arise within the retroperitoneum.
- In this location, the most common histologic subtypes are liposarcoma and leiomyosarcoma. Most patients present with a large abdominal mass.
- Abdominal pain is present in about 50% of the patients.
- Other symptoms are related to organ compression from the tumor and include early satiety, nausea, vomiting, constipation, weight loss, and lower extremity edema.
- Symptoms due to nerve compression by the tumor, such as lower extremity paresthesia and paresis, are also reported.
- IOC is CECT Abdomen
- Liposarcoma is diagnosed by variable fat density. No need of Image guided Biopsy

154. Which of the following are used to arrest the Variceal Bleeding?

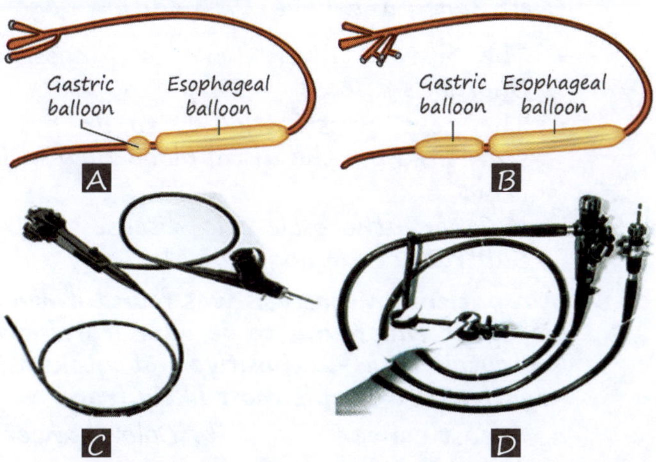

1. A, B, C, D
2. A, B, C
3. A, B
4. A and D

Ans. 1. A, B, C, D

(Ref: Sabiston 21st edition page 1159)

The gadgets shown in image are:

- Image A—Old Sengstaken-Blakemore tube with 3 lumens
- Image B—Modified Sengstaken-Blakemore tube (MINNESOTA Tube) with 4 lumens (4th One to aspirate Esophageal contents)
- Image C—Upper GI Scopy for Sclerosant injection.
- Image D—Upper GI Scopy with Band applicators.

155. A 40-year-old female patient underwent cholecystectomy, post-op she is complaining of pain in abdomen. Which test is performed to identify bile leak?

a. HIDA
b. MRCP
c. ERCP
d. CECT

Ans. c. ERCP and d. CECT

(Ref: Sabiston 21st edition page 1514 and Bailey 27th edition page 1204)

- If bile duct injury is suspected, CT Scan should be performed which shows Ascites or Right Upper Quadrant Collection consistent with Bilooma**
- Immediate PCD placement is done to control the infection.
- Electively ERCP is done to know the site and pattern of injury, for which we have a classification known as Strasberg Classification.
- HIDA scanning may be helpful as it can confirm the presence of a leak or biliary obstruction.
- It can be used to identify and quantitate the leak.
- If available, ERCP should be considered because this is both diagnostic and potentially therapeutic.
- The most common bile leak following cholecystectomy is from the cystic duct. This can be treated by a gastroenterologist placing a biliary endoprosthesis (stent) in the common bile duct across the origin of the cystic duct.
- MRCP is also helpful in determining the level and degree of injury.

156. Bile leak from the aberrant right hepatic duct that is not communicating from the common bile duct comes under which type of Strasberg classification?

a. TYPE A
b. TYPE B
c. TYPE C
d. TYPE D

Ans. c. TYPE C

(Ref: Bailey and Love 27th edition page 1204)

Strasberg Classification:

A. Bile leak from cystic duct stump or a minor biliary radical in gallbladder fossa.

B. Occluded right posterior sectoral duct.

C. Bile leak from divided right posterior sectoral duct.

D. Bile leak from main bile duct without major tissue loss.

- E1: Transected main bile duct with a stricture more than 2 cm from the hilus.
- E2: Transected main bile duct with a stricture less than 2 cm from the hilus.
- E3: Stricture of the hilus with right and left ducts in communication.
- E4: Stricture of the hilus with separation of right and left hepatic ducts.
- E5: Stricture of the main bile duct and the right posterior sectoral duct.
- E6: Complete excision of the extrahepatic ducts involving the confluence

157. A 40-year-old male is a known case of varicose vein. On examination, eczema and lipodermatosclerosis were found. It comes under ___ of CEAP classification system:

a. C1 b. C2
c. C3 d. C4

Ans. d. C4

(Ref: Bailey and Love 27th edition page 974)

- C4b stands for Lipodermatosclerosis and Atrophie blanche

158. Which of the following is correct related to the image given below?

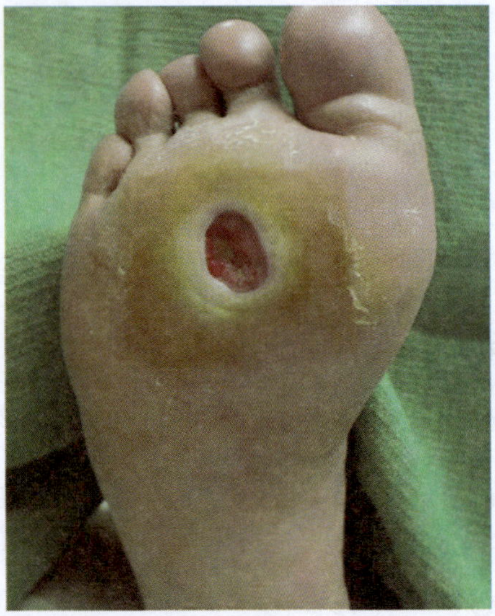

1. Peripheral neuropathy
2. Distal pulses not palpable
3. Restriction in movement of toes
4. Diabetes mellitus

a. 1, 2 and 3 b. 1 and 4
c. 1, 3, 4 d. 1, 2, 3 and 4

Ans. d. 1, 2, 3 and 4

(Ref: Short cases in Surgery by Dr RRM)

- This is a picture of trophic ulcer
- Multiple factors contribute to trophic ulcer like Neuropathy + Vasculopathy
- The major causes are – diabetes, leprosy, peripheral vascular disease, etc.
- The absence of pain perception and excess pressure result in such types of ulcers.
- Secondary infection may occur.

159. A 35-year-old male, which is a chronic smoker, came to OPD with right calf muscle pain and ulcer over the great toe with surrounding Black pigmentation. What is the next investigation you do to this patient?

a. CT angiography
b. Digital subtraction angiography
c. MR angiography
d. Duplex scan of lower limb vessels

Ans. d. Duplex scan of lower limb vessels

(Ref: Bailey and Love 27th edition page 946)

- The history given here is suggestive of Buerger's disease
- The next investigation is to do a Duplex scan to know the distal blood flow in lower limbs.
- IOC for atherosclerotic diseases is Digital Subtraction angiography**

160. In a patient, metastasis was found in liver. On biopsy, it was found to be adenocarcinoma. It was cytokeratin-20 positive and cytokeratin-7 negative. Primary is most likely from:

a. Breast cancer b. Colon cancer
c. Pancreatic cancer d. Lung cancer

Ans. b. Colon cancer

(Ref: Pathology Sources)

- The two most common cytokeratin stains used for Cancer of unknown Primary are CK7 and CK20, though they are not specific.
- **CK7-negative/CK20-positive** phenotype is often associated with carcinomas of colorectal origin.
- **CK7-positive/CK20-negative** phenotype is seen in a wide variety of carcinomas, including carcinomas of the lung, breast, thyroid, pancreas, and female genital tract.

FMGE JANUARY 2023

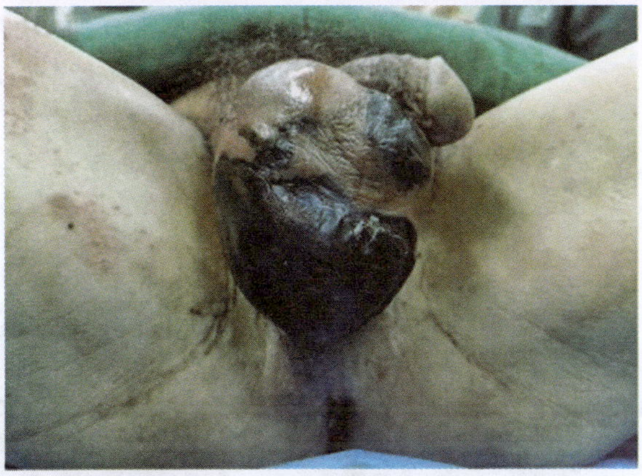

161. Which of the following is true about the given image seen in a diabetic patient suffering from fever?

a. Caused by *Staphylococcus aureus* only
b. Testes remain unaffected
c. Symptomatic management
d. Scrotal support is the treatment

Ans. b. Testes remain unaffected

(Ref. Bailey and Love 28th Edition page 58)

Necrotizing fasciitis will not affect the testes usually.

162. Identify the Stapler shown in the image.

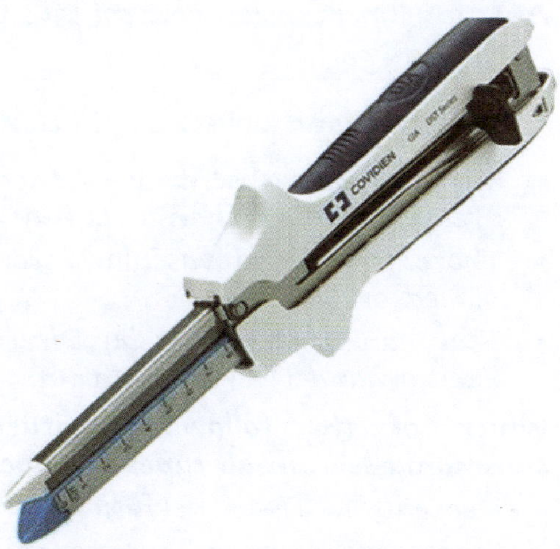

a. Linear stapler
b. Circular stapler
c. Skin stapler
d. Curved stapler

Ans. a. Linear stapler

(Ref. Surgery Sixer 6th Edition page 17)

Linear stapler is used for Side to Side anastomosis in bowel.

163. A 25-year-old male met with a bike accident and was brought to emergency department. On examination, his vitals are SBP <90 mm Hg, PR >140/min. Urine output starts decreasing from which stage onward?

a. Compensatory
b. Mild
c. Moderate
d. Severe

Ans. c. Moderate

(Ref. Bailey 28th Edition page 15)

Clinical features of shock

	Compensated		Uncompensated
	Mild	Moderate	Severe
Lactic acidosis	+	++	+++
Urine output	Normal	Reduced	**Anuric**
Conscious level	**Mild anxiety**	Drowsy	Comatose
Respiratory rate	Increased	**Increased**	Labored
Pulse rate	Increased	Increased	**Increased**
Blood pressure	Normal	Mild hypotension	Severe hypotension

164. In a Trauma patient, there is a sudden increase in respiratory rate of 26/min and his Systolic BP is 90 mm Hg. His GCS is 10. qSOFA score for this patient includes all; except:

a. Respiratory rate
b. Systolic BP
c. Confused status
d. LDH

Ans. d. LDH

(Ref. Surgery Sixer 6th Edition page 9)

qSOFA score includes Respiratory rate, Confused status and Low BP.

165. A 36-year-old female patient has recently undergone laparotomy. What will be the sure sign of wound dehiscence?

a. Copious serosanguineous discharge
b. Bleeding
c. Hypotension
d. Abdominal pain

Ans. a. Copious serosanguineous discharge

(Ref. Surgery Sixer 6th Edition page 31)

Salmon Sign - Sudden gush of fluid in burst abdomen

166. An army person after blast injury in a war was wounded with crepitations. He came to hospital on 2nd day. The patient had brick-shaped bacteria with spores. What is the organism associated?

a. Clostridium perfringens
b. Clostridium septicum
c. Clostridium novyi
d. Clostridium difficile

Ans. a. Clostridium perfringens

(Ref. Bailey and Love 28th Edition page 57)

- Gram-positive spore forming Bacilli
- Naturally found organism in soil and feces
- Immunocompromised patients will have greater risk
- Crepitus due to gas gangrene+
- Releases Collagenase and Hyaluronidase and alpha toxins
- Wound produces "Brown Sweet Smelling Exudate"

167. A 55-year-old male was brought to emergency with H/o Trauma. NCCT done is shown below, identify.

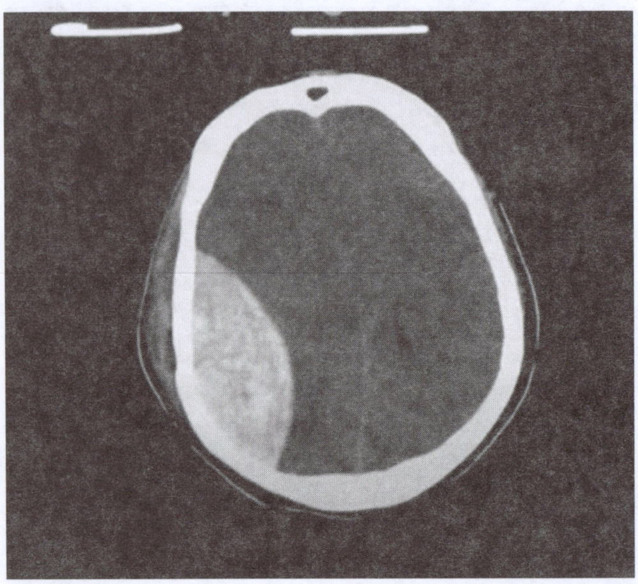

a. EDH
b. SAH
c. ICH
d. SDH

Ans. a. EDH

(Ref. Surgery Sixer 6th Edition page 61)

- EDH—Biconvex-shaped hematoma
- SDH—Concavoconvex hematoma

168. A patient has severe abdominal pain with nausea and shortness of breath. CT scan of the patient is given below. What is the next step in management of this patient?

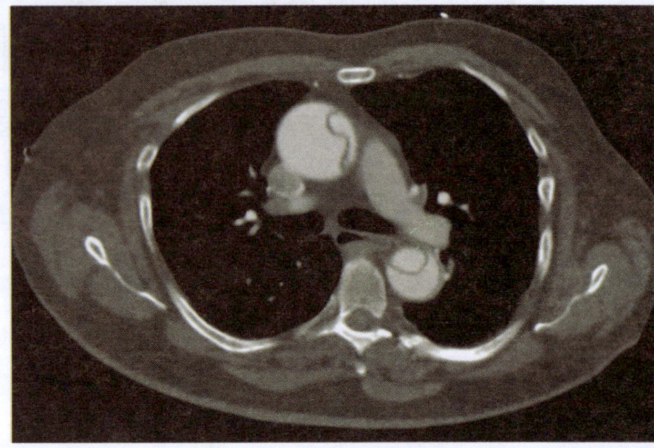

a. Hypertension control plus urgent surgery
b. Wait and watch
c. Give Antihypertensive Nicardipine and send home
d. Urgent Surgery

Ans. a. Hypertension control plus urgent surgery

(Ref. Bailey and Love 28th Edition page 376)

- Initial management is—Control Systolic pressure (to less than 120 mm Hg).
- Thereafter, Endovascular stent can be placed or
- Tear can be repaired by Direct repair or Excision and Dacron Grafting

169. Which of the following feature is most commonly seen in all types of Shock?

a. Decrease in Tissue perfusion
b. Increased Peripheral resistance
c. Decrease in RR
d. Hyperthermia

Ans. a. Decrease in Tissue perfusion

(Ref. Bailey 28th Edition page 11)

Shock is defined as a systemic state of Low Tissue perfusion that is inadequate for normal respiration.

Cardiovascular and metabolic characteristics of shock

	Hypovolemic	Cardiogenic	Obstructive	Distribute
Cardiac output	Low	Low	Low	High
Systemic vascular resistance	High	High	High	Low
Venous pressure	Low	High	High	Low
Mixed venous saturation	Low	Low	Low	High
Base deficit	High	High	High	High

170. Image of a baby with hemangioma on eye and face shows:

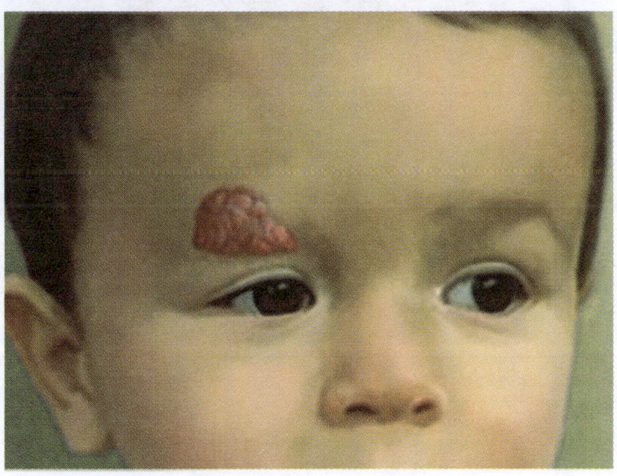

a. Macular stain
b. Capillary hemangioma
c. Cavernous hemangioma
d. Herpes simplex

Ans. b. Capillary hemangioma

(Ref. Bailey and Love 27th Edition page 660)

Capillary hemangioma (Strawberry nevus)

- Most common birthmark on head and neck
- 90% are seen at birth and 10% resolve in 1 year and 70% resolved by 7 years
- White skin affected commonly
- MC in girls
- It is a consequence of vascular thrombosis, fibrosis and mast cell infiltration.

171. Four patients came to hospital following a mass trauma. Which is the correct match?

a. EDH—Pinpoint pupil
b. Penetrating injury to Eustachian Tube—CSF otorrhea
c. Penetrating injury to eye—Battle sign
d. Gaze paresis—Midbrain

Ans. d. Gaze paresis—Midbrain

(Ref. Bailey and Love 28th Edition page 364)

- EDH—Fixed Dilated Pupil
- Penetrating injury to ET—Bleeding from ear (Not CSF otorrhea)
- Battle sign is a feature of Middle cranial fossa fracture
- **Midbrain or Brainstem dysfunction leads to:**
  - Gaze Paresis (Inability of eyes to look across midline)
  - Dysconjugate Gaze—Inability of eyes to work together
  - Roving Eye movements

172. Which of the following involvement is seen in the condition given below in image?

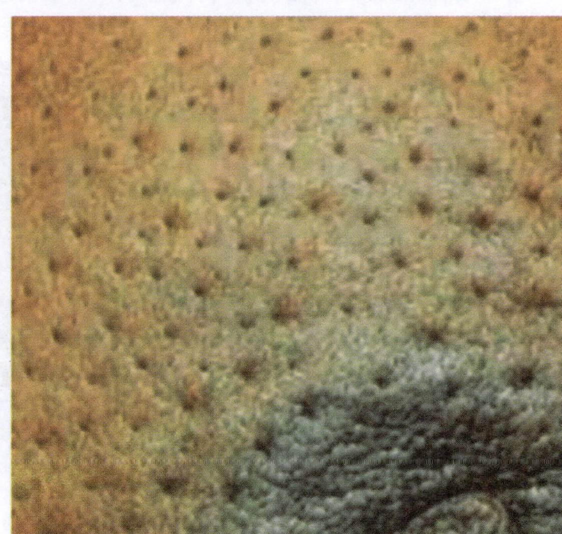

a. Superficial Lymphatics
b. Deep Lymphatics
c. Artery
d. Vein

Ans. a. Superficial Lymphatics

(Ref. Surgery Sixer 6th Edition page 157)

Subdermal lymphatics infiltration is Peau d'orange* (T4b)

173. Genetic testing for BRCA 1 and BRCA 2 should be checked in all the following; except:

a. Men with breast cancer
b. Women with breast cancer detected after 50 years of age
c. Bilateral Breast cancer
d. Breast and Ovarian cancer

Ans. b. Women with breast cancer detected after 50 years of age

(Ref. Bailey 28th Edition page 942, Table)

Genetic risk evaluation is advised for:

- Breast cancer <50 years
- Triple negative breast cancer <60 years of age
- Two breast cancer primary
- Male breast cancer
- One or more relatives had breast cancer
- List of other cancers including colon, stomach, ovarian cancers+ is also mentioned

174. A 50-year-old woman presented to hospital with complaint of mass in right breast. On examination, the mass was movable and further investigations showed—Left Axillary node involved, mass is >2 cm. No systemic involvement. She had been given neoadjuvant chemotherapy before. What will be the tumor staging?

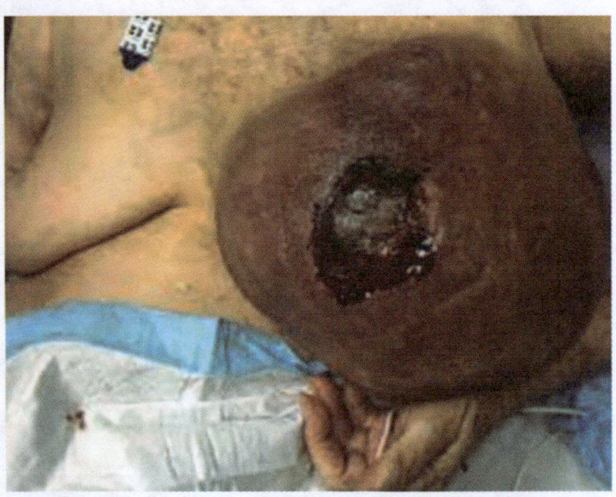

a. cT3N1MO
b. cT4N1MO
c. yT3N1MO
d. yT4N1MO

Ans. d. yT4N1MO

y stands for post Neoadjuvant therapy with Skin involvement is T4*

175. A patient presented to surgery OPD with complaint of a reducible mass felt near the left side of inguinal region with cough impulse seen with an expansile impulse. After further investigations, it was diagnosed as Inguinal hernia. What will be the management of this patient?

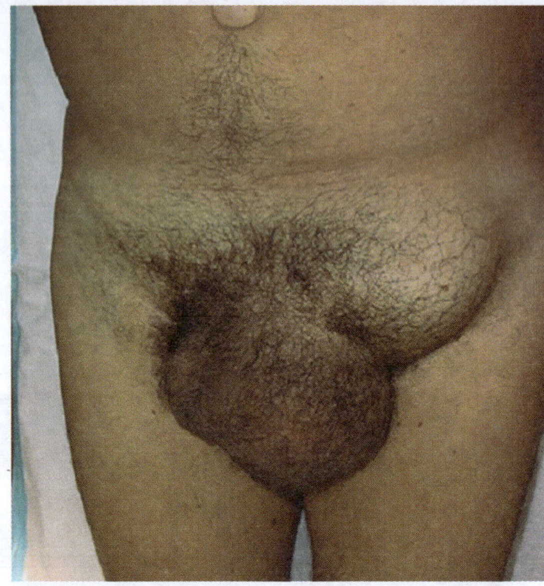

a. Hernioplasty
b. Herniotomy
c. Wait and watch
d. None of these

Ans. a. Hernioplasty

(Ref. Surgery Sixer 6th Edition page 179 Table)

- Indirect hernia—Herniorrhaphy or Hernio-plasty done
- Direct hernia—only Hernioplasty advised
- Spherical shape image implies it is Direct hernia**

176. Which of the following shape of pelvis will have recurrent hernia?

a. Tall and wide
b. Short and wide
c. Short and narrow
d. Tall and wide

Ans. b. Short and wide

177. A 65-year-old male patient presents with complaint of 7 months of white lesion between gingiva and buccal mucosa. He had H/o of Tobacco chewing more than 30 years. What is the management of this lesion?

a. Local excision and Biopsy
b. Stop tobacco chewing and do not bother of patchy lesion
c. Electrocoagulation with chemicals
d. Steroid and Vitamin supplements

Ans. a. Local excision and Biopsy

(Ref. Bailey and Love 28th Edition page 815)

- The risk of malignancy in oral leukoplakia is 0.13–34%
- Biopsy of lesions is advocated for accurate pathological diagnosis as well as to ascertain the degree of dysplasia or presence of malignancy in lesion.

178. A 60-year-old female patient diagnosed with papillary cancer is visiting you for an opinion after undergoing Total Thyroidectomy. What will you do regarding this patient?

a. Reassure and follow-up
b. Radio iodine study
c. Chemotherapy
d. Radiotherapy

Ans. b. Radio iodine study

(Ref. Bailey 28th Edition page 870)

For papillary cancers after Total thyroidectomy, RAIU study is done to look for metastasis.

179. A baby presenting with a condition shown below is due to nonfusion of:

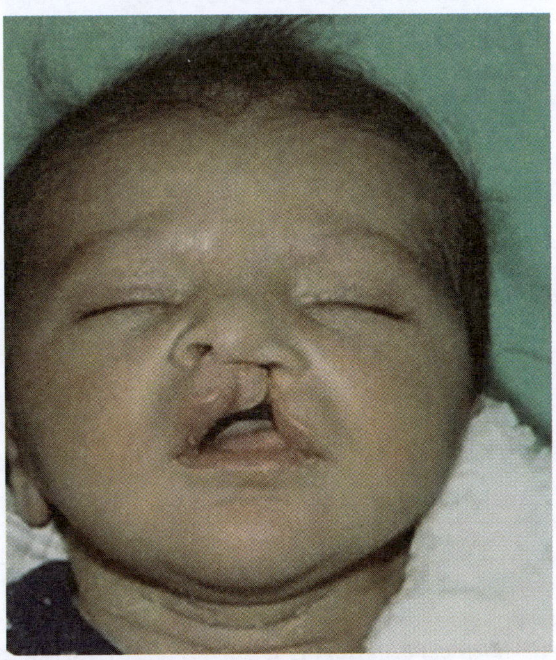

a. Medial nasal process and maxillary process
b. Lateral and medial nasal process
c. Maxillary and mandible process
d. Lateral nasal process and maxillary process

Ans. a. Medial nasal process and maxillary process

(Ref. Bailey and Love 28th Edition page 742)

- Cleft lip/nose is due to failure of fusion of medial nasal process+ Maxillary process
- Cleft palate is due to failure of descend of fusion of palatal shelves

180. Most important risk factor for acute mastitis:

a. Breast engorgement
b. Cracked nipple
c. Failure of lactation
d. Massage

Ans. b. Cracked nipple

(Ref. Bailey and Love 28th Edition page 927)

- Mastitis is due to bacteria entering the nipple via a cracked nipple or retracted nipple.
- No more Incision and Drainage advised for Abscess—Always USG guided Aspiration is done.
- If size >3 cm or 30 mL on USG, a vacuum suction catheter is inserted to drain pus.

181. Which of the following is the cause of constriction at 25 cm from incisor teeth?

a. Aortobronchial/Upper left bronchus
b. Arch of aorta
c. Right main bronchus
d. Upper right bronchus

Ans. a. Aortobronchial/Upper left bronchus

(Ref. Bailey and Love 28th Edition page 1107)

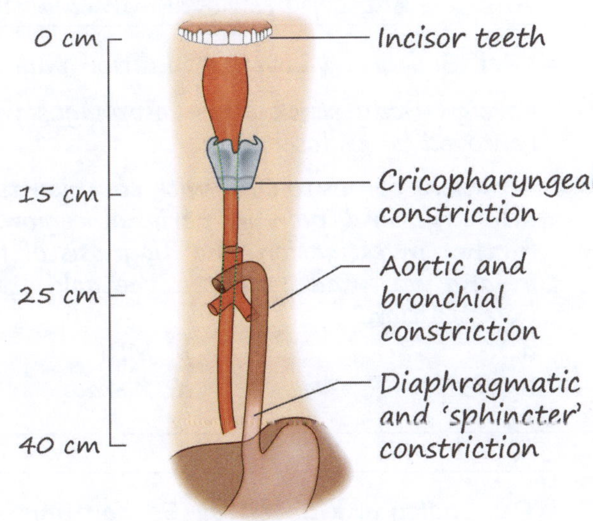

182. A 4-year-old child is brought to casualty with complaint of accidental ingestion of Coin while playing. Chest X-rays of child is given below. Which of the following is the management in this patient?

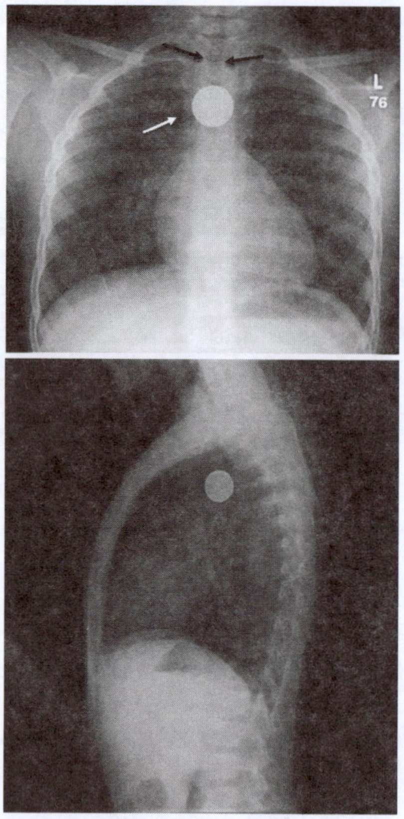

a. Endoscopy removal immediately
b. Bronchoscopy removal immediately
c. Heimlich maneuver
d. Tracheostomy

Ans. a. Endoscopy removal immediately

(Ref. Bailey and Love 28th Edition page 1132)

Foreign Body stuck up in esophagus must be removed by endoscopy

183. A patient comes to OPD with complaints of Pus discharge and pain in perianal region. After further investigation, the diagnosis of fistula-in-ano was made. What is the gold standard investigation?

a. CT
b. MRI
c. USG
d. X-ray

Ans. b. MRI

(Ref. Bailey and Love 28th Edition page 1436)

- MRI is Gold standard
- Short Tau Inversion Recovery (STIR) sequencing—A fat suppression technique is used.

184. Which of the following is Child-Pugh Score?

a. Albumin, Globulin and Creatinine
b. Albumin, Bilirubin, Thrombin
c. Bilirubin, Albumin, Ascites, Prothrombin time, Encephalopathy
d. APTT, Albumin, Ascites, Encephalopathy

Ans. c. Bilirubin, Albumin, Ascites, Prothrombin time, Encephalopathy

(Ref. Bailey and Love 28th Edition page 1196)

Mnemonic—BAAPE—Bilirubin, Albumin, Ascites, Prothrombin time and Encephalopathy

185. Which of the following procedure is having least chances of recurrence of Duodenal Ulcer?

a. TV + antrectomy
b. Truncal vagotomy
c. Gastrojejunostomy
d. High selective vagotomy

Ans. a. TV + antrectomy

(Ref. Bailey 28th Edition page 1161)

- Recurrence rates following various surgeries for duodenal ulcer
  - **TV + antrectomy:** 1%
  - **TV + GJ:** 2–7%
  - **HSV:** 2–10%

186. A homosexual man with painful defecation, not reduced and has foul smelling cauliflower like growth. On biopsy, diagnosis of squamous cell carcinoma was made. Which of the following is ideal treatment?

a. Wide local excision
b. Nigro regimen
c. Chemotherapy
d. APR with Colostomy

Ans. b. Nigro regimen

(Ref. Bailey and Love 28th Edition page 1444)

Nigro regimen is ChemoRT for Anal canal SCC*

187. A baby was brought to emergency on 2nd day of birth with excessive frothing and respiratory distress. X-ray shows Coiling of Ryles tube. What is the diagnosis?

a. Tracheoesophageal fistula
b. Cystic fibrosis
c. Hyaline membrane
d. Transient tachpnea of newborn

Ans. a. Tracheoesophageal fistula

(Ref. Bailey and Love 28th Edition Page 265)

Coiling of Ryle's tube is seen in Congenital TEF*

188. A 40-year-old diabetic female patient presents with DVT along with Necrolytic migratory erythema and Hyperglycemia. What is your diagnosis?

a. Somatostatinoma
b. Glucagonoma
c. Gastrinoma
d. Insulinoma

Ans. b. Glucagonoma

(Ref. Surgery Sixer 6th Edition page 365)

- Insulinoma—Whipple Triad
- Gastrinoma—Zollinger Ellison Syndrome
- Glucagonoma—Necrolytic erythema

189. Increased tone of LES in Achalasia cardia is due to:

a. Decreased Substance P in LES
b. Decreased ACh receptors in LES
c. Decreased NO in LES
d. Absent Myenteric plexus in esophagus

Ans. d. Absent Myenteric plexus in esophagus

(Ref. Bailey 28th Edition page 1121)

- Bailey writes, Etiology is uncertain but it is postulated that loss of inhibitory ganglion cells in myenteric plexus is possibly related to viral-induced autoimmune effect.
- Histology shows reduction in ganglion cells.
- The mismatch in excitatory and inhibitory neurons results in failure of LOS to open.

190. A baby presented with Projectile vomiting, Congenital Hypertrophic Pyloric Stenosis. False statement is:

a. Presents with Non-bilious vomiting
b. USG is 100% sensitive
c. Caused by Hypertrophy of Longitudinal muscles
d. Hypokalemic Hypochloremic alkalosis seen

Ans. c. Caused by Hypertrophy of Longitudinal muscles

(Ref. Bailey and Love 28th Edition page 260)

Hypertrophy of circular muscles seen in CHPS*

191. An alcoholic patient presents with epigastric pain radiating to back. Serum amylase is increased. What is the diagnosis?

a. Acute pancreatitis
b. Chronic hepatitis
c. Appendicitis
d. Fatty liver

Ans. a. Acute pancreatitis

(Ref. Bailey and Love 28th Edition page 1271)

Mohammed Prayer Sign—Acute pancreatitis

192. Identify the structure in following Barium image.

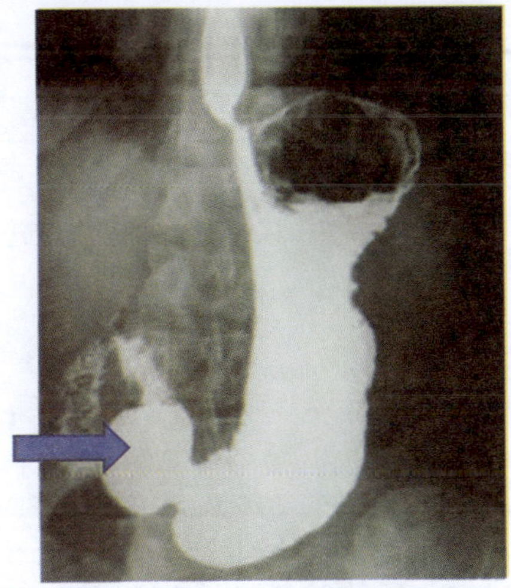

a. Duodenum
b. Jejunum
c. Colon
d. Ileum

Ans. a. Duodenum

(Ref. Surgery Sixer Page 244)

Duodenal cap is shown in the arrow

193. Most common indication for splenectomy in Hemolytic anemias:

a. ITP
b. G6PD
c. Hereditary spherocytosis
d. Hairy cell leukemia

Ans. c. Hereditary spherocytosis

(Ref. Bailey and Love 28th Edition page 1229)

- MC indication for Splenectomy—Trauma
- MC indication for Elective Splenectomy—Idiopathic Thrombocytopenic Purpura*

194. A 20-year-old male patient is a known case of Left Testicular carcinoma and presented to hospital for follow-up. Which of the following lymph node is first to be involved?

a. Iliac lymph node
b. Precaval node
c. Para-aortic node
d. Inguinal node

Ans. c. Para-aortic node

(Ref. Short cases in Surgery, RRM)

- Right side Testicular cancer drains to Inter aortocaval nodes
- Left side Testicular cancer drains to Para-aortic nodes.

195. Which of the following does not lead to bilateral hydronephrosis?

a. Phimosis
b. Urethral Stricture
c. Posterior urethral valve
d. Retrocaval ureter

Ans. d. Retrocaval ureter

(Ref. Bailey 28th Edition page 1467)

- Retrocaval ureter is due to anomalous development of IVC with persistent posterior subcardinal vein.
- Right ureter passes behind the IVC rather than lying on its right side.
- Only right side is involved and hence, right side obstruction only seen.

196. What is the ideal management of the case shown in the figure?

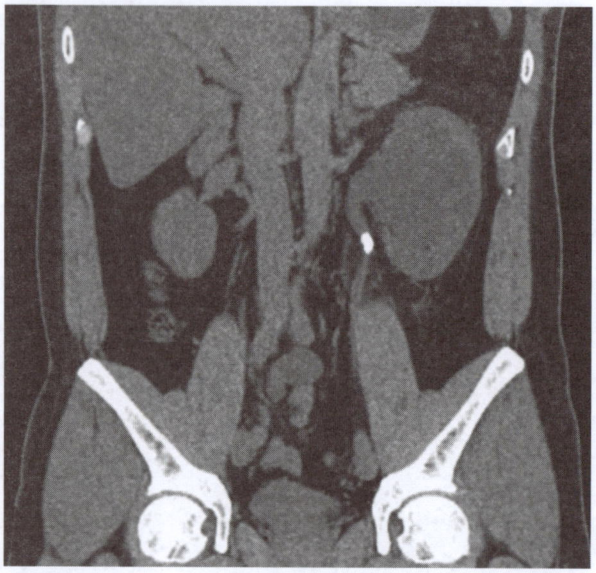

a. ESWL
b. Ureteroscopy
c. PCNL
d. Reassurance

Ans. b. Ureteroscopy

(Ref. Bailey 28th Edition page 1475)

This is a Left Ureteric calculus removed by Dormia Basket using ureteroscopy.

197. Identify the disease from the image shown.

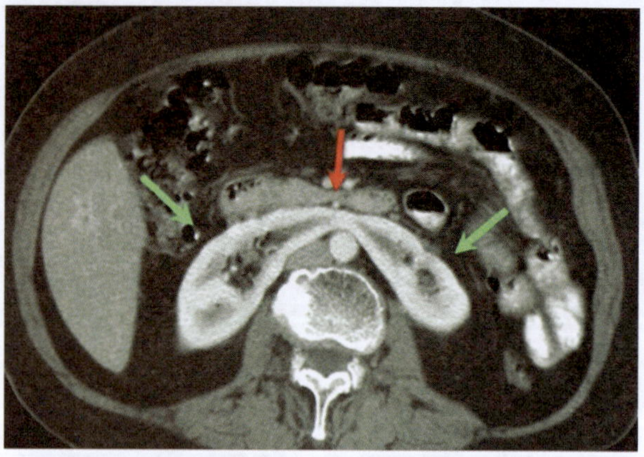

a. Horse-shoe kidney
b. Hydronephrosis
c. Pancake kidney
d. PCKD

Ans. a. Horse-shoe kidney

(Ref. Bailey and Love 28th Edition page 1467))

- In Horse-shoe kidney, lower pole is fused.
- If both upper and lower poles fuse, it is called pancake or doughnut kidney.

198. A 60-year-old patient presents with bladder cancer involving muscle layer. What is the management of this case?

a. Intravesical BCG
b. Cystoprostatectomy
c. Intravesical mitomycin
d. TUR

Ans. b. Cystoprostatectomy

(Ref. Bailey and Love 28th Edition page 1518)

For Bladder cancers involving the muscles, Radical Prostatectomy with removal of bladder, prostate and bilateral pelvic lymphadenectomy is done.

199. In BPH causing Urinary symptoms, first to do is:

a. Alpha blocker
b. TURP
c. Decrease water intake
d. Finasteride

Ans. a. Alpha blocker

(Ref. Bailey and Love 28th Edition page 1528)

- In BPH, the initial drug used is Alpha 1a blocker like Tamsulosin for immediate action.
- 5 alpha reductase (Finasteride) inhibitor takes 6 months to act.

200. All of the following are correct about Nephroblastoma; except:

a. Hematogenous spread is common
b. Early lung mets are seen
c. Chemotherapy is followed by surgery done always
d. Lymphatic spread is seen

Ans. c. Chemotherapy is followed by surgery done always

(Ref. Bailey 28th Edition page 1484)

- Wilms tumor (Nephroblastoma) is associated with hematogenous and lymphatic mets.
- Two modes of therapy are available; Chemo followed by Surgery and another is surgery followed by Adjuvant Chemotherapy

201. A 40-year-old female patient presented with pain in left flank and hypochondrium. On examination, a mass 4 cm was felt, which was ballotable on inspiration. On urine examination, malignant cells are seen. What will be the next line of management?

a. Do DTPA scan
b. Removal of cyst and envelope
c. Radical nephrectomy
d. Intravesical BCG followed by Chemotherapy

Ans. c. Radical nephrectomy

(Ref. Bailey 28th Edition page 1483)

- Tumors <4 cm can be treated by Nephron sparing surgery
- Tumors >4 cm usually Radical Nephrectomy done

202. Which of the following is the Gold standard treatment for Varicose veins?

a. Phlebotomy
b. SEPS
c. Stripping and Ligation
d. Endovenous Thermal ablation

Ans. d. Endovenous Thermal ablation

(Ref. Bailey 28th Edition page 1033)

Endothermal ablation techniques have completely replaced the conventional treatment of Ligation and Stripping as the GOLD STANDARD now.

203. Which of the following is the least commonly used Graft in CABG procedure?

a. LIMA
b. Long Saphenous vein
c. Radial artery
d. Intercostal artery

Ans. d. Intercostal artery

(Ref. Bailey 28th Edition page 951)

The graft materials used in Bypass are Internal mammary artery, Left (LIMA), RIMA, Radial Artery and Saphenous vein.

204. Which of the following is not a superior mediastinal tumor?

a. Thyroid
b. Thymus
c. Parathyroid
d. Lymphoma

Ans. b. Thymus

(Ref. Bailey 28th Edition page 992)

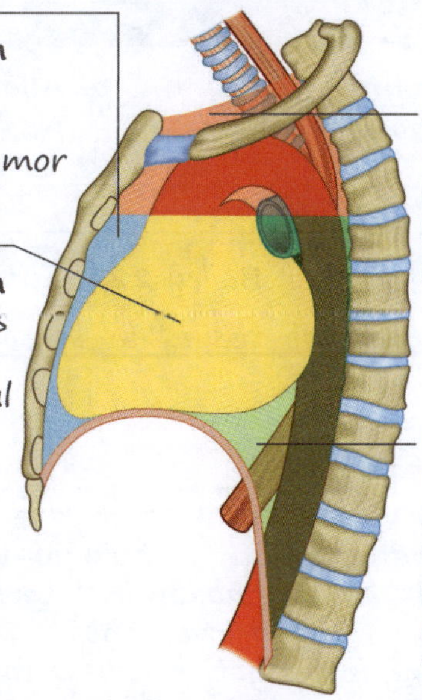

205. An 80-year-old man, smoker for more than 15 years has pain while walking. Comment your diagnosis based on given image.

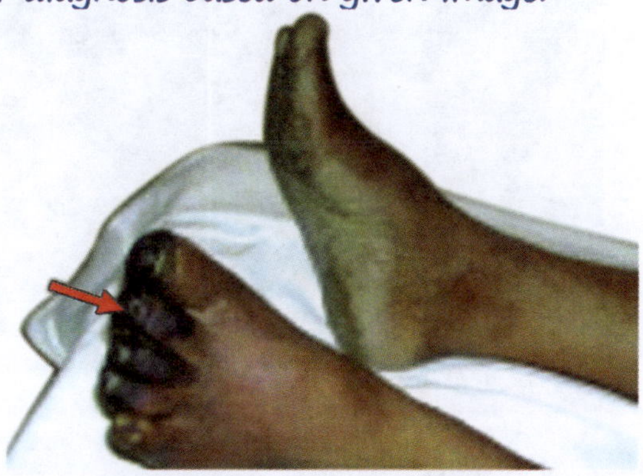

a. Buerger disease
b. Atherosclerosis
c. Giant cell arteritis
d. Raynaud disease

Ans. b. Atherosclerosis

(Ref. Bailey and Love 28th Edition page 997–999)

- Buerger's disease—Bilateral and seen in young age
- Atherosclerosis is seen in old age

206. A patient is done with the following procedure with his own skin graft. What is the type of skin graft?

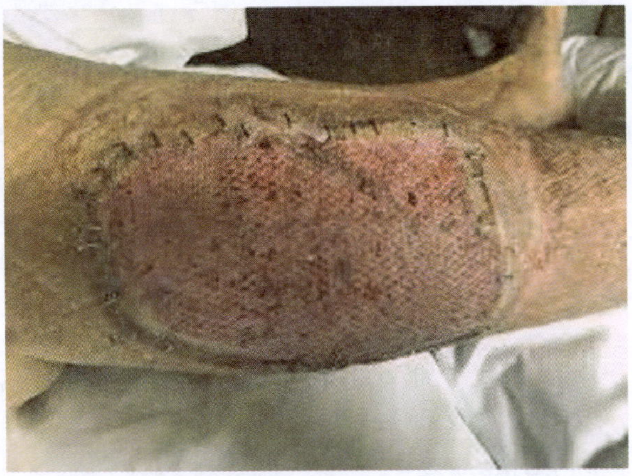

a. Autograft b. Allograft
c. Xenograft d. Homograft

Ans. a. Autograft

(Ref. Bailey 28th Edition page 687)

- Transfer of tissues in same individual is AUTOGRAFT
- Transfer of tissues in same species is ALLOGRAFT
- Xenograft—Different species

207. In a patient with history of kidney stones, painful bones, abdominal groans, psychic moans, fatigue overtones, which of the following investigation is used for diagnosis?

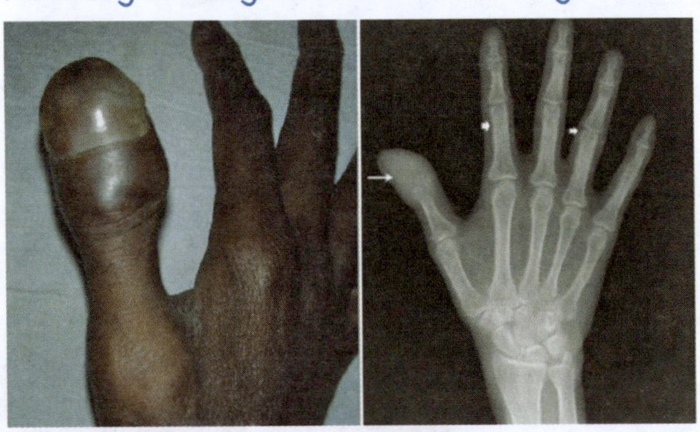

a. Tc 99m Sestamibi scan
b. USG Neck
c. CT scan
d. MRI

Ans. a. Tc 99m Sestamibi scan

(Ref. Bailey 28th Edition page 877)

Image shows Brown tumor and history is suggestive of hyperparathyroidism—Tc 99m Sestamibi scan is the IOC.

208. A patient is having severe thunderclap headache, which he has never felt in lifetime. There is no history of fever. Patient is on Antihypertensive medicines. Nuchal rigidity+. What is the diagnosis?

a. Encephalitis b. SAH
c. Meningitis d. Chronic Migraine

Ans. b. SAH

(Ref. Surgery Sixer 6th Edition page 61)

Thunderclap headache is suggestive of rupture of berry aneurysm causing Subarachnoid hemorrhage

209. A 35-year-old patient was having diaphoresis+ High BP and Palpitations. What is the diagnosis?

a. Pheochromocytoma
b. Adrenal cortical cancer
c. Episodic long term headache
d. Chronic migraine

Ans. a. Pheochromocytoma

(Ref. Bailey 28th Edition page 900)

Pheochromocytoma Triad—headache + palpitation + Sweating seen in 90%

FMGE JUNE 2022

210. What advice will you give to the female patient before laparoscopic surgery?

a. Eat full before surgery
b. Drink plenty of water before surgery
c. Enema in the night before surgery
d. NPO for specific hours before surgery

Ans. d. NPO for specific hours before surgery

(Ref. Bailey and Love 27th Edition page 259)

- Patients are advised not to take any solids within 6 hours and clear fluids (isotonic drinks and water) within 2 hours before General anesthesia to avoid risk of acid aspiration syndrome.
- Remember 6 Solid and 2 Water.

211. Patient's relative wants to donate the blood. Before transfusion, the blood is tested for all of the following; except:

a. Hepatitis A
b. Hepatitis B
c. Hepatitis C
d. HIV-1 and HIV-2

Ans. a. Hepatitis A

(Ref. Bailey and Love 27th Edition page 20)

- In UK, a person can donate blood 3 times/ year and each time 450 mL
- Each unit is tested for Hepatitis B virus, Hepatitis C virus, HIV 1 and HIV 2 and Syphilis.
- To prevent Creutzfeldt-Jacob disease, donated blood is leukodepleted.

212. Which of the following is the best method for hair removal to avoid surgical site infection?

a. Shaving with razor, the night before operation
b. Depilatory cream before operation
c. Hair clippers on table
d. None of the above

Ans. c. Hair clippers on table

(Ref. Bailey and Love 27th Edition page 52)

- Preoperative shaving is undertaken in Operating theater immediately before surgery as the SSI rate after clean wound surgery may be doubled if shaving is performed the night before as minor skin injury by the barbers will cause superficial bacterial colonization.
- Cream Depilation is messy and hence, hair clippers have the lowest SSI.

213. A 2-year-old pediatric patient presented in an unconscious state. He was having profound diarrhea and mild pneumonia. In the management of this baby, ABCDE is done. What does 'D' stand for?

a. Diarrhea
b. Dehydration
c. Disability
d. Developmental delay

Ans. c. Disability

(Ref. Bailey and Love 27th Edition page 325)

The patient in Primary survey protocol must follow:

- Airway
- Breathing
- Circulation
- Disability
- Exposure

The important thing done in Disability assessment is GCS calculation**

214. A patient undergone a surgical procedure for pathology wherein preoperatively the left lung was collapsed as shown. After the operation, the lung has expanded. What can be the diagnosis?

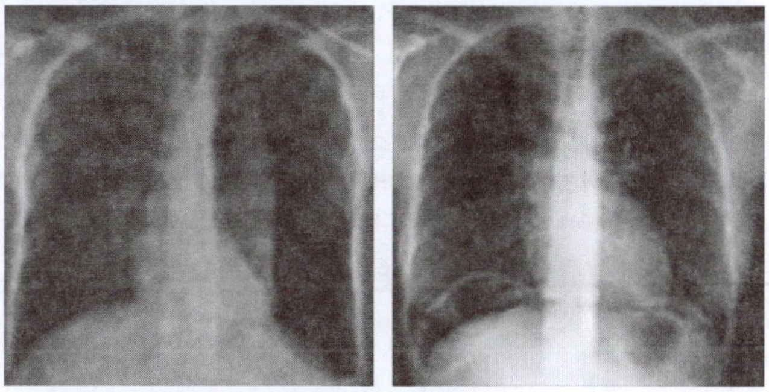

a. Right pneumothorax
b. Left pneumothorax
c. Cardiac tamponade
d. Pneumonia

Ans. b. Left pneumothorax

(Ref. Bailey and Love 27th Edition page 367)

The first picture shows Pneumothorax and the patient might have been taken for Needle thoracostomy or ICD placement and the lung has expanded now.

215. What should be the treatment in a patient who presented in the emergency with respiratory distress? He was having dilated large veins. Large amount of air was seen on the left side along with mediastinal shift as shown.

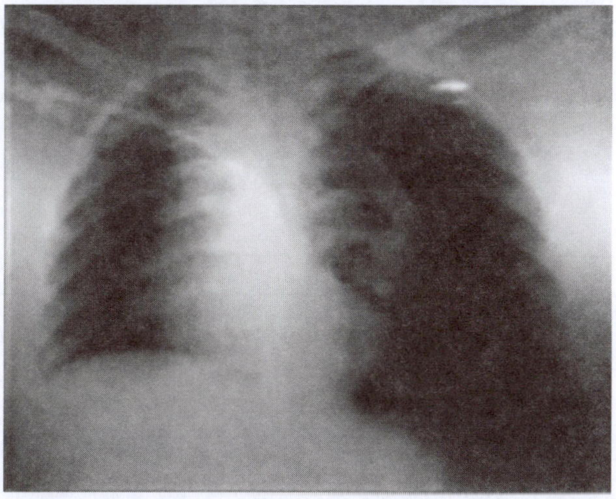

a. Wide bore needle insertion in intercostal space
b. Endotracheal intubation
c. Tracheostomy
d. Pericardiocentesis

Ans. a. Wide bore needle insertion in intercostal space

(Ref. Bailey and Love 27th Edition page 367)

This is a case of Tension Pneumothorax, and as per Bailey, the moment we see such case we have to put a needle in the 2nd ICS at Mid clavicular line and drain the gas.

216. A lady presented with burns from the neck to the lower back. What will be the preferred sequence of treatment in this lady?

a. First debridement, resuscitation, then autograft
b. First debridement then reconstruction and then resuscitation
c. First resuscitation then reconstruction and then debridement
d. First resuscitation, then debridement and then autograft or allograft

Ans. d. First resuscitation, then debridement and then autograft or allograft

(Ref. Bailey and Love 27th Edition page 628)

- In Burns case in protocol of ABCDE, we must do resuscitation, then do debridement and then reconstruction using Autograft by Split skin graft or if the skin loss is extensive Allograft from matched humans can be done.
- The basic concept in this question is we have to resuscitate the patient before doing any reconstruction.

217. What is not a component of splenic trauma based on AAST grading?

a. Parenchymal laceration
b. Vascular involvement
c. Adjacent organ involvement
d. Hematoma

Ans. c. Adjacent organ involvement

(Ref. Sabiston 21st Edition page 415)

As per AAST 2018 Revision Scale:

The following components in CECT abdomen are taken in grading the splenic injury to 5 grades:

1. Subcapsular hematoma
2. Parenchymal laceration
3. Intraparenchymal hematoma
4. Splenic vascular injury
5. Hilar or segmental vessels

218. Patient had trauma, GCS score of the patient was 10. What is the severity of injury?

a. Moderate b. Severe
c. Mild d. None of these

Ans. a. Moderate

(Ref. Bailey and Love 27th Edition page 329)

GCS classification:

- Minor—GCS 15 with no loss of consciousness
- Mild—GCS 14 or 15 with LOC
- Moderate—GCS 9–13
- Severe—GCS 3–8

219. In a 35-year-old pregnant female with hyperthyroidism, which antithyroid drug should be given in the first trimester?

a. Methimazole b. Carbimazole
c. Propylthiouracil d. Lugol's iodine

Ans. c. Propylthiouracil

(Ref. Bailey and Love 27th Edition page 813)

- For preop preparation of Toxicosis patients, the most commonly used antithyroid is—Carbimazole or methimazole.
- The major drawback of these drugs is decreasing WBC count and agranulocytosis.
- Another disadvantage is they cross Placental barrier and can cause congenital hypothyroidism to baby.
- Propylthiouracil is DOC in pregnant females.

220. A 30-year-old lady presented with mobile breast lump like a moving mouse feel. What is the diagnosis?

a. Phyllodes tumor
b. Fibroadenoma
c. Invasive ductal carcinoma
d. Breast abscess

Ans. b. Fibroadenoma

(Ref. Bailey and Love 27th Edition page 870)

- MC in the age of 15–25 years
- They arise from hyperplasia of a single lobule and usually grow up to 2–3 cm in size.
- Since they have a well-defined capsule, enucleation is enough. Excision is done only in cases of suspicious etiology.
- Giant Fibroadenoma >5 cm size
- Fibroadenomas have Indian rubber firm consistency and move like mouse in all quadrants of breast.

221. A female presented with pain and redness of the left breast. She is lactating for the last 3 months. On local examination, local temperature is raised and cracked nipple noted. Ultrasound of breast was suggestive of significant liquid collection. What should be the next line of management?

a. Antibiotics
b. Multiple needle aspirations
c. Incision and drainage
d. Breast support

Ans. b. Multiple needle aspirations

(Ref. Bailey and Love 27th Edition page 866)

- If antibiotic is used in undrained pus, an antibioma will form which is large, sterile, brawny edematous swelling that may take weeks to resolve.
- Old treatment for breast abscess was incision and drainage, but recent concept is to do repeated aspirations under antibiotic cover using USG guidance if necessary.
- Pus in the syringe is sent for Culture and sensitivity.

222. Which of the following is considered having better prognosis in a lady presenting with breast lump in the lower outer quadrant of the breast with axillary node involvement diagnosed as invasive breast cancer?

a. Over expression of Her2neu gene
b. High mitotic index
c. Axillary lymph node involvement
d. Mucinous or colloid breast cancer

Ans. d. Mucinous or colloid breast cancer

(Ref. Bailey and Love 27th Edition page 872)

- Among the pathological types of breast cancer, Colloid or Mucinous type carries the best prognosis and Medullar cancer carries bad prognosis.
- Her2 overexpression and high Mitotic index are bad prognostic factors.
- Most important prognostic factor in Cancer breast is Axillary node involvement.

223. A young girl presented with reflux and retrosternal discomfort. Best investigation for this is?

a. 24-hour ambulatory pH monitoring
b. Upper GI endoscopy
c. CECT
d. MRI

Ans. a. 24-hour ambulatory pH monitoring

(Ref. Bailey and Love 27th Edition page 1077)

- Gold standard investigation for diagnosis of GERD is 24-hour ambulatory pH monitoring.
- DeMeester score >14.7 calculated by this test is said to be confirmed GERD.

224. A patient undergone surgery as shown in the image. After the surgery, after 30 minutes of taking the meal, patient develops light headedness, tachycardia, dizziness, epigastric fullness and sweating. What this could be?

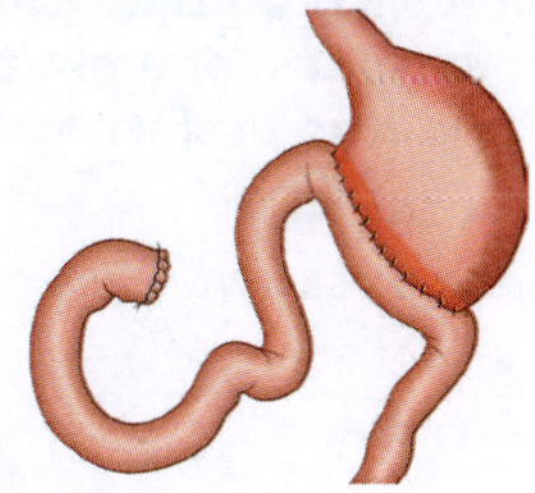

a. Reflux gastritis
b. Dumping syndrome
c. Post vagotomy diarrhea
d. Frey's syndrome

Ans. b. Dumping syndrome

(Ref. Bailey and Love 27th Edition page 1124)

- Any case of Gastrojejunostomy will lead to Dumping syndrome.
- The image shown here is Billroth 2 reconstruction.
- The clinical features mentioned are seen in early dumping.
- Early dumping is due to massive fluid shift happens in half an hour.

225. A 34-year-old female with history of alcohol intake was taking NSAIDs for abdominal pain. She developed severe pain in the whole abdomen. Radiograph is given below. What is the diagnosis?

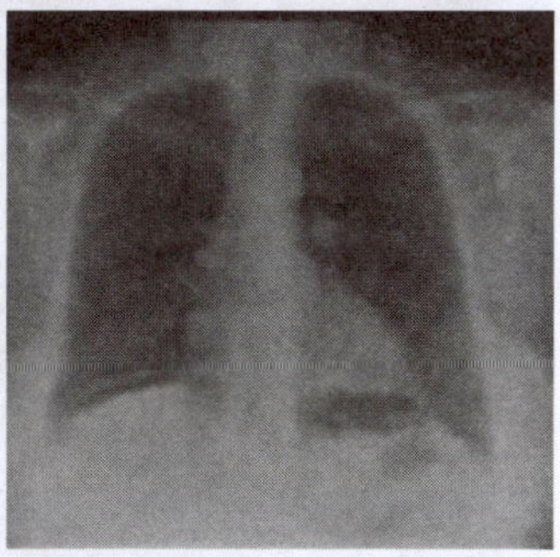

a. Acute pancreatitis
b. Liver abscess
c. Acute cholecystitis
d. Hollow viscus perforation

Ans. d. Hollow viscus perforation

(Ref. Bailey and Love 27th Edition page 1125)

- This is hundred times asked MCQ; showing X-ray of air under diaphragm
- This is most commonly caused by Duodenal ulcer perforation causing peritonitis.
- H/o of NSAID can cause severe erosions and acid secretion resulting in perforation of Duodenal ulcer which is already present for this patient

226. A 35-year-old male with gastric outlet obstruction presented to emergency with multiple episodes of vomiting. Which of the following fluid is preferred for this patient?

a. Normal saline
b. 20% dextrose with water
c. Ringer lactate
d. 5% dextrose

Ans. a. Normal saline

(Ref. Bailey and Love 27th Edition page 1130)

- Patients with GOO will develop Hypokalemic, Hypochloremic, Hyponatremic, Hypocalcemic metabolic alkalosis with paradoxical renal aciduria*
- They are treated by Isotonic Normal saline with Potassium supplementation.

227. This patient after surgically removing of given image from her stomach should be referred to whom?

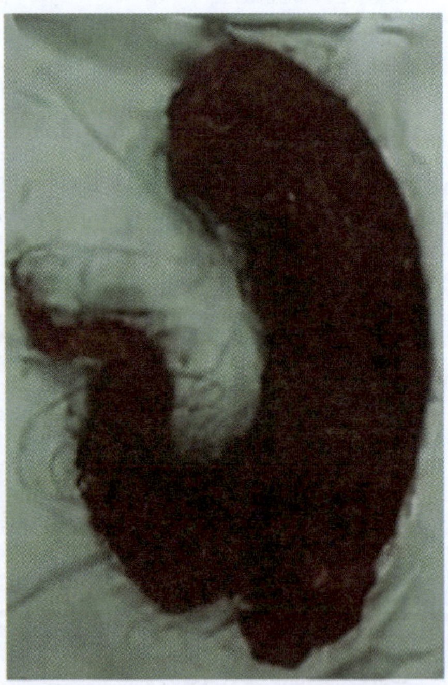

a. Pediatrician b. Psychiatrist
c. Cardiologist d. Dermatologist

Ans. b. Psychiatrist

(Ref. Bailey and Love 27th Edition page 1142)

- This is the image of Gastric Trichobezoar.
- Very common in female young psychiatric patients plucking the hair and eating them.
- After removal of the bezoar by surgical treatment, they must be referred to psychiatrist.

228. Which of the following incisions is preferred for appendicectomy?

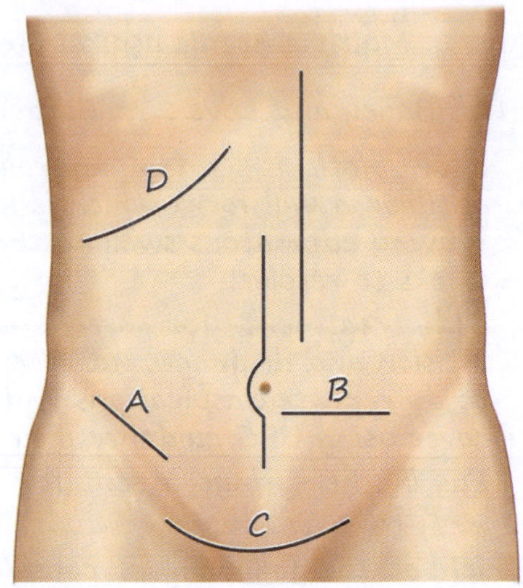

a. A b. B
c. C d. D

Ans. a. A

(Ref. Bailey and Love 27th Edition page 1309)

- The incision A shown is Grid iron incision for appendectomy
- B is transverse incision for pediatric surgery
- C is Pfannenstiel incision for LSCS
- D is Kocher incision for cholecystectomy

229. A patient presented with history of bronchospasm. Tumor was present in the ileum with increased 5-hydroxy indole acetic acid in urine. What is the diagnosis?

a. Carcinoid syndrome b. Neuroblastoma
c. Pheochromocytoma d. Leiomyoma

Ans. a. Carcinoid syndrome

(Ref. Bailey and Love 27th Edition page 1251)

- From increased 5-HIAA in urine sample, we can confirm this can be Carcinoid tumor.
- Features of Bronchospasm, Diarrhea and Flushing are all findings seen in Carcinoid syndrome developing in Metastasis to liver.

230. Identify the pathology in the newborn baby as shown in the image.

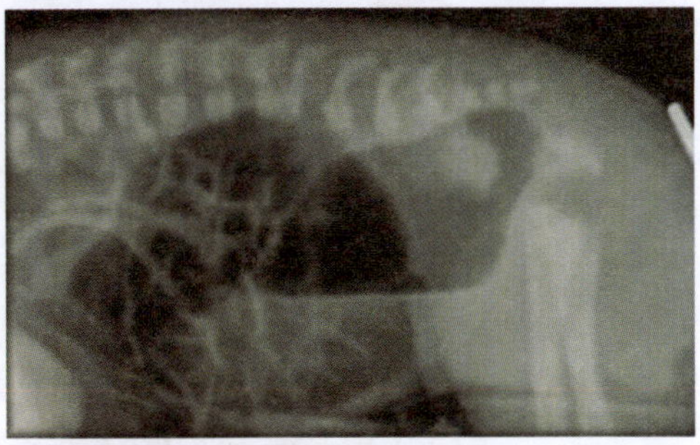

a. Meningocele
b. Congenital megacolon
c. Imperforate anus
d. Pyloric stenosis

Ans. c. Imperforate anus

(Ref. Bailey and Love 27th Edition page 137)

- This is the image of Invertogram in which imperforate anus causes distal opening of the colon.
- No contrast is used, the swallowed gas of the baby reaches the distal colon and the gas acts as a contrast.
- The test is done usually after 24 hours.

231. Chronic alcoholic female patient with chronic liver disease presents with hematemesis. What is the most common cause?

a. Mallory Weiss tear
b. Boerhaave syndrome
c. Bleeding varices
d. Perforated ulcer

Ans. c. Bleeding varices

(Ref. Bailey and Love 27th Edition page 1163)

- Chronic liver disease cases develop varices in the esophagus most commonly due to portal hypertension.
- Bleeding from esophageal varices is the 2nd common cause of death in liver failure patients.

232. Patient has undergone cholecystectomy few days back and now the patient has presented with upper abdominal pain. MRCP was done which showed leaking of bile from the cystic duct stump. Patient is hemodynamically stable. Which of the following should be the next line of management?

a. Roux-en-Y hepaticojejunostomy
b. ERCP and stenting
c. Exploratory laparotomy
d. Conservative treatment with antibiotics

Ans. d. Conservative treatment with antibiotics

(Ref. Bailey and Love 27th Edition page 1203)

- This is the case of Bile duct leak; Strasberg Type A (Cystic duct leak)
- Since patient is hemodynamically stable, we can manage by conservative treatment with antibiotics.
- If patient is hemodynamically unstable with toxic features, we can do next USG and look for Bilioma collection.
- If Bilioma is seen, we will put a Percutaneous Catheter
- If patient is having persistent leak after two weeks, we will go for ERCP and stenting. But please remember in many patients, the leak settles in two weeks.

233. According to Bismuth Corlette classification, which of the following is type III bile duct Cancer?

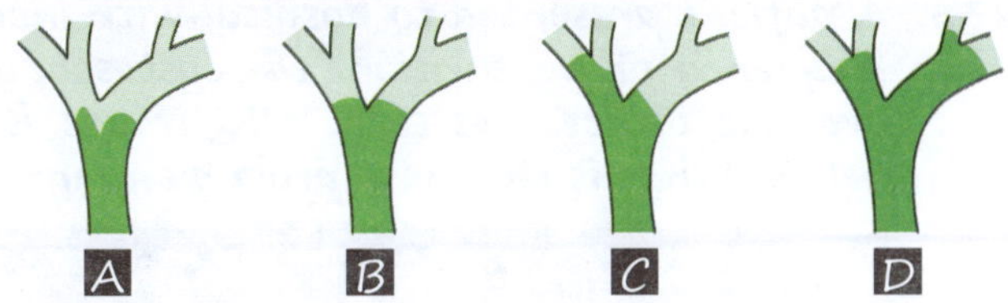

a. A
b. B
c. C
d. D

Ans. c. C

(Ref. Bailey and Love 27th Edition page 1210)

As per Bismuth-Corlette classification, Cholangiocarcinoma is having the following types:

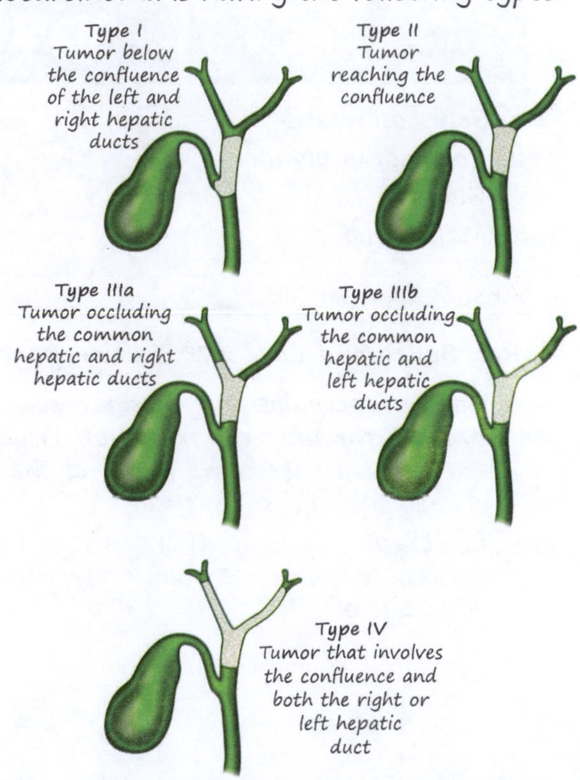

234. Neuroendocrine tumor of pancreas associated with necrolytic erythema migrans is:

a. Insulinoma
b. Glucagonoma
c. Somatostatinoma
d. VIPoma

Ans. b. Glucagonoma

(Ref. Bailey and Love 27th Edition page 849 Table 52.3)

- Glucagonoma—Incidence is 4% of Pancreatic neuroendocrine tumors
- 80% are malignant
- Characterized by Migratory necrolytic erythema, glossitis, stomatitis, angular cheilitis, diabetes and weight loss with diarrhea.

235. A patient presented to hospital with increased frequency of micturition. On cystoscopy, pale ureteric orifice was seen. MRI image is given below. What is the most probable diagnosis?

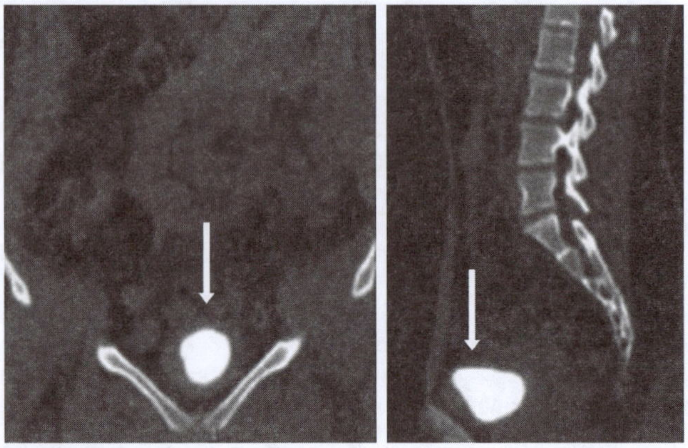

a. Schistosomiasis
b. Carcinoma bladder
c. Bladder TB
d. Malakoplakia

Ans. c. Bladder TB

(Ref. Bailey and Love 27th Edition page 1442)

- Early Tuberculosis of Bladder starts from around the ureteric orifice or Trigone, the earliest evidence being Pallor of the mucosa due to submucosal edema.
- In chronic cases, there may be small contracted Thimble bladder seen as shown in image of MRI.

236. Identify the type of fistula shown in the image.

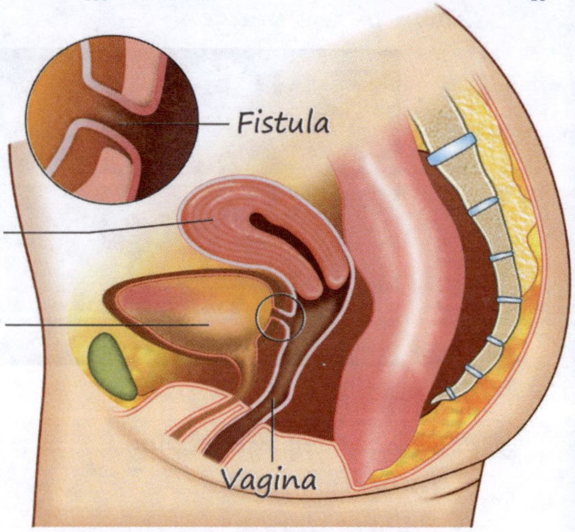

Vesicovaginal fistula

a. Vesicoureteric fistula
b. Vesicovaginal fistula
c. Rectovaginal fistula
d. Uterovaginal fistula

Ans. b. Vesicovaginal fistula

- The most common cause of Vesicovaginal fistula is following a difficult labor that causes pressure necrosis at the junction of Bladder and Vagina.
- It can happen in Violent Rape, some congenital syndromes like VACTERL syndrome

237. A one and half year male child is having problem urinating from last 3 months. Contrast dye is introduced from urethra to visualize which is shown in the image. What could be the investigation?

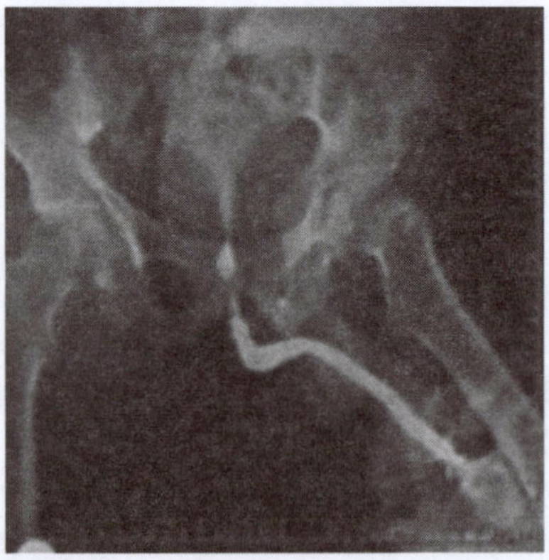

a. Micturating cystourethrogram
b. Retrograde urethrogram
c. Antegrade pyelography
d. Retrograde pyelography

Ans. a. Micturating cystourethrogram

(Ref. Bailey and Love 27th Edition page 1477)

- Posterior urethral valve is the most common cause of urinary obstruction in male child.
- Obstruction is seen distal to the Verumontanum.
- They function as flap valves and so they are obstructive to antegrade urinary flow but a urethral catheter will easily pass retrogradely.
- IOC is MCU as shown in image.
- Treatment is endoscopic destruction of the valves.

238. What is the pathological grading used for prostate cancer?

a. Bloom-Richardson grading
b. Gleason score
c. Fuhrman nuclear grading
d. Leibovich score

Ans. b. Gleason score

(Ref. Bailey and Love 27th Edition page 1469)

- Gleason score: Prostate cancer
- Bloom and Richardson grade: Cancer Breast
- Fuhrman Grade and Leibovich score: Renal cell cancer

239. Which of the following isotope is used in the treatment of prostate cancer?

a. I-131
b. I-125
c. I-123
d. I-121

Ans. b. I-125

(Ref. Bailey and Love 27th Edition page 1473)

- Brachytherapy for Prostate cancer is passed via a transperineal needle
- Radioisotopes commonly used are Iodine-125 and Palladium-103.
- These isotopes deliver an intense, confined radiation dose.

240. What is this investigation?

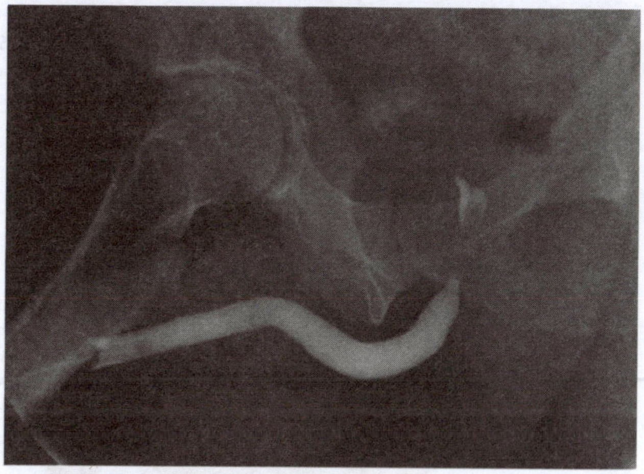

a. Intravenous pyelogram
b. Retrograde urethrogram
c. Micturating cystourethrogram
d. Ureterogram

Ans. b. Retrograde urethrogram

From the picture, you can observe a cannula/Catheter is inserted at penile tip and dye is injected retrograde to look for urethral injuries. This is known as RGU.

241. A 14-year-old boy presented to OPD has left scrotal sac empty. On clinical examination, the left testis was found in the superficial inguinal pouch. What is the most likely diagnosis?

a. Cryptorchidism
b. Left undescended testis
c. Left ectopic testis
d. Retractile testis

Ans. c. Left ectopic testis

(Ref. Bailey and Love 27th Edition page 1499)

- The major difference between Ectopic and Undescended testis is the location.
- In UDT, the location of the testis is along the normal path somewhere in Inguinal canal to lumbar region.
- In Ectopic testis, the location is along some of the ectopic tails like in Superficial inguinal pouch, Femoral canal, Pubic region, Perineal region, etc.

242. A young male presented with slight dragging sensation in the scrotum. On examination, a bag of worm feel was noted in the left side of scrotum. However, testes were normal. What is the diagnosis?

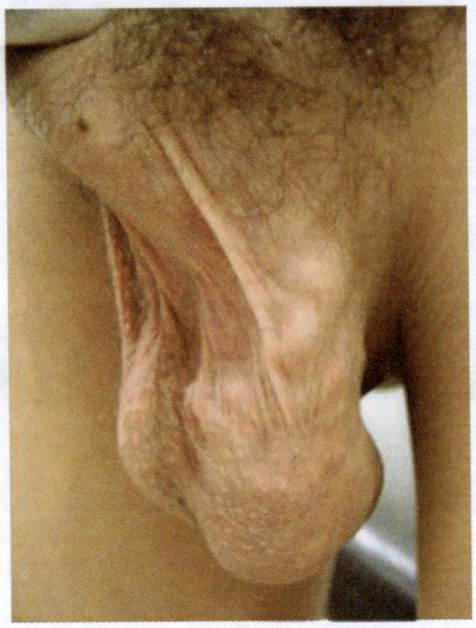

a. Left hydrocele b. Inguinal hernia
c. Epididymo-orchitis d. Left varicocele

Ans. d. Left varicocele

(Ref. Bailey and Love 27th Edition page 1502)

- Bag of worm sensation+ Cough impulse+ Reduced on Lying down are features of Varicocele testis.
- If the varicocele on left side is not getting reduced, you must think of RCC infiltrating the left renal vein.

243. A chronic young smoker starts having pain in the calf on walking distance of 400 meters initially. Gradually, he starts developing pain on walking distance of 200 meters only and then he starts having pain even during sleeping so decides to sleep in sitting position which makes him feel better. What is the likely diagnosis?

a. Venous claudication
b. Neurological claudication
c. Sciatica
d. Rest pain

Ans. d. Rest pain

(Ref. Bailey and Love 27th Edition page 957)

- This case can be a Buerger's disease seen among smokers.
- The history given is Claudication pain (pain on walking due to spasm of vessels in lower limb)
- In extreme cases as per BOYD Classification–Grade 4, Rest pain happens.

244. A female who is washing clothes sees her hands in cold water exhibit color changes from white to red. Which of the following drugs is best suited for this patient?

a. ACEI
b. CCB
c. Thiazides
d. Alpha blockers

Ans. b. CCB

(Ref. Bailey and Love 27th Edition page 967)

- This is a case of Raynaud disease in which on exposure to cold there is vasospasm and episodes of Color change from White fingers to Blue to crimson red on reflow occurs.
- Advise her to avoid cold and CCB like Nifedipine may have a role.

245. A 50-year-old male, chronic smoker, came to OPD with cough, dyspnea and difficulty in swallowing. Palpable lump was present in the neck. What is the most common cancer found in smoker?

a. Adenocarcinoma
b. Squamous cell carcinoma
c. Large cell carcinoma
d. Adenoid cystic carcinoma

Ans. b. Squamous cell carcinoma

(Ref. Bailey and Love 27th Edition page 925)

- Cigarette smoking is the major risk factor of Lung cancer—85–95% of all cases have smoking history.
- SCC is associated with smoking more commonly.
- The palpable lump in neck may be due to metastatic nodes.
- Common symptoms are Cough+ Weight Loss+ Dyspnea+ Chest pain
- Dysphagia can happen when there is mediastinal involvement compressing the esophagus.
- Hoarseness is due to involvement of recurrent laryngeal nerve.

246. Long-lasting results in CABG are obtained by:

a. Long saphenous vein
b. Internal mammary artery
c. Polytetrafluoroethyl
d. Gastroepiploic artery

Ans. b. Internal mammary artery

(Ref. Bailey and Love 27th Edition page 890)

Patency rates of:

- LIMA- 98% and hence, LIMA is the conduit of choice during CABG
- LSV- 50-60% patency at 10 years

247. What does the following X-ray depict?

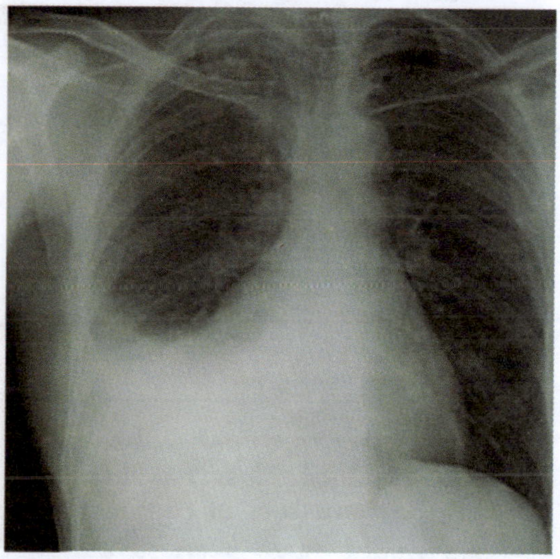

a. Pleural effusion
b. Pericardial effusion
c. Pneumothorax
d. Pneumonia

Ans. a. Pleural effusion

(Ref. Bailey and Love 27th Edition page 921)

X-ray findings are Blunting of Costophrenic angle, Cardiophrenic angle and haziness like shape of meniscus is seen. (Some physicians call this as S-shaped curve of Ellis)

248. Split skin graft is composed of:

a. Only epidermis
b. Epidermis and partial dermis
c. Epidermis and deep dermis
d. Epidermis, dermis, subcutaneous fat

Ans. b. Epidermis and partial dermis

(Ref. Bailey and Love 27th Edition page 634)

- Split skin graft is a partial thickness graft in which only epidermis and part of dermis is taken.
- Full thickness Wolfe graft both epidermis and dermis are taken.

249. A patient suffering from injury 3 days ago following which he was brought to hospital as shown in the image. What would be the likely treatment in this patient?

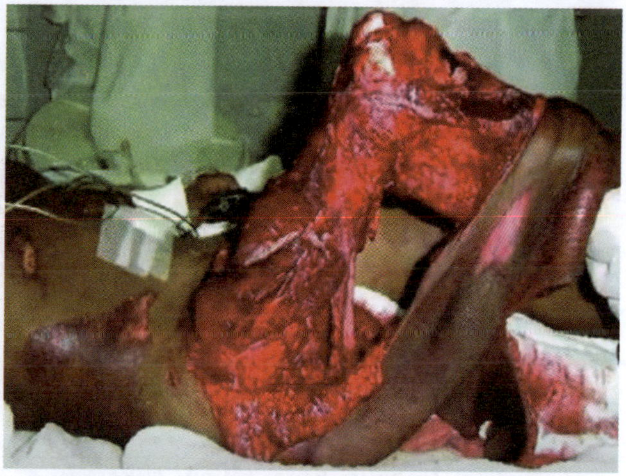

a. Debridement and rotational advancement flap
b. Debridement and primary closure
c. Debridement and hyperbaric oxygen
d. Amputation

Ans. a. Debridement and rotational advancement flap

(Ref. Bailey and Love 27th Edition page 637)

- Wounds which have so much of tissue loss cannot be closed by primary closure.
- Unless the tissues are compromised and gangrenous, no need to do amputation.
- This patient is not infected with Clostridium botulinum and hence, does not need Hyperbaric oxygen therapy there is no clue given to say this is Clostridium (like crepitus in muscles)
- Hence, for such extensive tissue loss, Flaps will be ideal to closure.

250. A 50-year-old male patient presents with palpitations, episodic headache and sweating episodes. Work-up shows small left sided suprarenal mass. Which of the following would be done for confirmation?

a. Urinary vanillylmandelic acid levels
b. Blood 5-HIAA levels
c. Urine myoglobin
d. Stool trypsin levels

Ans. a. Urinary vanillylmandelic acid levels

(Ref. Bailey and Love 27th Edition page 845)

- This is a case of Pheochromocytoma from the history.
- IOC to confirm the diagnosis is to measure urinary metabolites of norepinephrine like Metanephrines and Urinary VMA

251. A newborn child presented with bilious vomiting. What will be the most appropriate test to diagnose the condition in this baby?

a. Barium swallow
b. Barium meal
c. Barium meal follow through
d. CECT abdomen

Ans. c. Barium meal follow through

(Ref. Bailey and Love 27th Edition page 135)

The various causes of Bilious Vomiting in newborn:

- Duodenal Atresia
- Jejunal Atresia
- Malrotation of Gut

252. Grade of glioblastoma multiforme is:

a. I
b. II
c. III
d. IV

Ans. d. IV

(Ref. Bailey and Love 27th Edition page 664)

- Gliomas are divided into: WHO 4 grades:
- Grade IV is the worst of all gliomas and it is Glioblastoma multiforme and is the most common primary brain tumor in adults.

253. In an old patient after complete excision of Glioblastoma, what should be done next?

a. Chemotherapy with Temozolomide
b. Radiotherapy
c. Nothing to be done
d. Chemoradiation

Ans. d. Chemoradiation

(Ref. Bailey and Love 27th Edition page 665)

- After surgery for Glioblastoma multiforme, we must give high-dose-focused radiation therapy, and chemotherapy administered locally as carmustine wafers at time of resection.
- Systemically Oral Temozolomide is given**

FMGE DECEMBER 2021

254. An alcoholic patient who is diagnosed with chronic hepatitis has been admitted to emergency room for vomiting of blood since last 2 days due to variceal bleeding. Patient is in shock. You are the doctor and you have started the first-line treatment, but the patient died. What is the underlying cause of death in this patient?

a. Hepatic failure
b. Variceal bleeding
c. Chronic Hepatitis
d. Hypovolemic shock

Ans. d. Hypovolemic shock

- This is due to Upper GI hemorrhage causing massive blood loss > 2 liters from Varices and patient dies of Hypovolemic shock.
- He might have been saved by Endoscopic Banding and Blood Transfusion.

255. A patient was brought to the emergency in hypotension with cold extremities. Blood pressure was 90/60 mm Hg. Most likely cause of shock in this patient is:

a. Cardiogenic
b. Neurogenic
c. Hypovolemic
d. Septic

Ans. c. Hypovolemic > a. Cardiogenic

- Both Cardiogenic and Hypovolemic shock can cause Low BP and Cold peripheries due to peripheral vasoconstriction.
- Since Most likely cause is asked we will go with Hypovolemic shock.
- Septic shock will have warm peripheries**

256. Central line was being put in the Subclavian vein and the patient collapsed during insertion of the central line. On examination, breath sounds suddenly were found to be absent on the side of insertion of central line. On Percussion, hyperresonance sounds were heard

on the same side of insertion of central line. Most likely cause in this patient is:

a. Pneumothorax
b. Hemothorax
c. Tension pneumothorax
d. Neurogenic shock

Ans. c. Tension pneumothorax > a. Pneumothorax

- This patient is having a clear cut complication of SCV catheter insertion causing pneumothorax.
- From the symptoms – Patient collapse is due to tension pneumothorax causing Shock due to mediastinal shift.
- Immediate needle insertion must be inserted which can save the patient (Bailey says to insert in MCL 2nd ICS)

257. Pressure to cause the pressure sore is:

a. 10 mm Hg
b. 20 mm Hg
c. 25 mm Hg
d. 30 mm Hg

Ans. d. 30 mm of Hg

- Bedsore or Pressure sore is due to chronic immobilization causing Ischemia in capillaries (This happens when Capillary pressure is above 30 mm Hg)
- The more common sites in order are- Ischium> Greater Trochanter>Sacrum.

258. What should be the treatment for the pathology as shown in the given image?

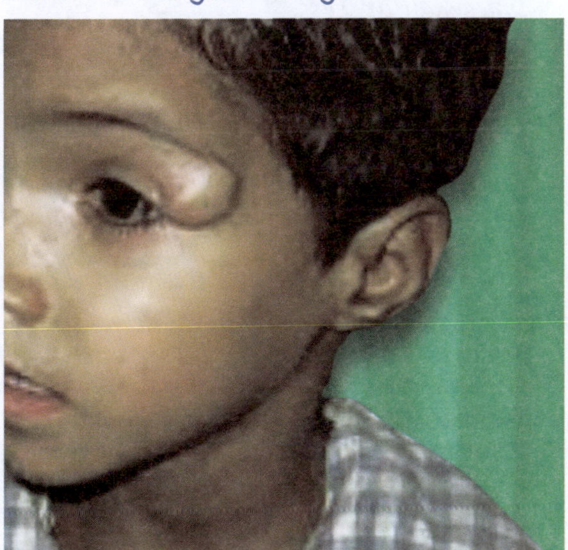

a. Incision and drainage
b. Sclerotherapy
c. Radiotherapy
d. Surgical excision

Ans. d. Surgical excision

- Typical image of External angular Dermoid cyst is shown here.
- Clinically you can see bony indentation and firm consistency.
- Ideal to do surgical excision.

259. A 55-year-old man underwent an operation for lipoma. 11 months after surgery he felt itching and burning on the operated site where a scar is formed which is limited to the wound boundary. What is the nature of this lesion?

a. Hypertrophic scar
b. Keloid
c. Subserous lipoma
d. Granulation tissue

Ans. a. Hypertrophic scar

Major difference between Keloid and Hypertrophic scar is:

- In Hypertrophic scar, the Scar will be limited to the wound.
- In Keloid, it will extend beyond the wound.

260. A patient was brought to the emergency with hypotension, raised JVP, heart sounds were not properly audible, neck veins were engorged. He died in the hospital and autopsy was done which showed the following image. Most likely cause of death in this patient would be:

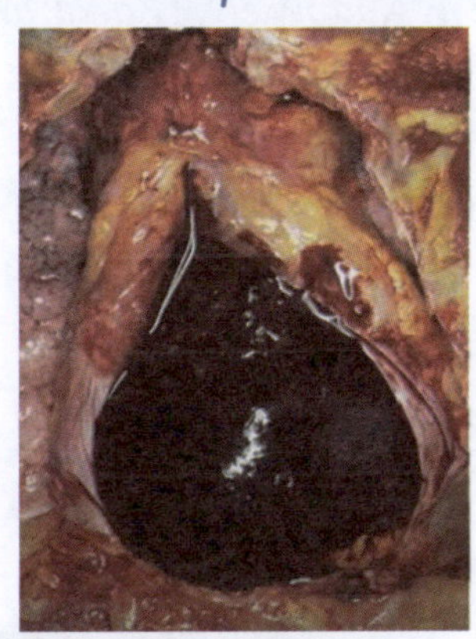

a. Fat necrosis
b. Cardiac tamponade
c. Perforation of intestine
d. Pneumonia

Ans. b. Cardiac tamponade

- The image is opened pericardium showing Blood in pericardial cavity causing BECK's TRIAD symptoms and Cardiac tamponade.
- Beck's Triad = Raised JVP + Low BP and Muffled S1 and S2

261. Lucid interval is seen in:

a. Extradural hematoma
b. Subdural hematoma
c. Subarachnoid hemorrhage
d. Scalp hematoma

Ans. a. Extradural hematoma

- EDH causes a normal period of consciousness before patient falls unconscious. (Lucid interval).
- SDH has loss of Consciousness from time of injury.

262. A patient was brought to the emergency following a car accident. His Blood Pressure is 90/60 mm of Hg, his Glasgow Coma Scale is 9. He is having visceral injuries. Least likely cause of hypovolemia in this patient is:

a. Splenic injury
b. Subdural hematoma
c. Retroperitoneal hematoma
d. Hemothorax

Ans. b. Subdural hematoma

- GCS 9/15 implies there is head injury, but in head injury there won't be fall in BP as blood loss will be meagre.
- Hence, it must be due to injuries elsewhere like in Abdomen, Thorax or Retroperitoneum

263. Battle's sign is seen in:

a. Bruise over mastoid
b. Bitemporal bruises
c. Bruises around the eye
d. Bruises in the neck

Ans. a. Bruise over mastoid

In Base of Skull Fractures – there will be bruising over mastoid region known as Battle's sign

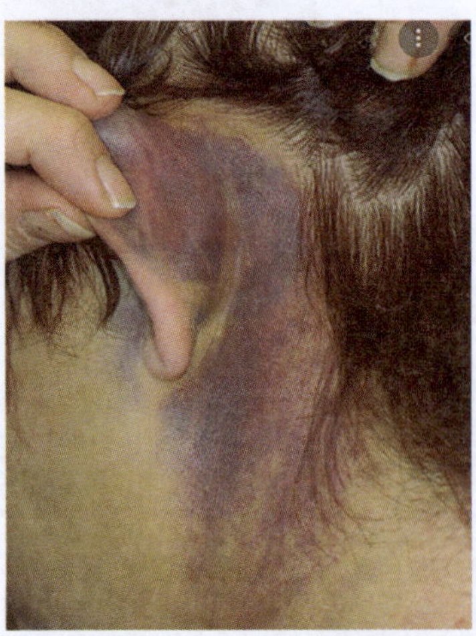

It's a feature of middle cranial fossa fracture.

264. A patient suffered from Blunt trauma to the abdomen and was brought to the Emergency room. He is unstable having Blood pressure of 90/60 mm of Hg. You are the doctor, basic resuscitation is done with intravenous fluids, FAST is positive. He is not improving despite intravenous fluids. Next step in the management is:

a. CECT
b. Exploratory laparotomy
c. Laparoscopy
d. MRI

Ans. b. Exploratory laparotomy

- E-Fast Positive – Unstable Cases – Emergency Laparotomy advised
- E-Fast Positive – Stable Cases – CECT abdomen advised

265. A lactating woman comes in the hospital with 3 days history of painful, red, fluctuant, 2 cm mass in the breast. USG shows fluid collection. What will you do in the management of this patient?

a. Antibiotics and Follow-up after 3 days
b. Incision and Drainage
c. Hot fomentation
d. Empty the breasts every 3 hours

Ans. a. Antibiotics and Follow-up after 3 days

- Lactating women + Painful red fluctuant – 2 cm mass in breast is more suggestive a small abscess.
- Such a small abscess doesn't need incision and drainage.
- Also, nowadays, newer treatment is to do Needle aspiration via USG guidance and no incision and drainage done.
- Antibiotic of choice is Cloxacillin. If abscess is increasing in size after 3 days we will do aspiration (Not incision and drainage)

266. A 32-year-old lady, 2 cm single, mobile, asymptomatic breast lump with well-defined margin, noticed by the patient herself on self-breast examination, presented to the OPD. She was diagnosed with a benign lesion in FNAC. You are the doctor and what would you recommend to this patient?

a. Reassure and continue to follow-up the patient
b. Surgical Excision
c. Biopsy
d. Give Danazol

Ans. a. Reassure and continue follow-up the patient

- From the history—painless mobile mass with well-defined margin is suggestive of Fibroadenoma.
- On mammography, there will be popcorn calcification
- FNAC will show it as benign lesion.
- It is not premalignant
- Just follow-up is enough for such cases.

267. Best prognosis is of which of the following Breast cancer:

a. Luminal A
b. Luminal B
c. Triple Negative Breast cancer
d. Her2 neu enriched

Ans. a. Luminal A

- Most common is Luminal Type A- ER+, PR+ and HER 2 negative. This has the best prognosis
- Worst prognosis is Basal type

268. A patient has presented with herniation of intestinal loop which passes along the spermatic cord and reaches till scrotum/cremaster muscle:

a. Femoral hernia
b. Direct inguinal hernia
c. Indirect inguinal hernia
d. Paraumbilical hernia

Ans. c. Indirect inguinal hernia

- The anatomy of Indirect hernia is the contents descending from Deep ring to Superficial ring.
- The sac descends from Deep ring and enters the canal and exits Superficial ring in Indirect hernia.
- In Direct hernia, the contents enter from Hesselbach triangle and exit via the Superficial ring (most times it will be limited to canal and we call them as incomplete direct hernia)

269. Identify the pathology in the given image:

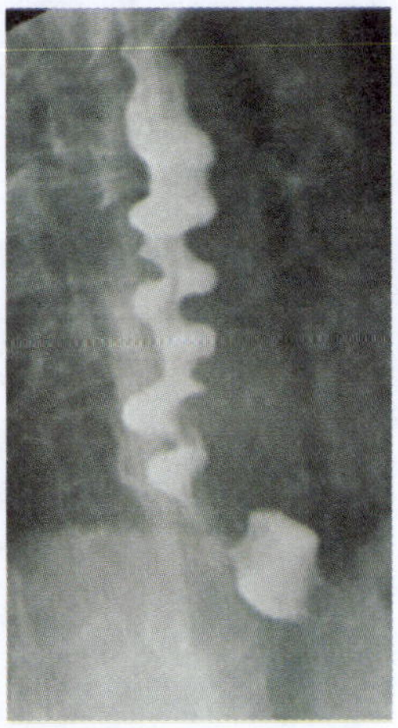

a. Achalasia cardia
b. Cancer esophagus
c. Nutcracker esophagus
d. Diffuse esophageal spasm

Ans. d. Diffuse esophageal spasm

- This is a Barium swallow showing—Cork Screw appearance in esophagus. This is seen in Diffuse Esophageal spasm.
- Bird Beak—Achalasia
- Rat tail—Cancer
- Feline esophagus—Eosinophilic esophagitis

270. Patient is having retching pain, vomiting and retrosternal burning. Most likely cause in this patient is?

a. Esophagitis
b. Intestinal obstruction
c. Pyloric stenosis
d. Peptic ulcer disease

Ans. a. Esophagitis

- Vomiting with retrosternal pain is classically seen in GERD
- Due to esophagitis—patient may develop Heart burn, Retrosternal discomfort and Retching pain.

271. A child had difficulty in gobbling (shout) and he was able to speak. Identify the site of foreign body as shown in the image.

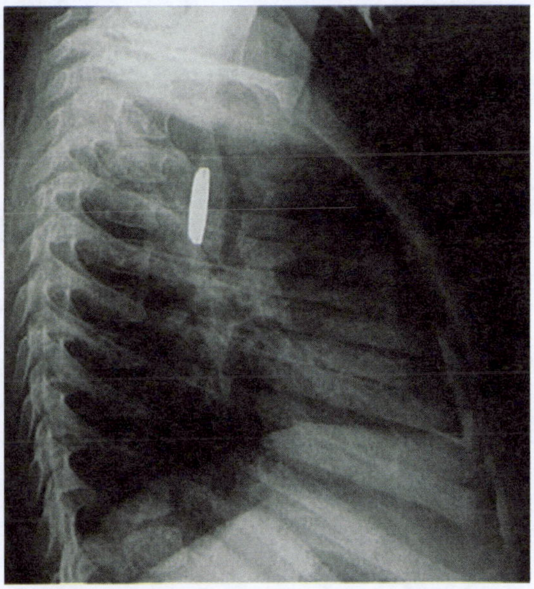

a. Trachea
b. Esophagus
c. Mediastinum
d. Pleural cavity

Ans. b. Esophagus

- This is the image showing Coin seen in Esophagus posterior to Trachea.
- The image of Tracheal shadow is shown anteriorly
- An AP View cannot detect the exact location of coin. So, we need a lateral image as shown.

272. A patient underwent Total Gastrectomy. Which of the following deficiencies would be seen in this patient?

a. Vitamin B_{12}
b. Vitamin A
c. Vitamin B_1
d. Vitamin C

Ans. a. Vitamin B_{12}

- After gastrectomy, there is a deficiency in intrinsic factor.
- Intrinsic factor is an essential component to absorb vitamin B_{12} in terminal ileum.
- Therefore, severe B_{12} deficiency happens post gastrectomy.
- But the most common malnutrition is Iron deficiency anemia**

273. A female who was taking NSAIDs for long period of time for her arthritis presented to the emergency with severe pain abdomen. Abdominal Radiograph done is given below. Most likely diagnosis is:

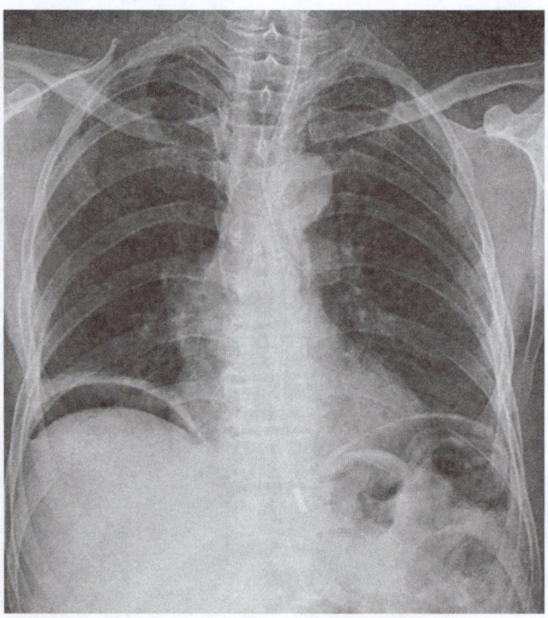

a. Pericardial effusion
b. Pneumothorax
c. Peptic ulcer disease
d. Perforation of peptic ulcer

Ans. d. Perforation of peptic ulcer

- X-ray showing air under diaphragm
- Cupola Sign—Moustache like air at xiphisternal area in perforation
- Rigler Sign—Air inside and outside the Lumen of bowel in perforation

274. A 5-year-old baby having constipation. We are giving stool softeners also but is still able to pass only one stool in one week. There is a history of passage of meconium after 48 hrs of birth. What investigation would you do initially in this baby?

a. Ask mother to give high fiber diet
b. Plain X-ray of abdomen
c. Barium enema and anorectal manometry
d. CECT abdomen

Ans. c. Barium enema and anorectal manometry

- Delayed passage of meconium is the clue here for a baby with severe constipation. Such features are seen in Hirschsprung disease*
- Initial diagnosis is made by Barium enema which will show dilated colon and constricted rectum.
- Anorectal manometry will show Absent Rectoanal inhibitory reflex.
- Investigation of Choice is Full-thickness rectal biopsy.

275. Identify the investigation shown below.

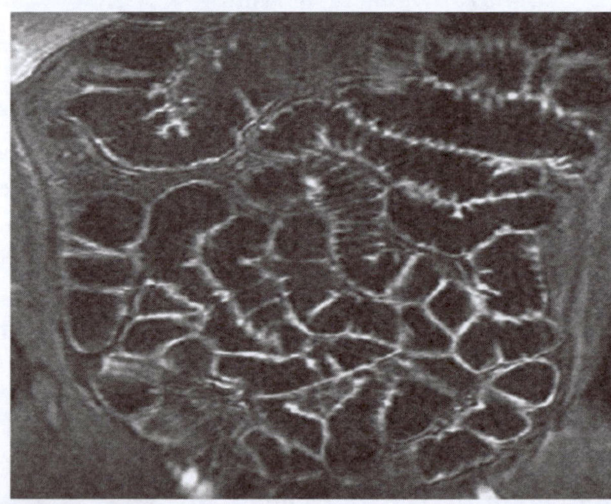

a. Barium meal follow through
b. Enterography
c. CT enteroclysis
d. MR enteroclysis

Ans. d. MR enteroclysis

- This is an image showing Fluid-filled Bowel-MR enteroclysis
- In CECT enteroclysis, there will be bright bone image.

276. Lady is in first trimester of pregnancy, presents to ER, with acute abdominal pain. She is diagnosed with acute appendicitis. Next step in the management will be:

a. Terminate the pregnancy
b. Give Antibiotics and wait till 2nd trimester
c. Do appendectomy
d. Wait and watch

Ans. c. Do appendectomy

- In pregnancy-Acute appendicitis is most common in 2nd trimester
- Acute appendicitis is the most common non obstetric surgical emergency in Pregnancy.
- Whatever the trimester is- if appendicitis is confirmed, we must do Appendectomy.

277. A patient suffering from Inflammatory bowel disease presented with Peritonitis following ileal perforation. Exploration is done. You as a doctor would prefer to do which of the following?

a. Ileostomy and definite surgery later
b. Ileal pouch anal anastomosis
c. Resection of the diseased segment and anastomosis of normal segment
d. Right hemicolectomy and ileotransverse anastomosis

Ans. a. Ileostomy and definite surgery later

- Any case of peritonitis with sepsis, we must not try to do any anastomosis- this is a general rule.
- In this patient with IBD and peritonitis- the ideal option is to do a temporary ileostomy and plan definitive surgery later.

278. The internal opening in Anal fistula usually begins at:

a. Crypt at dentate line
b. Perineal body
c. Anal verge
d. Anorectal junction

Ans. a. Crypt at dentate line

- Anal crypts of Morgagni are seen in Dentate line.
- They have glands which infected cause Cryptoglandular abscess.
- The cryptoglandular abscess ruptures outside resulting in Fistula.
- MC cause of Fistula in ano is Cryptoglandular abscess

279. After 3 days of cholecystectomy, patient developed severe abdominal pain with fever. Her LFT was Normal, Serum Amylase was also Normal. What is the most likely cause of her condition?

a. Bile leak
b. CBD stone
c. Acute pancreatitis
d. Liver abscess

Ans. a. Bile leak

- The history is clear, there is a history of Cholecystectomy done and patient has pain on 3rd day.
- Pain along with fever in postoperative cases of cholecystectomy we must think of CBD stone or leak.
- If CBD stone is the issue, LFT will be increased.
- Amylase normal rules out pancreatitis.
- LFT is raised in Liver abscess cases.

280. A lady was incidentally diagnosed with a 0.5 cm solid mass in her Gallbladder on USG which was nonmobile, diagnosed as GB polyp. She is asymptomatic. Next step in the management is:

a. Reassure the patient and follow-up
b. Laparoscopic Cholecystectomy
c. Open Cholecystectomy
d. CECT abdomen

Ans. a. Reassure the patient and follow-up

- USG shows nonmobile mass means more suggestive of Polyp
- USG will show stone as mobile mass with posterior acoustic shadow.
- Such small polyp of size of <1 cm can be managed by follow-up alone.
- Indications for surgery for polyps

281. What do you expect in a lady after GB removal most commonly?

a. Weight loss
b. Steatorrhea
c. High cholesterol
d. Hypoglycemia

Ans. b. Steatorrhea

- Bile salts are essential components of Fat Digestion.
- They are concentrated from Gallbladder and secreted into Duodenum.
- Initially for a few months after cholecystectomy the storage function is lost and patient has mild steatorrhea. Gradually the Bile ducts themselves take the function and steatorrhea is absent after few months.

282. A patient has an USG finding of a gallstone abutting the cystic duct with dilatation of Common Hepatic Duct. What is the most likely diagnosis?

a. Acute cholecystitis
b. Porcelain GB
c. GB polyp
d. Mirizzi syndrome

Ans. d. Mirizzi syndrome

- Mirizzi syndrome is a condition in which the Stone in Cystic duct or Hartman's pouch of Gallbladder compresses the CBD causing Jaundice and in USG shows Dilated CBD*

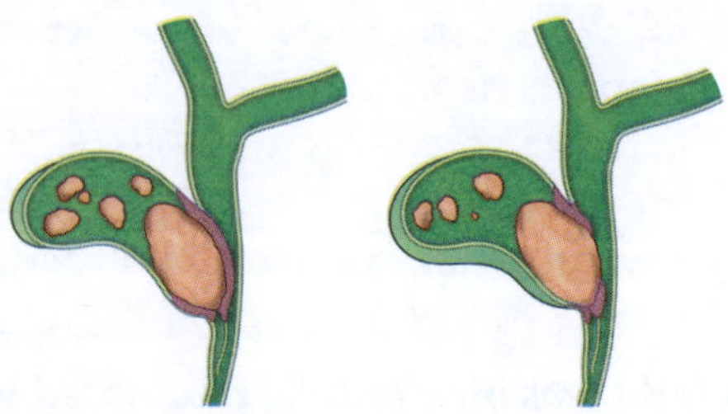

283. A female presents with epigastric pain and right hypochondrial pain radiating to back with guarding and rigidity in right hypochondrium. She has similar episodes past 1 year on and off. Most likely diagnosis is:

a. Acute pancreatitis
b. Acute cholecystitis
c. Hydatid cyst
d. Liver abscess

Ans. b. Acute cholecystitis

- Biliary colicky pain is the classical symptom of pain in the right hypochondrium radiating to back.
- The symptom is intermittent and follows fatty food consumption.
- The pain is not typical colicky but may extend from 1–24 hours until the obstructing stone moves away.

284. A patient presents with pain in right hypochondrium. Blood investigations showed AST- 22 IU/L and ALT- 27 IU/L. Serum Bilirubin levels – 5 mg/dL and also ALP- 200 mg%. What should be the initial investigation in this patient?

a. USG abdomen
b. CECT abdomen
c. HBsAG
d. HIDA scan

Ans. a. USG abdomen

Please don't get confused- in an obstructive jaundice patient

- 1st done- USG
- IOC- MRCP
- Gold standard for CBD stone- ERCP

285. Miss X, 35 years old presented to the emergency with upper abdominal pain radiating to the back. On X-ray Colon, cut-off sign is seen. Most likely diagnosis is:

a. Acute cholecystitis
b. Acute appendicitis
c. Acute pancreatitis
d. Acute cholangitis

Ans. c. Acute pancreatitis

Due to Ileus and fluid secretion inside abdominal cavity -which happens due to pancreatic enzymes from damaged pancreas- the following signs are seen on Plain X-ray:

- Sentinel loop sign
- Colon cut-off sign
- Gasless abdomen

286. A 25-year-old alcoholic male presents with pain epigastric region radiating to back. What is the most likely diagnosis from the image?

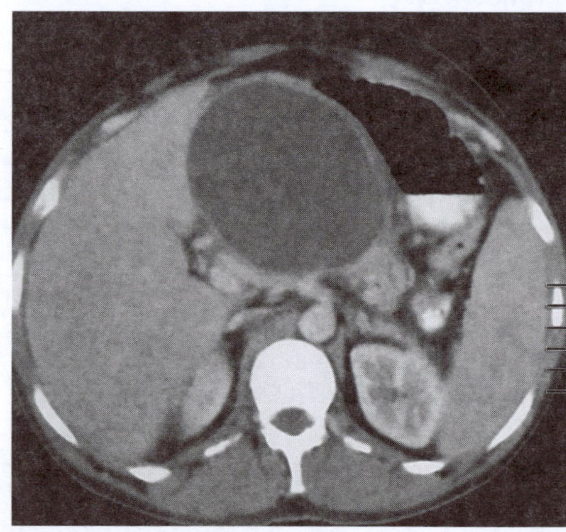

a. Amebic liver abscess
b. Pseudocyst of pancreas
c. Acute cholecystitis
d. Hydatid cyst

Ans. b. Pseudocyst of pancreas

H/o of alcohol + Pain radiating to back all suggests pancreatitis and the image shows a cyst behind the stomach and hence Pseudocyst pancreas.

287. A 5-year-old girl is having continuous dribbling of urine and also normal micturition. Most likely cause is:

a. Posterior urethral valves
b. Ureteric opening distal to external sphincter
c. Urinary tract infection
d. Vesicoureteric reflux

Ans. b. Ureteric opening distal to external sphincter

- Normal urination is also seen in history, dribbling of urine along with normal urination is suggestive of Ectopic ureter opening distal to External urethral sphincter.
- This phenomenon is known as Paradoxical urinary incontinency.

288. Most common type of kidney stone is:

a. Calcium oxalate
b. Triple phosphate
c. Uric acid
d. Cystine

Ans. a. Calcium oxalate

- MC type of Kidney stone- Calcium oxalate
- MC type of kidney stone in alkaline urine is Triple phosphate stone
- MC type of Stone in Infection – Triple phosphate stone
- Other name of Triple phosphate is- Struvite stone, Jack stone, Staghorn stone

289. Whitaker test is done in:

a. Posterior urethral valves
b. Hydronephrosis to compare intrarenal and urinary bladder pressures
c. Ureterocele
d. Benign prostatic hyperplasia

Ans. b. Hydronephrosis to compare intra-renal and urinary bladder pressures

- Done in cases of congenital PUJ
- Pressure transducers are introduced in Renal pelvis and bladder and pressure checked. There will be high pressure in renal pelvis compared to bladder.
- These are outdated tests and no one does them nowadays.

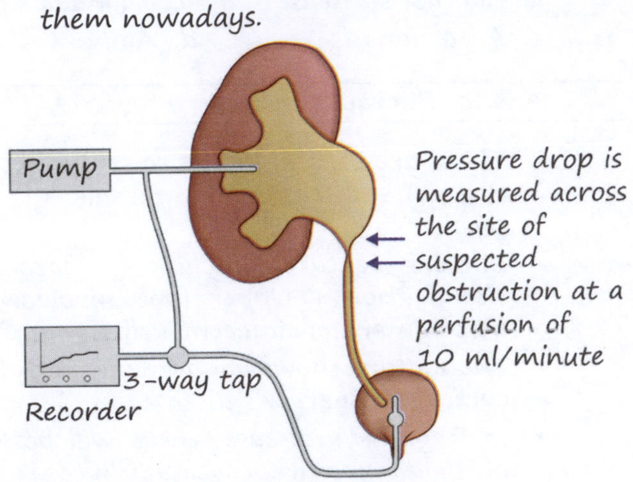

290. A 65-year-old male presented with a mass in the left lumbar region which was ballotable. He was having abdominal discomfort and on investigations, he was found to have a 7 × 5 × 3 cm which was confined within the kidney and diagnosed as Renal cell carcinoma. What would be the treatment in this patient?

a. Partial nephrectomy
b. Radical nephrectomy
c. Radiotherapy
d. Chemotherapy

Ans. b. Radical nephrectomy

It's a straight forward one liner:

- **Tumor in Kidney <7 cm:** Partial nephrectomy can be done
- **Tumor in Kidney >7 cm:** Radical nephrectomy is treatment of choice

291. Identify the following investigation and diagnosis.

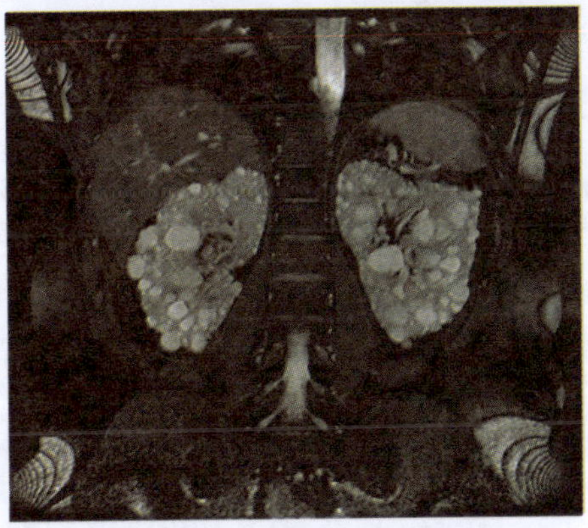

a. IVP of polycystic Kidney disease
b. CT of polycystic Kidney disease
c. MRI of polycystic Kidney disease
d. CT scan of horseshoe kidney

Ans. c. MRI of polycystic kidney disease

- T2-weighted image of MRI showing both kidney with Fluid-filled cysts in this case of PCKD
- CECT will show Bright Bones on imaging.
- Spider leg appearance is seen in PCKD

292. Mother while giving bath to her 7-day-old baby noticed that the scrotum of the baby is empty. You are the doctor, what treatment you will offer in this baby?

a. Wait and watch for spontaneous resolution
b. Give GnRH for 1 month, if testis does not descend down on its own, then do surgery before 2 years
c. Give GnRH for 1 month, if testis does not descend down on its own, then do surgery before 5 years
d. Do immediate Surgery

Ans. a. Wait and watch for spontaneous resolution

- Wait and watch is enough for this boy who is just 7 days old.
- Undescended Testis (UDT) is more common in preterm baby.
- UDT usually descends in 3 months of time. So, we have to wait and watch
- If testis is not descending, we will go for Orchidopexy in 6 months- 1 year of age.
- **GnRH analogs are tried for finding out whether there is secretion of testosterone, but not useful for this case** in many studies**

293. Three testicle appearance is seen in:

a. Vaginal hydrocele
b. Spermatocele
c. Epididymo-orchitis
d. Torsion Testis

Ans. b. Spermatocele

- Three testicle appearance on palpation– Spermatocele
- Chinese lantern transillumination– Epididymal cyst
- Transillumination– Vaginal hydrocele

294. An old age patient felt heaviness in the left scrotum, he was suspecting cancer, came to ER. There was no pain or tenderness and transillumination was negative, most likely diagnosis in this patient would be:

a. Varicocele
b. Hydrocele
c. Testicular torsion
d. Epididymo-orchitis

Ans. a. Varicocele

- History is very clear that there is no pain or tenderness. The conditions without pain in list given are Hydrocele and Varicocele.
- Hydrocele can be excluded as there is no transillumination.

295. A young male presented with enlargement of the scrotum along with lump in the paraumbilical region and swelling in the supraclavicular fossa. Most likely diagnosis is:

a. Testicular tumor
b. Hydrocele
c. Testicular torsion
d. Epididymo-orchitis

Ans. a. Testicular tumor

- Swelling in Testicular region, a young male with Nodal masses- like para-aortic and Supraclavicular are seen in Seminoma and Nonseminoma type testicular cancers.
- The metastatic nodes in Para-aortic region present as Mass in periumbilical region

296. A young male was found to have a testicular swelling. After evaluation, high inguinal orchidectomy was done. What will be the probable diagnosis?

a. Torsion
b. Seminoma testis
c. Fournier gangrene
d. Hematocele

Ans. b. Seminoma testis

- High Inguinal Orchidectomy is a surgery done for testicular tumors.
- To avoid tumor dissemination, surgery is done via inguinal incision

297. A 25-year-old male, a chronic smoker, presents with pain in the finger with changes as shown in the image. Most likely pathology in this patient would be?

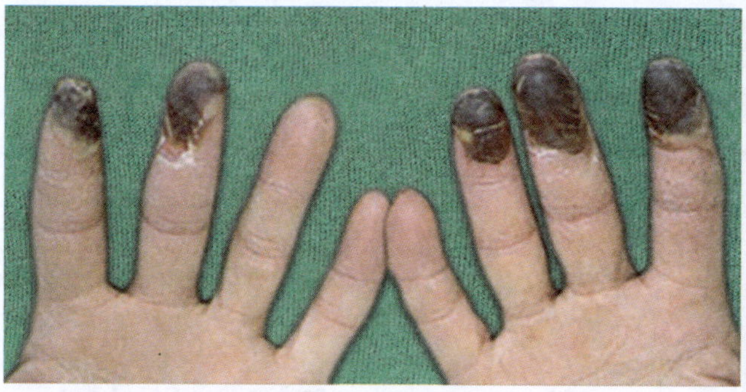

a. Buerger's disease
b. Raynaud's disease
c. Acrocyanosis
d. Ainhum

Ans. a. Buerger's disease

- There are clinical points to strongly suggest Buerger's disease (Young male + Chronic smoker)
- Clinical features include- Bilateral leg claudication + Upper limb involvement + Involvement of adjacent veins and nerves
- The picture shows gangrene in both fingers typical of Buerger's disease.
- In Raynaud's disease, there will be history of Cold exposure causing White + Blue + Crimson red color changes in fingers.

298. A patient admitted for pelvic fracture is under treatment. He suddenly developed breathlessness and died on 3rd POD. What's the reason probably?

a. Myocardial infarction
b. Venous thromboembolism
c. CVA
d. Pleural effusion

Ans. b. Venous thromboembolism

- DVT is a common complication in Pelvic fractures and surgeries.
- Patients with DVT have high risk of pulmonary embolism and high mortality.

299. Cannonball appearance is seen in:

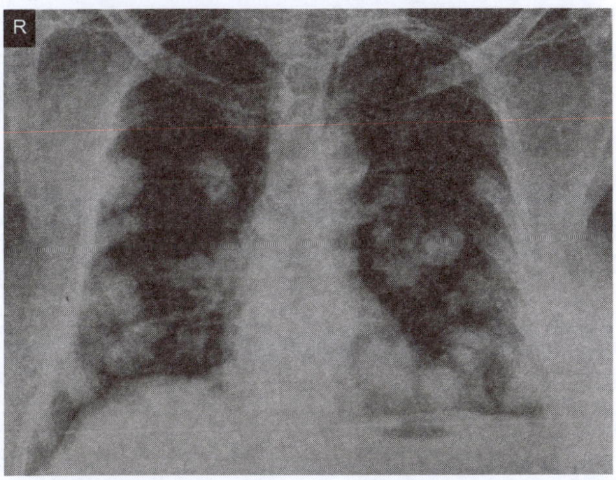

a. Lung metastasis
b. Tuberculosis
c. Sarcoidosis
d. Silicosis

Ans. a. Lung metastasis

- Lung mets will appear as Cannonball
- Seen in Seminoma, RCC, etc.

FMGE JUNE 2021

300. If a patient requires an emergency surgery to survive and no attenders are available to give consent. What will you do?

a. Will operate without consent
b. Will wait for attenders to reach the hospital for consent
c. Will not operate
d. Will get consent from hospital authorities

Ans. a. Will operate without consent

In case of emergency and if the surgery is needed urgently with intention to save the life of the patient, patient can be operated without consent if the patient is unconscious

301. Central Venous pressure is raised in which of the following shocks?

a. Neurogenic
b. Anaphylactic
c. Cardiogenic
d. Hypovolemic

Ans. c. Cardiogenic

CVP is raised in Cardiogenic shock and Septic shock and in fact the value is not accurate in these cases and hence, we must do Pulmonary Capillary Wedge pressure (PCWP) in these two shocks

302. A chronic smoker was undergoing major surgery under general anesthesia with oxygen and nitrous oxide. Suddenly he collapsed on table and breath sounds were not heard on left side of chest. What will be the cause?

a. Tension pneumothorax
b. Pulmonary edema
c. Cardiac tamponade
d. ARDS

Ans. a. Tension pneumothorax

Rupture of Pulmonary Bullae is a complication which can happen due to PEEP setting in ventilator and may present as sudden collapse due to Tension pneumothorax

303. A patient who had burns some years back now presents with ulceration over the burns area indicative of malignancy. What is it?

a. Basal cell cancer
b. Marjolin's ulcer
c. Rodent Ulcer
d. Verrucous cancer

Ans. b. Marjolin's ulcer

The malignancy arising from Burns scar is Marjolin ulcer (SCC)

304. A patient presents with Head injury and increased ICP with low BP. Which of the following drug is used?

a. Mannitol
b. Prednisolone
c. Dexamethasone
d. Frusemide

Ans. a. Mannitol

- Mannitol is the drug of choice to reduce the intracranial pressure in head injury patients
- Frusemide can be allowed if BP is normal
- In head injury, we must not use steroids to reduce ICP
- Please remember same time, steroids are the DOC for raised ICP due to Tumors

305. A patient presented to emergency after Blunt Abdominal trauma with low Blood pressure. What should be the initial step?

a. Start resuscitation with IV crystalloids
b. Immediate exploration with laparotomy
c. Get a CT-Scan done and start IV fluids later
d. Start resuscitation with Blood products

Ans. a. Start resuscitation with IV crystalloids

- Please remember, in any trauma patient with low BP, we must follow ABCDE protocol of primary survey
- As per the protocol since airway and breathing are not mentioned we go next to circulation
- The treatment for Hemorrhagic shock is to start minimum 2 Green (18G) cannulas in both upper limb and start Normal saline (crystalloids)
- Yes blood products are the best replacement for Hemorrhagic shock, but by the time, we arrange the blood we must infuse the IVF.

306. A patient following RTA was brought to hospital with high heart rate, very low Blood pressure and Respiratory rate > 22 /minute. What should be the next step in this patient?

a. Airway intubation b. FAST
c. CT scan d. IV fluids

Ans. a. Airway Intubation

This is the same as discussed in previous question. Airway is the first priority.

307. A patient with head injury was brought to casualty with GCS-12. CT scan was taken that is shown in the image. What is your diagnosis?

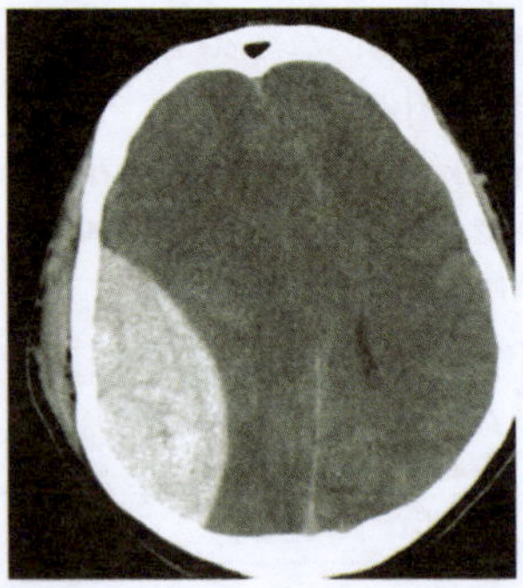

a. EDH
b. SDH
c. SAH
d. Intracerebral hemorrhage

Ans. a. EDH

Biconvex shaped hematoma in EDH*

308. Identify the lesion shown in the image.

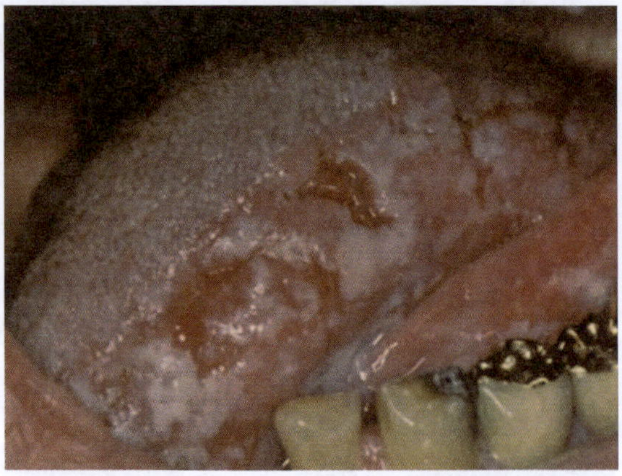

a. Leukoplakia b. Erythroplakia
c. Apthous ulcer d. Syphilic chancre

Ans. a. Leukoplakia

(Ref: Bailey and Love 27th Edition page 762)

White patch or plaque in oral cavity is known as Leukoplakia

309. Which of the following is the most common site of malignancy in head and neck?

a. Oral cavity b. Nasopharynx
c. Larynx d. Oropharynx

Ans. a. Oral cavity

(Ref: Bailey and Love 27th edition page 760)

- MC malignancy in Head and neck is oral cancer
- In oral cancer MC site in world is Tongue
- In oral cancer MC site in India is Buccal mucosa

310. Radio isotope used in Thyroid cancer treatment:

a. I-131 b. Tc 99 m
c. I-33 Cesium d. 89 Strontium

Ans. a. I-131

- I-131 is the Radioactive iodine used for therapeutic purpose to ablate the metastasis
- Its half-life is 8 days*

311. A patient comes with thyroiditis- has high TSH value and TPO antibody value. Diagnosis is:

a. Hashimoto's thyroiditis
b. Reidel's thyroiditis
c. De Quervain's
d. Subacute thyroiditis

Ans. a. Hashimoto's thyroiditis

- Thyroid peroxidase antibodies are elevated in Hashimoto's

- TSH receptor antibodies and Antithyroglobulin antibodies are also seen
- T4 and T3 will be low with TSH high

312. A patient comes with goiter swelling and T3 and T4 increased and a decreased TSH. What is the diagnosis?

a. Graves disease
b. Hashimoto's thyroiditis
c. Plummer disease
d. Physiological

Ans. b. Hashimoto's thyroiditis

Question is focusing on Hypothyroidism and the most common cause of Hypothyroidism is Hashimoto's

313. Pale Orphan Annie eyed nucleus is seen in:

a. Papillary cancer
b. Follicular cancer
c. Medullary cancer
d. Anaplastic cancer

Ans. a. Papillary cancer

Psammoma bodies and orphan annie eye nuclei are features of papillary thyroid cancer.

314. A 60-year-old lady with Hard Breast mass 6 × 4 cm in size is shown in image. There is a single node palpable. There is no evidence of mets. What would be the ideal treatment?

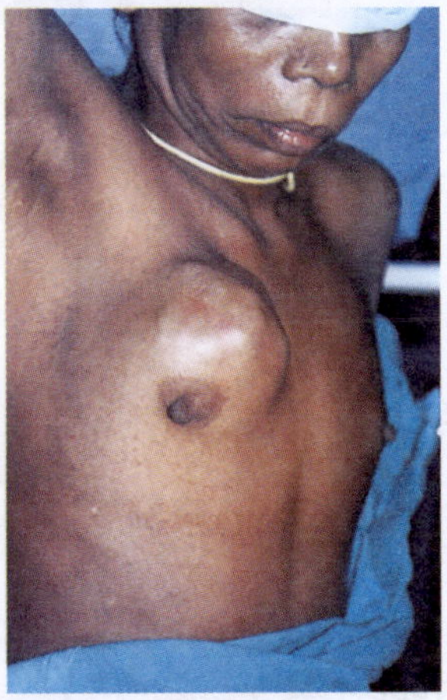

a. Radical mastectomy
b. Modified radical mastectomy followed by Adjuvant CRT
c. Neoadjuvant Chemotherapy followed by Surgery
d. Palliative mastectomy

Ans. c. Neoadjuvant Chemotherapy followed by Surgery

- Tumor size >5 cm: so T3
- Node- N1
- Mets- M0
- T3N1M0 will come under locally advanced cancer and hence treatment is Neoadjuvant Chemotherapy followed by Surgery

315. A postpartum lactating female presents with redness and swelling in the breast. Identify the pathology in the given image.

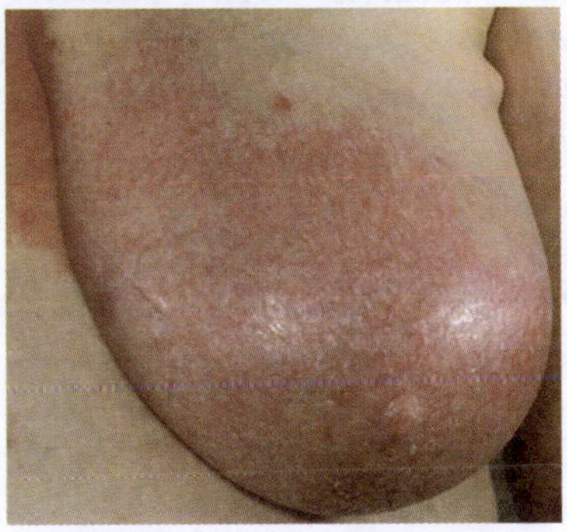

a. Breast abscess
b. Mondor
c. Fibroadenoma
d. Phyllodes Tumor

Ans. a. Breast abscess

Tender fluctuant swelling in lactating women is suggestive of Breast abscess

316. Following image is suggestive of which stage of Breast cancer?

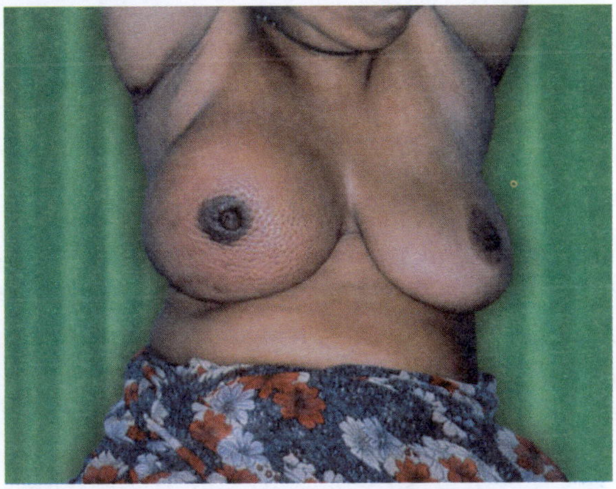

a. T4a
b. T4b
c. T3
d. T2

Ans. b. T4b

Peau d' orange is T4b- Skin Involvement

317. A 30-year-old female presented with a mass in inguinal region, which produced a gurgling sound on reduction and the mass completely disappears on pressing it through the deep inguinal ring. What is your diagnosis?

a. Indirect inguinal hernia
b. Direct inguinal hernia
c. Femoral hernia
d. Strangulated hernia

Ans. a. Indirect hernia

Indirect hernia is entering via Deep ring to Superficial ring and hence, it gets reduced via the deep ring on compression

318. After Binge drinking of alcohol, a young male presents with sudden vomiting and hematemesis. What is your diagnosis?

a. Duodenal ulcer perforation
b. Boerhaave syndrome
c. Mallory Weiss Tear
d. Tension pneumothorax

Ans. c. Mallory Weiss Tear

- Sudden vomiting after an alcoholic binge and subsequent Hematemesis is due to tear in mucosa at OG junction level known as Mallory Weiss tear.
- All 90% times it is self limiting and no treatment is needed
- 10% cases may need endoscopic coagulation

319. Kilian's Dehiscence is seen between:

a. Thyropharyngeus and stylopharyngeus
b. Thyropharyngeus and cricopharyngeus
c. Cricopharyngeus and stylopharyngeus
d. Inferior and middle constrictor

Ans. b. Thyropharyngeus and Cricopharyngeus

- Kilian's dehiscence is a triangular defect between the Cricopharyngeus muscle (horizontal) and Thyropharyngeus (Oblique)
- This is the defect via which Zenker diverticulum happens

320. A 9-year-old boy was having dinner with his parents and after swallowing a food bolus, he had a choking sensation. Next step done is:

a. Hyperextension of neck to look for airway
b. Large sips of water or fizzy drinks to push it down
c. Upper abdominal thrusts to force vomiting
d. Endotracheal intubation

Ans. b. Large sips of water or fizzy drinks to push it down

- Sudden occlusion of food bolus in esophagus is common in children due to dry food, and they must be advised to drink large sips of water or some fizzy drinks like Pepsi or cola to push the food down.
- Such intermittent episodic aphagia can also occur in Schatzki ring after a heavy meal and may need proteolytic enzymes to dissolve.

321. A 60-year-old man has presented with chronic projectile vomiting and significant weight loss. Which of the following electrolyte abnormality is seen in this patient?

a. Hypokalemic hypochloremic Metabolic alkalosis with Hyponatremia
b. Hypokalemic hypochloremic Metabolic alkalosis with Hypernatremia
c. Hypokalemic hypochloremic Metabolic alkalosis with Hypercalcemia
d. Hypokalemic hypochloremic Metabolic alkalosis with Hypomagnesemia

Ans. a. Hypokalemic hypochloremic Metabolic alkalosis with Hyponatremia

Electrolyte imbalance in GOO:

- Hypochloremia
- Metabolic alkalosis
- Hyponatremia
- Hypokalemia
- Hypocalcelmia
- Paradoxical renal aciduria

322. The following staging is done for which of the following cancers?

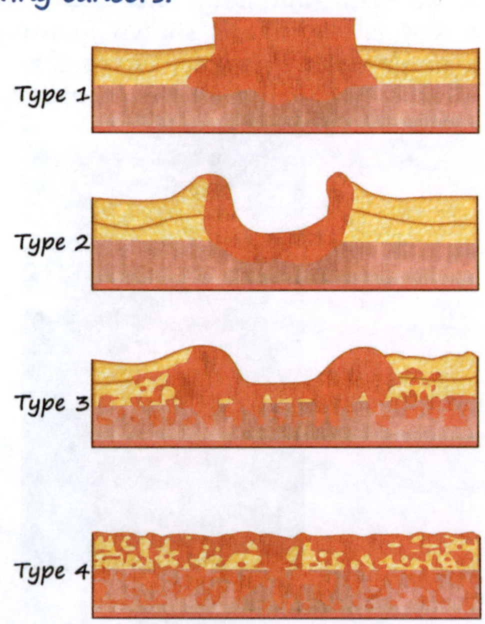

a. Oral cancer- AJCC
b. Bladder cancer- WHO
c. Gastric cancer- Borrmann
d. Colon cancer- Duke

Ans. c. Gastric cancer- Borrmann

- This is Borrmann classification for Gastric cancers*
- It's a morphological classification based on appearance grossly
- Lauren's is a microscopic classification

323. A 36-year-old male presents with low grade fever and anorexia and weight loss past 1 year. During the investigation following image is obtained on a contrast study. What is your diagnosis?

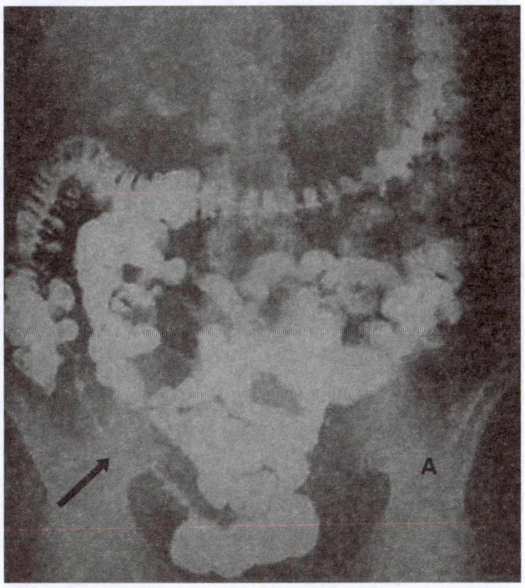

a. Ileocecal TB
b. Cancer colon
c. Volvulus
d. Diverticulosis of colon

Ans. a. Ileocecal TB

- In this Barium meal follow through, we can see the String sign of Kantor* which is seen in Crohn and Ileocecal TB
- In Ileocecal TB, we can also see sometimes pulled up subhepatic cecum

324. A 45-year-old male presents with complaints of pain in abdomen, vomiting on and off and diarrhea. Measurement of Serum creatinine is high. What is the probable diagnosis?

a. Lymphoma
b. Carcinoid tumor
c. Adenocarcinoma
d. GIST

Ans. b. Carcinoid Tumor

- Explosive watery diarrhea with abdominal pain is a feature of Carcinoid tumor of GIT
- The vomiting is seen due to partial obstruction caused by the tumor.
- Patient may go for Renal failure due to Fluid loss and hence, there is serum creatinine elevation
- Octreotide is the DOC for this case to start with.

325. An elderly woman who had not taken food for past few days now presented with bilious vomiting. Her X-ray is shown below. What is your diagnosis?

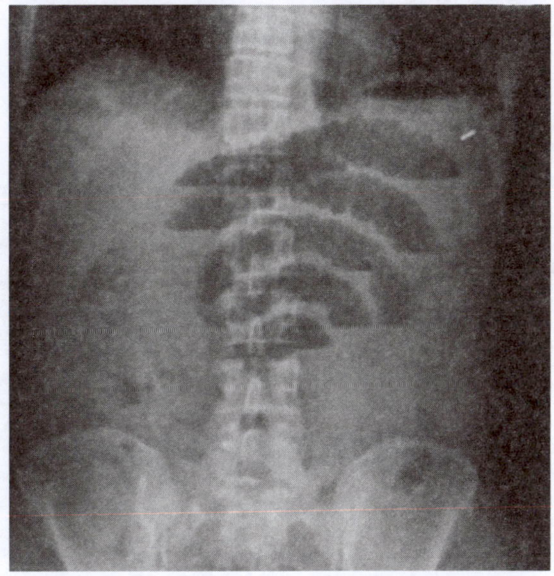

a. Distal obstruction in small intestine
b. Proximal obstruction in small intestine
c. Pseudo obstruction
d. Distal colonic obstruction

Ans. a. Distal Obstruction in small intestine

In this X-ray, we can see dilated Jejunum (due to Valvulae Conniventes) and that means the obstruction is in Ileum level.

326. A 25-year-old female who had pain in the right iliac fossa with vomiting was managed conservatively. She was stable for two days after which she had worsening of the symptoms for which extra peritoneal drainage done by USG guidance. What is the diagnosis?

a. Perinephric abscess
b. Appendicular abscess
c. Ruptured ectopic
d. Acute cholecystitis

Ans. b. Appendicular abscess

- History is clearly suggestive of Acute appendicitis, gone for appendicular abscess.
- In appendicular abscess, we do extra peritoneal drainage.

327. Which is the site of maximum pain in Acute appendicitis?

a. Mc Burney's point
b. Left flank
c. Suprapubic region
d. Umbilicus

Ans. a. Mc Burney's Point

Junction of medial 2/3rd and Lateral 1/3rd of Spino-umbilical line is known as Mc Burney Point.

328. Barium enema image shows:

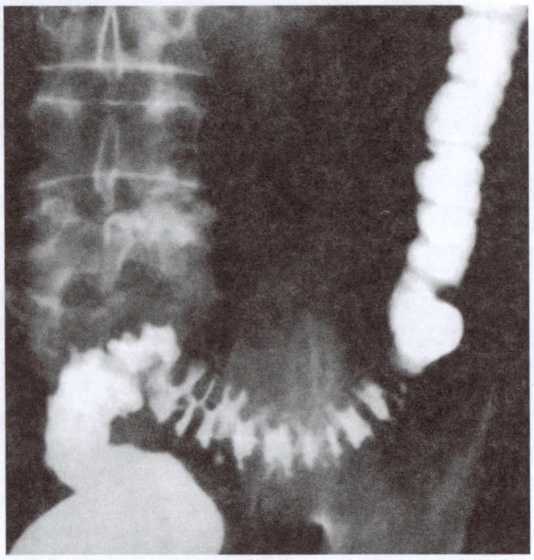

a. Meckel's diverticulum
b. Sigmoid Diverticulosis
c. Sigmoid volvulus
d. Colon cancer

Ans. b. Sigmoid Diverticulosis

Saw tooth appearance seen in Sigmoid diverticulosis is Barium enema

329. Identify the pathology shown in the image.

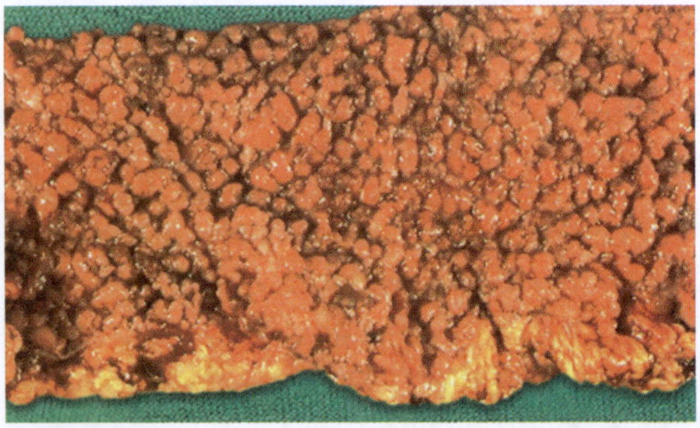

a. Familial hereditary non polyposis syndrome
b. Familial adenomatous polyposis syndrome
c. Colon cancer
d. Juvenile polyposis

Ans. b. Familial adenomatous polyposis syndrome

- This is a case of FAP, where >100 polyps are seen in Colon
- It is 100% premaligant and needs Prophylactic Total proctocolectomy + ileal pouch anal anastomosis before High school joining

330. In a 70-year-elderly male presents: on rectal examination, a mass was found suspicious of cancer. He had normal bowel habits and he actually visited to your hospital for a regular Master health checkup. What will you advise him next?

a. CT scan abdomen
b. Flexible sigmoidoscopy and biopsy
c. Full colonoscopy and biopsy
d. Barium enema

Ans. b. Flexible sigmoidoscopy and biopsy

- For cancer rectum, the immediate next step should be to confirm it by doing a Proctoscopy/sigmoidoscopy and take a biopsy
- Definitely he has to undergo full colonoscopy before surgery to rule out any synchronous cancers before surgery

331. A 65-year-old male presents with painless Hematuria. He has a Ballotable mass in left flank. On examination; RBC is present in urine, while WBC is absent in urine. Most likely diagnosis in this patient:

a. Hydronephrosis
b. Pyelonephritis
c. Renal Cell cancer
d. Polycysic Kidney disease

Ans. c. Renal Cell cancer

- Ballotable mass + Hematuria is a feature of RCC.
- Since it is painless, Hydronephrosis and Pyelonephritis are ruled out
- PCKD present in early age with Renal failure.

332. A young male presents with rupture of bulbar urethra—where is the accumulation of urine seen?

a. Subcutaneously in chest
b. Perineum
c. Peritoneum
d. Bladder retention

Ans. d. Bladder retention

- In Bulbar urethral injury, there will be full bladder and will need SPC
- In Extraperitoneal rupture of Bladder, we have subcutaneous extravasation up to chest level above and Holden's line below.

333. Mr Gupta working in a dye industry presents with Bladder cancer. What is the common type of bladder cancer seen?

a. Squamous cell cancer
b. Transitional cell cancer

c. Adenocarcinoma
d. Adenosquamous cancer

Ans. b. Transitional Cell cancer

MC bladder cancer in Dye workers is Transitional cell cancer

334. A patient's mother while bathing her child noticed there was no testes in the scrotum and on examination—the right testis was in Inguinal region and left was in perineum. What is the diagnosis?
a. Bilateral undescended testis
b. Bilateral ectopic testis
c. Right undescended and left ectopic testis
d. Left undescended and right ectopic testis

Ans. c. Right UDT and Left Ectopic testis

- Undescended Testis—Testis found in the normal path due to failure of descent.
- Ectopic Testis—Testis is found in abnormal path due to predominant Ectopic Tails (Superficial Inguinal pouch, Perineum, Femoral, Pubic region)

335. Which of the following Virus causes Orchitis?
a. Mumps b. Measles
c. Adenovirus d. Herpes

Ans. a. Mumps

(Ref: Bailey and Love 27th edition page 1506)

- Mumps orchitis, most common form of Orchitis
- Develops in 20–30% of post pubertal patients as Parotitis which shows waning.
- IgM antibodies support the diagnosis.
- Mumps can cause testicular Atrophy, which leads to infertility if bilateral.

336. A 20-year-old young male presents with sudden onset of pain in the inguino scrotal region following a sports activity. On Examination the right testis is in higher position and tender on palpation. What is your diagnosis?
a. Right side Epididymo-orchitis
b. Right side Torsion testis
c. Strangulated Inguinal hernia
d. Right side hydrocele

Ans. b. Right Side Torsion testis

(Ref: Bailey and Love 27th edition page 1500)

Prehn Sign—Differentiates Torsion and Orchitis
- In Torsion—Testis on lifting up increases pain
- In Orchitis—Testis on lifting up relieve the pain

337. A young boy presented with scrotal enlargement. On investigations, LDH is increased, HCG and AFP are normal. Histopathology of the testis is shown after orchidectomy. What is your diagnosis?

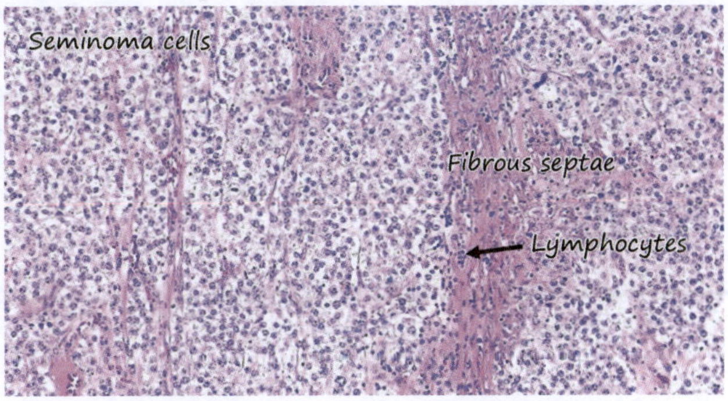

a. Yolk sac tumor b. Seminoma
c. Choriocarcinoma d. Teratoma

Ans. b. Seminoma

- Though this is a Pathology image question, which even I don't to diagnose seeing the cells, I can make the diagnosis from the other clues
- LDH is increased, HCG and AFP are normal in pure seminoma
- In Nonseminomas—HCG and AFP will be increased

338. A newborn baby is presented with absent testes in scrotum. Testes are found in retroperitoneum above deep ring. Which of the following may help in descent of testes?
a. GnRH analogues
b. Testosterone
c. Cold Compresses
d. Surgical method of bringing the testes down

Ans. d. Surgical method of Bringing the testes down.

(Ref: Bailey and Love 27th edition page 1498)

- About 4% of boys are born with one or both testes incompletely descended.
- About two-thirds of these reach the scrotum during the first 3 months of life, but full descent after that is uncommon.
- The incidence of testicular maldescent at the age of 1 year is around 1%
- Surgery should be done before 12 months.

339. A patient underwent surgery for which she was immobilized for prolonged period. The surgeon examined her lower limb and found Homans sign positive. What is your diagnosis?
a. Deep vein thrombosis
b. Peripheral vascular disease

c. Lymphangitis
d. Abdominal aortic aneurysm

Ans. a. Deep vein thrombosis

Homans sign and Moses sign are old signs of DVT, no more used in practice.

340. An old lady, known case of Atrial fibrillation, developed sudden arterial occlusive disease. Which of the following is having poorest prognosis?

a. Pain
b. Pallor
c. Pulselessness
d. Paralysis

Ans. d. Paralysis

The five (P) signs of Acute limb ischemia:
1. Pain
2. Pallor
3. Paralysis
4. Pulselessness
5. Paresthesia

341. A baby is born with Scaphoid abdomen and breathlessness. X-ray chest is shown below. What is your diagnosis?

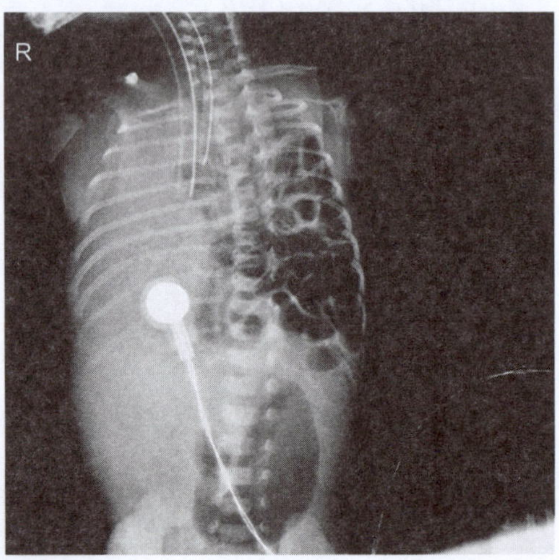

a. Hiatal hernia
b. Pneumothorax
c. Congenital diaphragmatic hernia
d. Pneumonia

Ans. c. Congenital diaphragmatic hernia

- X-ray clearly shows—Diaphragmatic hernia in the left side.
- This is Bochdalek hernia

342. A young male has both sides L1 ganglion removed during Lumbar sympathectomy. What will be the side effect?

a. Retrograde ejaculation
b. Urinary disturbance
c. Paralysis of lower limbs
d. Erectile dysfunction

Ans. a. Retrograde ejaculation

- The L1 ganglion is nervi erigentes involved in antegrade ejaculation of sperm.
- If both sides are removed, there will be retrograde ejaculation and infertility.

343. What is the diagnosis from the image shown?

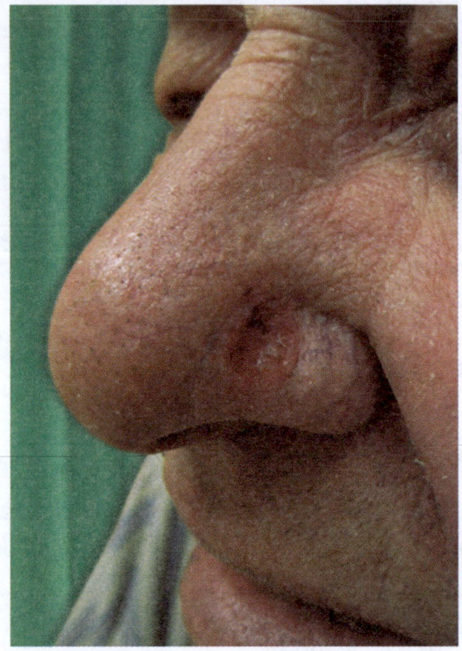

a. Basal cell cancer
b. Keratoacanthoma
c. Sebaceous horn
d. Squamous cell cancer

Ans. a. Basal cell cancer

(Ref: Bailey and Love 27th edition page 604)

- BCC grows slowly and is more of local spread only (hence known as Rodent ulcer)
- It is most common on face in tear flow area (hence known as tear cancer)
- Rolled out edges are seen

344. An old man presents with metastasis in bone and vertebra. What is the most likely diagnosis?

a. Testicular cancer
b. Lung cancer
c. Prostate cancer
d. Colon cancer

Ans. c. Prostate cancer

- MC cause of Bone metastasis in men-Prostate cancer
- MC cause of Bone metastasis in women-Breast cancer
- Prostatic mets are osteoblastic in nature